ESSENTIALS OF ACCIDENT AND EMERGENCY MEDICINE

Edited by **Ahmed Subhy Alsheikhly**

Essentials of Accident and Emergency Medicine
http://dx.doi.org/10.5772/intechopen.71634
Edited by Ahmed Subhy Alsheikhly

Contributors

Ahmad Subhy Humadi Alsheikhly, Nor'Azim Mohd Yunos, Abdulnasir Al-Jazairi, Ekanem Philip-Ephraim, Ehab Aki, Galal Alessai, Waleed Awad, Laura Galdamez, Rasha Buhumaid, Irma Faruqi, Maryam Siddiqi, Shahzad Anjum, Aml Yousif Elemamali, Agata Kawalec, Rana Hussein, TJ FitzGerald

First published in London, United Kingdom, 2019 by IntechOpen
IntechOpen is the global imprint of INTECHOPEN LIMITED, registered in England and Wales, registration number: 11086078, The Shard, 25th floor, 32 London Bridge Street
London, SE19SG – United Kingdom
Printed in Croatia

British Library Cataloguing-in-Publication Data
A catalogue record for this book is available from the British Library

Additional hard copies can be obtained from orders@intechopen.com

Essentials of Accident and Emergency Medicine, Edited by Ahmed Subhy Alsheikhly
p. cm.
Print ISBN 978-1-78984-832-8
Online ISBN 978-1-78984-833-5

Meet the editor

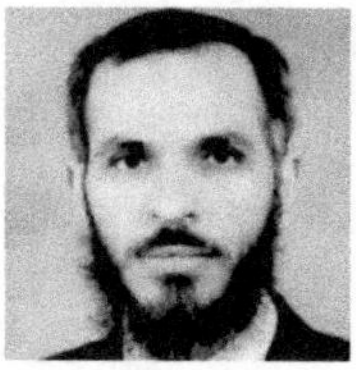

Professor Ahmed Subhy Alsheikhly, MD, FRCSI, CABS, MESICM, MACEP, graduated from Salahuddin Medical college in 1983, trained in Baghdad Teaching Hospital (Baghdad University Teaching Hospital) in the departments of pathology and general surgery, then specialized in general and emergency surgery from the Arab Board Council of Health Specializations, followed by fellowship from the Royal College of Surgeons in Ireland. His expertise includes general and emergency surgery, traumatology, and emergency medicine. He is a highly respected surgeon and emergency physician, teacher, and researcher, in addition to being an active member in the European Society of Intensive Care Medicine (ESICM), American College of Emergency Physicians (ACEP), World Sepsis Day Organization and many other local and international societies. He is the author of more than thirty peer-reviewed medical articles. He is currently a consultant in the Emergency Department of Hamad Medical Corporation and Weill Cornell Medical College (Qatar).

Contents

Preface

As physicians, we have a constant passion for improving and maintaining patient's care and safety. Our journey in providing safe patient care in an accident and emergency setting has always been, and still is, one of the greatest challenges of health services. On a regular basis, healthcare professionals are facing sudden, unexpected, and potentially life-threatening conditions. These situations don't give much time for in-depth reflection, but they need thoughtful actions despite the demand for swift decisions. This, as known for most of us, is a time-critical pressure full of uncertainty, stress, high stakes, erratic team process, and organizational shortcomings intermingling in an environment where good decisions and successful management is of paramount importance.

Acute surgical and medical care is not delivered by one person; instead it is provided through the combined efforts of professionals from various disciplines and specialties cooperating for a patient's sake. Thus, knowledge of successful strategies for improving team performance will create a safer and more effective clinical environment.

This book focuses on the general concepts, essentials of diagnosis and treatment in addition to basic training principles for accidents and emergency medicine. It presents an effort to collect substantial and up-to-date existing knowledge and skills involving recent development in the acute care settings management. The chapters selected for this book are written by an excellent group of recognized emergency surgeons and physicians from different countries and cultures facilitating a comprehensive and interesting approach to the problems of emergency treatment. All of them have their defined set of clinical and human factors-related skills that enable them to manage critical situations.

There are two ways to read the book; the first way is to follow through the text according to its inner logic, while the second way is to read selected chapters. The book has a modular character in that every chapter stands alone and can be read without knowledge of previous ones. To avoid excessive redundancy, basic concepts are explained once at the start of the book and then cross-referenced.

The first part of the book addresses basic concepts and principles needed to understand and manage problems in the emergency department. While the second part follows structural and systematic basic cognitive architecture and essential thinking patterns of diagnosing and treating emergency cases in the acute care units. The last part focuses on the perspectives that organize performance of healthcare providers.

For us, this book has been a team effort. The process of writing has been a challenging yet fruitful time for each of us. We were grateful to learn a great deal from the different perspectives clinicians and colleagues have on the same problem and from the divergent approach in problem solving. I hope that the reader will benefit from this process as well.

We hope this book will be helpful and used worldwide by medical students, clinicians, and researchers enhancing their knowledge and advancing their objectives by a book that intends to become a reference text for research and practice within accident and emergency medicine.

Ahmed Subhy Alsheikhly
Hamad Medical Corporation / Weill-Cornell Medical College
Qatar

Section 1

General Principles

Chapter 1

Essentials in Accident and Emergency Medicine Radiation Injury: Response and Treatment

Thomas J. FitzGerald, Maryann Bishop-Jodoin, Killian Dickson, Yuan-Chyuan Lo, Carla Bradford, Linda Ding, Jessica Hiatt, Harry Bushe, Jonathan Saleeby, I-lin Kuo, Elizabeth Bannon, Kenneth Ulin, David DeSantis, Sherri L. Shul, Bashera Nochomowitz, Julie Trifone, Thomas Quinn, Catherine Whelan, Joshua Taylor, Maureen Britton, Shannon Higgins, Karen Morano, Jean Quigley and Kathleen Briggs

Additional information is available at the end of the chapter

http://dx.doi.org/10.5772/intechopen.76863

Abstract

The discovery of radiation has enabled great healthcare advances as well as catastrophic injury. This paper reviews major historical incidents of public radiation exposure and the evolution of standards affecting today's public and health care workers. Current patient care and response assessment to radiation exposure are reviewed. The strengths of modern radiation therapy and the need for continuous process improvements to ensure optimal patient care and secure safe environments are identified. The discovery of radiation has brought significant scientific achievements as well as catastrophic injury.

Keywords: radiation, exposure, injury, therapy, safety

1. Introduction

Despite safety precautions and application of modern standards of radiation protection, injury from radiation can be generated from both intentional and unintentional situations and events. Injury can be catastrophic, immediately life-threatening, and survivors of exposure remain with a lifetime risk of secondary events including chronic health changes and malignancies. Even with the development of radiation protection standards and oversite organizations, accidents and misadministration of radiation deviant from intent continue to haunt daily application of radiation therapy. There is no antidote to radiation exposure and the fingerprints of injury remain for a lifetime. In this chapter we will review major incidents of public radiation exposure and accidents in history including cause and effect. We will review the application and evolution of standards and how this affects both the public and healthcare worker in modern care. We will review modern patient care and response assessment to radiation exposure including agents that may protect or mitigate radiation damage from radiation exposure. We will identify strengths of modern radiation therapy and the need for continuous process improvements to ensure optimal application of X-ray in a safe environment.

2. History

X-rays were discovered in 1895 by William Roentgen. In part due to the century old use of electricity in medicine, X-rays were rapidly assimilated into the medical armamentarium portfolio as beneficial applications of X-ray treatment were identified by early radiologists. Due to protracted exposure times and minimal knowledge of risk, early practitioners of the application of X-rays to treatment situations became victims themselves. Friedrich Otto Walkoff took the first dental radiograph in 1895 by placing a photographic plate between his teeth and tongue. He was able to generate an image with a 30-minute exposure time. He applied similar techniques to patients and reported epilation and skin blistering. Walkoff developed the first dental imaging laboratory in 1896 with Fritz Geisel. Geisel died in 1927 of metastatic carcinoma caused by heavy exposure of radiation to his hands. In 1896, a child was accidently shot in the head and was brought to a laboratory at Vanderbilt University (Nashville, TN). Investigators sought the location of the bullet by X-ray and a plate holder was tied to the head of the patient. The X-ray tube was placed at the patient's head. The exposure was 1 hour. About 21 days after exposure there was epilation at the site of X-ray application. In 1896, HD Hawkes gave a demonstration of an X-ray unit in New York City. He had to discontinue work after 4 days due to injury to the skin of his hand and chest. Within 2 weeks he had significant skin injuries, his fingernails deteriorated, and he exhibited systemic signs of radiation injury. In the same year, William Levy sought out to localize a bullet that had been lodged in his skull for 10 years. He was warned about the potential of injury; however, chose to move forward. Images were created over a 14-hour period from three static positions at his forehead, his open mouth, and behind his right ear. Within 24 hours, the dermal surfaces of his head were blistered and within days his mouth and lips had sores and epilation occurred within 3 weeks. The bullet was found within an inch of the occipital protuberance. In this circumstance, the absorbed dose by the victim was at least 15 Gray (Gy). Clarence Dally worked at the Edison laboratory and had the role of being a glassblower for Thomas Edison. He is thought to be the first individual to die from chronic radiation workplace exposure in 1904 from metastatic carcinoma at the age of 39. It is thought that his exposure was at least 30 Gy. Numerous deaths were reported in X-ray manufacturers and workers with noted deaths of Nobel Laureates Marie Curie and her daughter

Joliot Curie from radiation-associated diseases during the discovery of radium in 1898 and the near immediate application of radium to treat cancer.

While the benefits of the application of radium and X-rays were moving forward, the risk of injury was continually recognized at an international level. At the second international congress of radiology in 1928 held in Stockholm, Sweden, participating countries developed standards for radiation protection. These were centered on recommendations from the United Kingdom as guidelines for radiation protection had been employed for the previous decade. The congress established the International X-Ray and Radium Protection Committee which was remodeled after World War II (WWII) into two commissions that are active today. These are the International Commission on Radiological Protection (ICRP) and the International Commission on Radiation Units and Measurements (ICRU). In the United States today, the Environmental Protection Agency (EPA) is charged with the responsibility for providing guidance to federal agencies. The Nuclear Regulatory Commission (NRC) formulates rules for application of product materials and the Department of Energy is responsible for radiation safety regulations through the NRC. Multiple international agencies participate in radiation safety activities and help shape policy including health applications and strategy for nuclear energy [1–4].

3. Intentional injury

As the benefits and power of X-rays and radium matured, the use of nuclear tools for weapons of mass destruction came to power. During WWII, efforts for harnessing nuclear power for destruction reached application on August 6, 1945 with the use of a 9000-pound uranium-235 bomb known a "Little Boy" over the manufacturing city of Hiroshima, Japan. The bomb was dropped with a parachute and detonated 2000 feet above the city with blast equal to 15 kilotons About 2–3 days later, a plutonium-239 bomb known as "Fat Man" was dropped over the city of Nagasaki. The primary target was Kokura; however, clouds shrouded the primary target area. The plutonium bomb was more powerful than the bomb used on Hiroshima. The bomb weighed 10,000 pounds and produced a 22-kilotons blast. The topography of Nagasaki limited the radius of impact as the city is in a narrow valley between mountains. Initial destruction and death was due to heat and fire as well as associated trauma related to building damage and other structural/public health-related matters; however, those not at the epicenter of the blast were exposed to radiation as a function of distance from the epicenter. Early impact resulted in microcephaly and mental retardation in the most vulnerable unborn and young population with lifelong health risks including chronic health issues in multiple organ systems and cancer risks affecting all survivors. We have earned much about studying the population of survivors and have been able to apply this knowledge to risk assessment for the general population, healthcare workers, and pregnant/potentially pregnant patients [5–7].

4. Unintentional injury: nuclear power

After WWII, there was a significant interest in accelerating the production of nuclear weapons as well as promoting the use of nuclear energy in lieu of fossil fuels and other sources of non-renewable energy reserves. While we knew individual risk of the indiscriminate use of radiation, despite the application of nuclear weapons, little was known about the impact of risk upon the general population about accidents in the application of nuclear power and the secondary development of nuclear weapons.

The International Atomic Energy Agency (IAEA) maintains as website reporting nuclear accidents. As of 2014, there have been more than 100 serious accidents associated with the use of nuclear power. It is worrisome that more than 50% of the accidents have occurred since the accident at Chernobyl (1986) and that more than 60% of the accidents reported have occurred in the United States. These accidents have occurred over time due to many circumstances including poor design of the reactor and human judgment error in the attempt to prevent and mitigate the problem. Many of the most serious events will be described as follows [5–7].

4.1. Louis Slotin

In 1946, Canadian investigators evaluating nuclear weapons brought two hemispheres of neutron-reflective beryllium around a plutonium core. The hemispheres were only separated by a screwdriver which was against policy. The screwdriver slipped which set off a chain reaction filling the room with radiation validated by the presence of blue light. Louis Slotin (physicist) rapidly separated the hemispheres preventing further exposure to co-workers; however, he died of radiation exposure 9 days later [5].

4.2. Kyshtym

This event was a radioactive decontamination accident in 1957. The accident occurred at Mayak which was a plutonium production site in the eastern Ural Mountains in the Soviet Union. The actual site was not marked on topographical maps, therefore the accident is named after a nearby town.

Because the Soviet Union was behind the US in the development of uranium and plutonium nuclear weapons, the facility was constructed over a short period of time between 1945 and 1948. Initially, high levels of radioactive material were dumped into a nearby river which flowed into the Arctic Sea. The reactors (six) were located on a lake which was used for the cooling cycle. The primary lake was Lake Kyzyltash which became quickly contaminated and a secondary lake, Lake Karachay, also quickly became contaminated. A storage facility for liquid waste was built in 1953. It was a simple design with steel tanks mounted in concrete base 27 feet underground. Because the nuclear waste generated heat, a cooling system was built around each tank. Facilities for monitoring the operation were primitive.

On the day of the event, the cooling system failed in one of the tanks containing 80 tons of liquid radioactive waste. The liquid evaporated, and an explosion ensued estimated at 1 kiloton. A 160-ton concrete lid was thrown into the air and an estimated 20 Millicuries (mCi) of radioactivity was released. Although most of the contamination was near the explosion, there was a plume of radionucleotides that spread over hundreds of miles through the air. The long-term contamination area is estimated to be more than 7000 square miles including cesium 137 and strontium 90. It is estimated that 22 villages were affected, and more than 10,000 people were evacuated from the site over a 2-year period. Due to secrecy surrounding the incident

http://dx.doi.org/10.5772/intechopen.76863

and limitations in obtaining documentation, estimates of health damage, cancer, and current conditions can only be estimated. It is known that the East Ural region remains contaminated to this day and there were scores of documented cases of chronic radiation syndrome with an elevated cancer rate including a high rate of death due to malignancy.

In this situation, limited knowledge of reactor safety coupled with poor risk assessment resulted in an accident of significant magnitude, third only to the accidents at Fukashima and Chernobyl [5, 6, 8].

4.3. Windscale

In a similar manner, the British government initiated a nuclear weapons program after WWII using a plutonium-based platform. British physicists were involved in the Manhattan project and two reactors were built near the village of Seascale, UK, a few hundred feet apart from each other. The core of the reactors consisted of a large block of graphite with channels built for transport of uranium cartridges which would be pushed posteriorly into the back channel for cooling in a water filled channel. This was different from previous designs which had a constant supply of water that poured through the channels housed in the graphite. The first design was chosen because of fear of malfunction of the need for the constant water source. Filters were placed in situ in case one of the cartridges broke entering the water. Without water in the channels, cartridges did break and despite filters, radioactivity was documented around the site but not indicated to staff. One of the reactors was prone to heating and this was believed to be related to the graphite. It was known that neutrons created small fractures in the graphite which in turn could be annealed with increasing the heat of the system. This was known as the Wigner effect, named after physicist Eugene Wigner.

There was considerable political pressure for quickly producing a weapon and the decision was made to generate Tritium which required augmented heating in the reactor. To produce Tritium, the cooling fins on the plutonium cannisters decreased in size to increase heat exchange. Windscale was modified by adding enriched uranium and lithium-magnesium to the fuel rods making the situation more vulnerable to combustion.

On October 7, 1957, one of the reactors was heating more than norm and an additional Wigner annealing release was performed. This had the anticipated result except for one channel. A second Wigner release was performed which appeared to stabilize the situation. On October 10, 1957, a radiation detector in the chimney indicated a release of radiation. It was assumed that a rod had fractured. What was not recognized was the presence of a fire in the same channel likely started on October 7. To provide cooling, fans were augmented which unintentionally made the situation worse. Carbon dioxide and water did not extinguish the fire. It was estimated that 11 tons of uranium was ablaze. Leaders ordered evacuation and shut off all ventilation entering the reactor. This was successful and water flowing through the reactor was cold within 24 hours.

Radioactive material including Iodine 131 (740 Terabecquerel (TBq)), Cesium 137 (22 TBq), and Xenon 133 (12,000 TBq) was released. The presence of scrubbers and filters in the chimney proved to be important and likely limited damage. Both reactors were deemed unsafe for continued use and fuel was removed in 2012 [5, 6].

4.4. Stationary low-power reactor number 1 (SL-1)

SL-1 was a US Army nuclear power reactor located at the national reactor testing station 40 miles west of Idaho Falls, Idaho. The reactor became operational in 1958. The reactor used enriched uranium fuel and was cooled by water flowing through plates of uranium/aluminum alloy. The design relied on a primary central fuel rod. The reactor was closed for maintenance on January 3, 1961 and was being prepared to restart after the 11-day shutdown. Procedures that required the central rod be withdrawn to connect to the central drive mechanism. The rod was withdrawn too far, and the reactor instantly became critical. Within 4 milliseconds, the heat generated by the power excursion caused water to vaporize and explode. Radioactive water became a pressure wave striking the ceiling and a loose metal pin impaled one of the workers to the ceiling structure. It was determined on review that the 26,000-pound internal vessel had moved more than 9 feet in the superior direction and the control rod mechanisms struck the ceiling. There were three workers on site who each died quickly of their injuries. Their radiation exposure would also have been lethal, if they survived physical trauma. Review of the incident suggested that the central rod may have become fixed in position and one of the workers was able to free it; however, in the process the rod moved too far which generated the reaction.

Even without a containment structure, the reactor contained most of the radioactivity. In late 1961, the cleanup process began and all core and building materials were buried approximately 1600 feet from the site of the reactor. One of the conclusions was that design focus on a single central structure created untoward risk that could not be easily mitigated. First responders may have received significant compounded radiation dose due to increased radiation dose in the environment and during removal of the waste and remains of those who died. Those involved in the response were awarded certificates for heroism [5, 6].

4.5. Three Mile Island, Pennsylvania

During the evening of March 27, 1979, one reactor at Three Mile Island nuclear station was running at near full capacity, while a second reactor was shut down for re-fueling. The root cause of the accident occurred 11 hours prior to the declaration of the emergency, when the cooling system filters were cleaned with air compression and cooling water. A valve that was thought to be shut was open and water entered an instrument airline which caused a turbine trip. Three auxiliary pumps should have been activated when heat and pressure increased due to lack of cooling; however, these pumps were closed due to re-fueling. This was not NRC policy. A third valve opened to relive pressure; however, did not close when pressure was released, therefore coolant escaped and became root cause in core disintegration. Human factors delayed recognition of the problem as a light indicated that the open valve was closed and secondary safety procedures were not followed. Even though there was persistent loss of coolant, water levels increased through the open valve creating bubbles of steam in the liquid. At 4:15 am on March 28, 1979, the pressurizer in the relief tank ruptured and radioactive coolant leaked into the containment structure. In a series of activated pumping mechanisms, the coolant was then pumped beyond the containment area. At 6 am on March 28, 1979, the temperature in a pilot valve was noted to be excessive by an employee beginning his work shift and a back valve was used to stop the flow of coolant. However, by that time 32,000 gallons of coolant had leaked, and radiation levels were 300 times expected. The containment building was significantly damaged; however, the radioactive material remained in situ as it did not extend beyond the reactor vessel despite that approximately half of the core uranium melted during the incident.

The incident became an example of managing authority and responsibility in the nuclear industry. Lines of authority between private plant ownership, state authorities, and the NRC were not clear and accordingly in the early phase of the accident, it was difficult to obtain accurate information for risk assessment. This resulted in delayed evacuation. Clean up was not completed for more than a decade and long-term risks remain not well defined. Most of radioactive gas release was xenon, which was not considered significant; however, radioactive iodine was also released and the impact of increase in thyroid cancers remains uncertain [5, 6].

4.6. Chernobyl

The Chernobyl accident is one of the two most significant nuclear events in the history of unintentional radiation injury. The incident occurred on April 26, 1986. The irony of the event is that it occurred during a safety procedure evaluation and safety systems were intentionally disabled as part of the intended procedure. The reactor was brought to minimal activity with the expectation that cooling systems would manage the heat generated by thermal decay. The systems onsite unfortunately required more than 1 minute to activate and running the reactor at minimal power (below safety standard) resulted in the crisis. A series of events triggered by flaws in reactor design and poor decisions made by onsite personnel created situation where reactor cooling was inefficient and two steam explosions generated from thermal decay exposed the graphite core to air, which fueled the massive explosion. Exposure to oxygen fueled the explosion. The fires were extraordinary and sent radioactive elements and gas into the air for a week. Plumes of radioactive gas extended well into Western Europe for an extended period of time. Casualties were significant including first responders attempting to put out the fires as those involved were exposed to lethal levels of radiation. Scores of people were affected by radiation syndrome and estimates include thousands who will develop secondary cancers due to exposure. Cleanup continued for decades. It is estimated that more than 350,000 people relocated as part of a series of evacuations. Unfortunately, many evacuated during the initial phase of the accident were exposed to medically significant radiation as the exit road was directly under the parallax of the radioactive plume from the reactor fires. Reactor fires were eventually attenuated by helicopter droppings of cement, clay, sand, and boron to absorb neutron activity. The government decided to place a cover over the remains of the reactor and today this is referred to as a sarcophagus. Full understanding of risk and damage remains elusive due to limited access to information and lack of full disclosure for years by government sources [5, 6].

4.7. Fukashima

The nuclear power plant at Fukashima sustained damage from a massive Tsunami 50 minutes after the Tohoku earthquake in 2014. At the time of the earthquake, a mandatory shutdown of the reactor took place; however, decay heat, despite the elimination of the fission component of the reactor energy generation, needed to be managed and cooled with backup generators and power. The secondary backup cooling systems were damaged in three of the reactors and consequently, heat generated explosions contaminated the environment with radioactive particles and gas. Unlike Chernobyl, three had no direct deaths associated with the explosions and radiation exposure; however, issues with the cleanup continue until today. In the construction of Fukashima, more advanced backup systems existed in modern construction sites and these withstood the injury. The affected reactor had an older cooling design. Deaths occurred as part of the evacuation process, due in part to damage to facilities and inability to move rescue supplies into the region. This also compromised restoring the cooling mechanisms to the backup systems as batteries and generators that may have been helpful could not be transported to the site. The damage to the environment continues to today. Fukashima and Chernobyl are considered as two most powerful nuclear accidents in our history [5, 6].

4.8. Aftermath

The experiences listed depict the extraordinary damage created by nuclear accidents to people and the environment. Reactor design, poor secondary cooling backup systems for failure, poor response by onsite providers with decisions made in panic, and natural disasters with poor preparation have created an uncertain future for the safety and durability of nuclear power. Injuries for onsite providers are related to explosions, thermal and high dose radiation. The incidents can occur in fractions of seconds and the injuries and environmental impact can last generations. It is sobering to see the radiation injuries sustained by first responders and those who attempted to mitigate the disasters. Information for these people arriving onsite for disaster management was not clear and in retrospect was inaccurate. Their brave and self-sacrificing response could not overcome the power and danger imposed by the situation. The impact on the nearby population and environment will not be resolved for decades and the disaster at early accidents continues to haunt the environment. The impact on the lives of the victims has no clear limit or statute of limitations. We need improved safety, infallible design, and protective strategies moving forward. In the upcoming sections, we will describe what information is currently available for those involved in the triage of radiation injury for both acute and long-term injuries [5–11].

5. Unintentional injury: nuclear submarines

With the interest in nuclear power, efforts were developed to use nuclear power for transportation. Submarine technology for nuclear power was developed as it limited the need to refuel and missions could be extended for a significant period. However, as such issues and safety within the nuclear power community, safeguards, and measures of protection could not be provided with security. In the Soviet submarine fleet, many accidents occurred which limited the safety and security of the power source. In 1961, similar to a nuclear power plant, the cooling system failed on the K-19 Soviet nuclear submarine and the temperature rapidly rose as a result of decay heat. The captain ordered a secondary cooling built and sailors/engineers in the process of building a cooling system were exposed to lethal doses (LDs) of radiation in the process of building the system. More than 20 died of radiation injury. In 1968, nine sailors died during an explosion that released radioactive gas. In 1985, 10 died in an explosion caused by malfunction of a lid designed to keep fuel rods in position and 49 people were exposed to significant radiation, many of whom were first responders to the explosion and subsequent fire. These events demonstrated that safety precautions including well understood policy and procedure were and remain essential to mission if nuclear energy sources were being used [5].

5.1. Unintended injury from the application of radiation therapy and use of diagnostic X-ray equipment

In this section, we will describe a series of events that imposed injury to people and the environment from applications of therapeutic radiology and unintended overuse of imaging equipment. These events have significant consequence to unintended victims of equipment, safety measures, and human error.

5.2. Radiation accident in Morocco

In 1984, an Irridium-192 radioactive source became dislodged from the safety container. A worker unintentionally took the source back to his residence which exposed himself, his family, and visitors to high doses of radiation with three people sent to the Curie institute for treatment. It is believed that eight deaths were caused by the accident and there is a report that some deaths were due to pulmonary hemorrhage. Similar injuries have been reported in patients with myeloma undergoing total body radiation therapy as part of preparation for bone marrow transplant noted at doses of less than 10 Gy [5, 11].

5.3. Goiania, Brazil

In 1985, a Cesium-137 source was inadvertently left behind when a private radiation oncology clinic moved to a new facility. The source was found 2 years later by two people who brought the source and source carriage home and eventually ruptured the capsule of the source. During this time, hundreds of people were exposed and at least four died of radiation-related injuries. Cleanup processes took 6 months and at least 300 people were identified as having exposure to Cesium [5].

5.4. Zaragoza, Spain

On December 7, 1990, maintenance was performed on a linear accelerator at the radiation therapy clinic at Zaragoza, Spain and it returned to patient care service on December 10. What was not known was the accelerator (14 years in service) was incorrectly repaired and there was a breakdown in the internal control mechanism, therefore not detecting that patients were receiving much higher doses than specified with a higher beam energy. Initially, after 10 days of treatment, patients were identified as having accelerated dermal injuries. The first death associated with radiation injury was in February 1991. In total, 25 patients died in the first year after the event and 11 were attributed to injuries imposed by the incident [5].

5.5. San Salvador, El Salvador

In 1989, an accident occurred in a facility using a Co-60 source to sterilize medical products. The device became frozen in the on position. The worker by-passed safety measures and entered the room with two other workers to try and free the equipment. The exposure was so high that one worker died within 6 months of exposure and the two other workers sustained injuries requiring amputation [6, 7, 9].

6. Modern accelerator safety issues

The modern linear accelerator has a vast array of safety features including computer override systems which prevent improper application of therapy and internal monitoring diodes which monitor dose application. Safe operation of linear accelerators is a challenging task and users of modern equipment have to assume greater responsibilities for safe execution of patient care. Complex treatment plans and delivery system require thorough hands on understanding of machine operations and safety systems. Continuous process monitoring ensuring safe delivery of care is essential to mission to prevent abhorrent behavior of equipment. This includes well trained staff who can detect potential issues and report concerns to appropriate individuals for next step action to mitigate potential problems. Nevertheless, significant errors have occurred which continue to haunt patient care delivery. Advancement in therapy application often require tools that are developed by different companies and the tools must be harmonized through hardware and software adjustments to provide appropriate patient care. This has led to serious and life-threatening injuries when not applied appropriately. The most common errors in computer override situations are software flaws that indicate that a situation is safe when it is unsafe. Examples of software flaws include unintentionally reporting that multileaf jaws are moving appropriately during treatment when they are not and assuring the individual delivering therapy that system delivery is compliant to plan and calculation when the situation may be less secure. Treatments now require thousands of dynamic motions of individual leaves hidden in the gantry of the machine. Linear accelerators and radiation therapy treatment planning have become exceptionally complex. Treatment delivery capability has become exceptionally precise in its capability to deliver very high doses of treatment to small areas with submillimeter precision. The power of the new equipment is extraordinary; however, the power is often used as a marketing tool and does not recognize that new systems including training of personnel have not been appropriately vetted. This represents both the strength and weakness of modern care. The instrument is powerful; however, if not applied appropriately can cause significant harm. If not calibrated and executed properly, life-threatening injuries occur. In recent reporting through the New York Times, Walter Bogdanich accurately reported on misadministration of radiation therapy to multiple patients in several separate situations causing severe injury and death including injuries to tissues that could not be repaired. These are the innocent victims of our technology and their injuries are a sobering reminder that we must maintain a culture of safety [12].

Although software matters can be addressed, we must improve on right patient and right treatment. Human error remains too frequent in treatment delivery. Technology cannot resolve all causes of error and department processes including double identification and time out must be documented and validated to ensure patient safety. More sophisticated digital identification processes may be implemented into clinical operation including iris and fingerprint strategies for identification, similar to modern computer identification technologies. Written policies and validation that processes have been followed are crucial to successful clinical operation. Recent review of adverse events of radiation oncology devices from 1991 to 2015 revealed that adverse events increased over time and peaked in 2011. During this period of time, there was significant change in practice strategies including enterprise application of intensity modulation and the application of image guidance into daily therapy. About 50.8% of adverse events involved external therapy, 24.9% of events involved brachytherapy, 20.9% were mechanical, and 20.4% involved user error. While a department will perform 100 times more teletherapy treatments than brachytherapy applications, it was interesting to note that brachytherapy adverse events were only half of those reported for teletherapy, therefore potentially more prone to misadministration. Brachytherapy is done less often, and accordingly departmental processes may not be repeated frequently enough for flawless reproducibility and execution of care. Our department is responsible for more than 50,000 external treatments every year and each individual treatment and brachytherapy application must be correct. Injuries can be imposed by diagnostic X-ray equipment especially in situations requiring interventional radiology and the use of fluoroscopy. The radiation dose cannot be extracted once delivered and the injuries imposed often have no cure [6, 7, 9, 13, 14].

7. Impact of radiation therapy on normal tissues

7.1. Accidents and weapons: unintended exposure

In these circumstances, injuries imposed are related to strength of the radiation source and distance to the source of radiation. Thermal and mechanical injuries are immediately life-threatening. Within 15 minutes of exposure, victims exposed to high dose radiation can experience symptoms associated with the event. These symptoms are manifest with high exposure by neuromuscular changes and gastrointestinal effects. At very low-level exposure, the victim may appear well; however, gastrointestinal and bone marrow symptoms may become more visible in the upcoming month post exposure. Intermediate dose exposure results in upper abdominal symptoms and lassitude seen within hours of the exposure. High dose exposure results in more extreme symptoms including rapid fluid loss and hypotension associated with more pronounced neuromuscular symptoms. Often normal tissue sequelae associated with exposure can be divided into acute injury, sub-acute injury, and chronic injury. Unintentional exposure requires evaluation by a trained group of experts who can assess both injury to the victim and risk to others with continued exposure of radioactive sources either on or inhaled/ingested by the victim. The initial screening of victims requires evaluation by trained radiation safety officers and members of emergency services who can begin to apply best supportive care. In the initial phase of the evaluation, it is important to ascertain as accurate assessment of dose exposure as possible. Lymphocyte counts due to intermitotic death and chromosomal damage assessment can be qualitative surrogates for exposure in the early phase of response assessment. Healthcare workers will likely be monitored for exposure; however, the general public will not be monitored, therefore involving experts in radiation exposure early in response assessment is essential to mission in order to appropriately define the extent of the damage and risk of injury [7, 9, 15].

Acute injury occurs within 90 days of exposure, sub-acute injury occurs from 90 days to 2 years after exposure, and chronic injury occurs 2 years after exposure. All organ systems are affected by radiation exposure. At very high exposures of 10 Gy, death will occur within 24–48 hours due to unrelenting swelling within the central nervous system which compromises all neural processes. At exposure of 5–10 Gy, death will occur within 1–2 weeks due to de-population of gastrointestinal stem cells and bone marrow progenitors. Profound and uncontrollable fluid losses compounded by infection are the cause of death. Victims have survived exposures to this level if they can afford maximal supportive care with fluid replacement and bone marrow support. The term LD 50/30 is a term initially used in pharmacology to determine lethal dose (LD) in 50% of the population within 30 days. Historically, the LD 50/30 for radiation exposure was believed to be 2 Gy; however, with modern support services it is believed that this can be increased to 5 Gy.

If the exposure is determined to be at or below 5 Gy, most experts recommend no immediate intervention other than best supportive care and symptom management. The victim will need to be carefully monitored for manifestations of acute and sub-acute injury as well as chronic events that can appear at any point in later life including the development of malignancy. If the exposure is determined to be greater than 5 Gy, then death by hematopoietic syndrome including loss of bone marrow progenitors becomes a visible concern. Intervention with barrier nursing and appropriate blood product support is needed to move the victim through this phase into recovery. Recent nuclear accidents have suggested that infection control and vigorous supportive care may help victims survive an exposure dose of up to 7 Gy. The role of bone marrow transplantation in this effort remains to be established. It is likely of benefit in selected patients [15–17].

7.2. Response applications

Since the development of nuclear weapons and need for response metrics to injury, there is been a scientific interest in identifying compounds that can protect normal tissue from the effects of radiation exposure. Protectors are given either prior to or immediately thereafter exposure. Mitigators are compounds given after exposure to influence and diminish the impact of the exposure to normal tissue. Therapeutic compounds are applied when the event has occurred. After WWII, it has been known that sulfhydryl groups can function as radiation protectors with the simplest compound being cysteine which contains a natural amino acid. Sulfhydryl groups are toxic which can be decreased by the addition of a phosphate group. Once the compound enters the cell, the phosphate group is released, and the sulfhydryl group becomes a free radical scavenger. Sulfhydryl groups have been shown to protect mice from lethal doses of total body radiation. The only compound approved by the US Food and Drug Administration is amifostine (WR-2721). It is sold as ethyol and has been used to prevent xerostomia in patients treated with radiation therapy for head and neck malignancies. In clinical trials, the use of the compound has been shown to improve quality of life scores for patients undergoing radiation therapy. It has also been used to protect other mucosal surfaces (rectum) and pulmonary parenchyma in patients undergoing total body radiation therapy in preparation for bone marrow transplant. To date, there has been no defined tumor protective effect assigned to amifostine. There are complexities to outpatient clinical application which can be manifested as hypotension and nausea, therefore patients need to be carefully monitored both before and after administration. It is unusual in clinical practice for patients to receive every assigned dose each day. The success is well documented; however, with improvements in radiation dose delivery across salivary tissue, amifostine is not as commonly used in clinical practice as it was a decade earlier. Citron and colleagues have identified nitroxides as agents for protection. These function as well through a free radical scavenger mechanism. Superoxide dismutase (SOD) compounds with gene therapy applications have also been explored. The gene therapy vector has been used in animal models to enhance intracellular accumulation of SOD with SOD functioning as a free radical scavenger [18–21].

Mitigators are compounds that potentially limit damage of radiation exposure once the event has occurred without clinical manifestation of injury. These compounds influence the metabolic cascade of events that occur post exposure. These compounds include those that can stimulate bone marrow and dermal progenitors. These include granulocyte stimulating growth factor (G-CSF) and keratinocyte growth factor (KGF). KGF also appears to influence the recovery of mucosal surfaces as well as improve dermal integrity. Mitigators of late toxicity center around limiting fibrosis and the primary target is transforming growth factor beta (TGF beta) and interruption of the signaling pathway that promotes expression. Investigators at the University of Massachusetts have evaluated the use of interleukin 1 alpha to limit neutrophil infiltration into the site of radiation injury to limit the extent of injury in damaged dermal tissue. Knockout mice deficient in IL-1 alpha demonstrated both decreased dermal injury to radiation and more rapid time to repair injury. In another series of experiments, investigators at the University of Massachusetts studied optical imaging as a tool to evaluate radiation injury and determine if changes in metrics associated with oxygenation and deoxygenation can be related to dose. Optical imaging demonstrated that changes in dermal tissue associated with radiation within 12 hours of exposure and imaging defined consistent metrics for acute and chronic injury. In a separate patient breast cancer treatment protocol optical imaging successfully defined radiation dose and dose asymmetry (hot spots) in patients undergoing serial imaging during breast cancer radiation therapy. Chronic changes were likewise well defined on images obtained post treatment [18, 22, 23].

With increased risk of nuclear weapons and exposure to radiation through accident and future air/space travel, it is of increasing importance that emergency services become more familiar with the management of radiation exposure and injury. Radiation experts and safety officers likewise need to be aware and available to support colleagues in emergency services to optimize care for those affected by unintended exposure in time of crisis. There have been numerous incidents of unintended radiation exposure with victims exposed to both partial and total body X-ray. The Medical Science Division of the Oak Ridge Institute for Science and Education operates a Radiation Emergency Assistance Center for the US Department of Energy. The center is a 24-hour consultation service with both medical and health physics support for issues associated with radiation and X-ray exposure. The resources are comprehensive and include expertise for dose assessment, computation of dose from radionucleotides, and laboratory support. The 24-hour emergency telephone is 865 576 3131 and the website is http://www.orau.gov/reacts [9, 13–16, 24, 25].

7.3. Injury with diagnostic and therapeutic X-rays

There is an increasing number of cancer survivors. It is estimated that in each primary care practice by 2025 that 20% of the panel of patients in every primary care practice will be a cancer survivor. This creates a challenge for both the primary care and oncology community as management of the normal tissue imprint of therapy on the survivor does not have clear definition as providers differ in their perceived responsibilities and expertise. Historically, the focus of cancer management was driven to tumor control as a sole endpoint. Today, success brings new challenges. With survivorship improving, more patients now live in symbiosis with the known and unknown sequelae of management. Accordingly, cancer survivorship is beginning to mature as a sub-specialty service defined in oncology and executed through primary care. Gaps in both anticipation of injury and responsibility of management often are initially recognized in crisis by emergency services and often are not easily recognized as sequela of management. Unfortunately, electronic medical records are often insufficient in providing necessary information to facilitate problem solving and management. Most radiation therapy equipment and radiation therapy planning volumetric archives reside in proprietary software systems that are used to operate and validate daily treatment operations. Commercial electronic record systems do not have access to this information as the information in radiation oncology resides in proprietary systems. Although interfaces can be built to facilitate note transfer and medical billing documentation, in evaluation of a patient, the volumetric imaging, and radiation dose information is an essential aspect of problem solving in the emergency environment. For example, in the cancer survivor being evaluated for new onset chest pain, it is essential that dose/volume relationships to cardiac subsegments be available for review for analysis of risk assessment. The evolving field of oncocardiology requires an accurate record of radiation dose volume analysis to specific subsegments including pericardium, vessels, myocardium, cardiac valves, and the electrical conducting system. Each area can be affected by specific dose volume review and this information becomes essential for evaluation of the modern patient. Radiation is not a drug and has specific residual fingerprints on the area treated. Modern management of the cancer survivor requires comprehensive understanding of the impact of treatment on normal tissue by those who evaluate the patient after treatment is completed. The imposition of therapy on normal tissue lasts for the lifetime of the patient, therefore information on treatment needs to be available and in an easily retrievable format for all providers. In the next section, we will evaluate injury to tissue that is both acute and chronic. Acute effects of radiation exposure affect cells of rapid self-renewal potential such as skin, bone marrow, and gastrointestinal progenitors. Every organ system can manifest a late effect from radiation exposure [9, 13, 14, 24–26].

7.4. Skin

Skin is the visible site of acute reactions to X-ray and harbors chronic changes from therapy. Dermal stem cells reside at the basement membrane of the epidermis and the self-renewal process for the epidermis is 3 weeks in tissues that are uninjured. Prior to the use of linear accelerators for patient care, diagnostic X-ray equipment was used to treat patients for malignancies. This resulted in a much higher dose to superficial tissues including skin. Both acute and late effects of radiation therapy are influenced by daily dose and fractionation. In this circumstance, the skin would receive significantly high dose to skin surfaces relative to target. This has importance because fluoroscopy used in interventional radiology and cardiology can deliver exceptionally high doses to skin surfaces, especially in procedures that are highly complicated. Patients would unintentionally receive higher daily dose and accordingly, dermal sequela of management was and still can be highly visible and a significant problem. Modern linear accelerator equipment delivers dose below the skin surface, therefore skin sequelae with traditional treatment fractionation models are less visible in the modern world. However, from an emergency services perspective, radiation beams resonate on dermal surfaces in skin folds and intertriginous regions. These include skin folds in the breast and regional lymph node regions and inguinal/gluteal regions of patients treated for pelvic and anal malignancies. Dose to these areas is higher daily, therefore may have desquamation, both moist and dry, as a consequence of management. Uninformed providers refer to this issue as a "burn". This is inaccurate. Daily treatment limits the self-renewal capacity of stem cells and injury to the basement membrane exposes the dermis to air with resultant moist changes. Although this can be a future site of infection, conservative treatment measures uniformly outpace any barrier application applied in thermal injury, therefore symptom management is often the best approach in this situation. With interest in compressed fractionation schedules for selected patients, the degree of injury during the acute management phase may be more pronounced, therefore from an emergency services perspective, it is important to ask what for the daily dose, not just whether the patient has been treated. The skin is often hyperpigmented during this phase of treatment. Chronic changes appear as hypopigmentation and thinning of dermal tissue associated with fragments of visible surface blood vessels known as telangiectasia. In the chronic phase, the skin is functional; however, if injured, repair may be more protracted. Modern intensity modulation techniques can limit both the extent and volume of radiation dose asymmetry, thus ameliorating the extent of acute and chronic dermal injury for modern patients. It is also to recognize recall of injury by many medications including antibiotics. Modern targeted therapies including epidermal growth factor receptor (EGFR), B-Raf Proto-Oncogene (BRAF), and mechanistic target of rapamycin (mTor) therapies also result in dermal injury and the integrated use of radiation therapy may augment the reaction, even in areas not irradiated. Radiation oncology is evaluating the use of more compressed treatment strategies for outpatient care including stereotactic therapy. There are reports of dermal injury to patients due to equipment augmenting dose to skin. Treatment planning needs to limit this risk [19, 21–23, 27–33].

7.5. Bone marrow

Acute effects of radiation therapy affect marrow elements with rapid self-renewal potential. Lymphocytes die an intermitotic death, therefore can be used as a highly qualitative biomarker for radiation dose during exposure. Neutrophils self-renew on a near daily basis, therefore are highly sensitive to X-ray exposure like platelets. Red cells do not have nucleus, therefore decreased red cell count requires further evaluation to rule out a source of cell loss or limitation in production. It is interesting that the use of intensity-modulated radiation therapy (IMRT) for patients with pelvic malignancies is demonstrating an increase in issues associated with blood counts in patients treated with standard chemotherapy for gynecologic and rectal malignancies. This is due to the fact that most radiation oncologists have applied tighter bowel constraints for attenuation of small and large bowel sequelae of management. This brings dose further into pelvic marrow elements and away from bowel. Radiation oncologists must be conscientious on these points. Modern investigators are using advanced technology MRI and metabolic imaging tools to distinguish between red and yellow marrow elements and use IMRT for conformal avoidance to address this point. Prior to the use of modern tools for image guidance, radiation oncologists used more generous planning target volumes, and this likewise contributed to the problem. Pancytopenia and bone marrow aplasia and dysfunction are becoming a common consequence of therapy including secondary liquid malignancies. Often, these are first identified in the acute care setting. Bone marrow deficiencies can often take years and decades to develop as a consequence of therapy, therefore vigilance remains important in this area as part of patient management moving forward [19–21, 33].

7.6. Gastrointestinal tract

The cells that line the gastrointestinal tract have a rapid self-renewal potential with gastric lining undergoing renewal every day and the small bowel every 3 days. The mucosa is dynamic and is responsible for absorption of nutrition and water. Without mucosal lining, body fluid is readily lost and with intermediate level total body exposure, repopulation of mucosa cannot keep pace with fluid loss, hence the genesis of gastrointestinal death from exposure. Infection is also an issue as the barrier is denuded and intestinal flora autoinfect the victim. Therefore, barrier nursing, blood and fluid support are essential to survival in victims who have received an intermediate dose of X-ray. Investigators have demonstrated that bone marrow progenitors may repopulate and differentiate in the gastrointestinal system, indicating a potential benefit to bone marrow transplantation in victims of radiological exposure.

Therapeutic X-ray impact on the gastrointestinal tract is influenced by several factors including co-morbidities and previous surgery. Sequelae can be seen in patients who receive intermediate therapeutic dose to large segments of bowel as well as those who receive high dose to small bowel segments. Strictures are not thought to be a direct effect from treatment; however, if a bowel segment is fixed in position by adhesions, if irradiated, this segment of the GI tract can be further injured and may require surgical removal if symptoms become too demanding and life-threatening. Late effects from management include every tissue component of the gastrointestinal tract. Atrophy of mucosa exposures underlying submucosal tissues to external injury can lead to chronic infection and malabsorption with pain as nerve roots become exposed in the unprotected internal environment. Insufficiency syndromes including the exocrine pancreas are now being observed [19–21, 33].

7.7. Liver

With the marked increase in viral- and diet-induced liver disease, there is a significant increase in primary hepatic malignancies. Coupled with the improved efficacy of radiation therapy for metastatic disease to the liver, hepatic and diaphragmatic injury from radiation treatment is now well described. Although hepatic parenchyma does not have a rapid self-renewal component, injury to the hepatic reticulum results in disorderly repair limiting blood flow to parenchyma. This limits filtration of both nutrients and toxins. With increased vascular stasis due to disorganized repair, veno-occlusive disease (VOD) becomes an insidious issue and serves to complicate the delivery of care. Metrics for the degree of pre-existing VOD influence the radiation therapy approach to radiosurgery for both primary and metastatic patients. This is important in assessing hepatic disease in the acute care setting. One of the more challenging issues for emergency room providers and primary healthcare delivery teams is the fact that radiation therapy volumetric objects do not reside in a standard electronic medical record (EMR). This makes communication to the patient/family as well as disease assessment problematic including the delivery of intravascular therapy. In a chaotic vascular system, one can never be certain that dose intent is dose delivered. Efforts are made with external radiation therapy to limit mean liver dose and in an otherwise healthy liver to 30 Gy to 30% volume [19–21, 33–35].

7.8. Renal

Similar to the liver, the kidney is a sensitive late responding critical organ. Radiation doses greater than 20 Gy in 2 Gy fractions can result in renal damage with downstream consequence of anemia and hypertension. Although not validated through clinical trials, the tolerance dose is lower is patients who have also received chemotherapy. With advanced treatment technologies, modern radiation oncologists can optimize dose to the kidney using intensity modulation; however, even modern technologies leave a footprint which can limit future function. In comparison with siblings, cancer survivors have a higher likelihood of renal failure. We need to be aware of the tolerance dose as we design care plans with imaging [19, 21, 33].

7.9. Lung

Similar to the liver and kidney, the lung is a sensitive intermediate to late responding organ. In extreme situations, radiation injury to the lung is life-threatening. The period of active inflammation generally occurs 2–6 months post completion of therapy. Fibrosis can occur years after therapy and this can create distortions in pulmonary anatomy relative for the region treated and dose delivered. During the active inflammatory period, changes consistent with inflammation are visible on thoracic imaging. Interestingly, changes on imaging are often more frequent than symptoms, nevertheless, when symptoms occur at times management is challenging. Injury outside the radiation treatment field is often ascribed to radiation therapy and often we dismiss this as an event without merit. Recent investigations have demonstrated that nitric oxide gas is produced as a by-product of treatment which may explain, in part, why changes in untreated lung can be seen. It is important for radiation therapy treatment objects be available for acute care providers. Although the most recognized metric for pulmonary injury is the volume of parenchyma receiving 20 Gy, in selected situations, the volume of parenchyma receiving 10 and 5 Gy may be of equal importance in determining root cause of pulmonary dysfunction. Oncology treatment records are important for review as chemotherapy agent, targeted therapies and immunotherapy can significantly contribute to pulmonary toxicity. Cancer survivors have a higher risk of chronic pulmonary disease compared to siblings; therefore need to be vigilant to their long-term pulmonary health [21, 33, 36].

7.10. Cardiovascular

Although historically, the heart and large vessels were thought to be a late responding tissue to injury, modern cardiovascular evaluation and imaging have demonstrated that radiation therapy has an impact on all cardiac structures including coronary arteries, valves, myocardium, and the electrical conduction system. Although efforts in planning radiation therapy now focus on cardiac avoidance and compartment dose volume analysis, there are multiple generations of patients treated with traditional technologies that may remain at higher risk for cardiovascular injury. Chemotherapy agents also contribute to this risk and targeted therapies may unintentionally add to risk. For example, breast cancer patients are often treated with Adriamycin on an adjuvant basis. This agent has an established history of cardiotoxicity. After administration of Adriamycin, the recovering myocardium expresses Her 2 Neu. Her 2 Neu positive breast cancer patients will receive Herceptin after initial chemotherapy, therefore these patients are at higher risk for cardiac injury without radiation therapy. Modern radiation technologies including optical tracking of position, breath hold, and intensity modulation contribute to decreasing mean heart dose and limit radiation dose to specific cardiac volumes including the left ventricle which is an issue for left breast patients. The field of oncocardiology is an important field of study. Cancer survivors have a higher risk of cardiovascular disease compared to siblings and introducing cardiac-oriented survivorship plans as patients complete their primary therapy needs to become the standard of care. Long-term radiation injury is noted to the microvasculature in all organ systems; however, large vessels were thought to be less susceptible to injury. However, as we move to treatments that include non-traditional fractionation protocols and overlap of previous areas of radiation therapy, evaluation of large vessels with surveillance imaging including the carotid vessels for patients treated for head and neck cancer. With more patients being retreated for secondary events, conformal avoidance to cardiovascular structures as part of primary management and avoidance of radiation dose asymmetry will be important to optimize outcome moving forward [37–43].

7.11. Central nervous system

The brain has multiple cell systems susceptible to injury uniformly viewed as late responding tissues. Necrosis can occur after radiation therapy, especially in circumstances of compressed fractionation and stereotactic radiosurgery and radiotherapy. Although highly unusual, demyelinating syndromes can occur both in the brain and spinal cord associated with both radiation dose and volume treated. Toxicity is also increased with chemotherapy agents including but not limited to Ara-C and Methotrexate, both used in multiple disease settings due to penetrance beyond the blood-brain barrier. There are injuries noted to tissues with end arterial vascular systems. The optic chiasm is susceptible to injury with radiation therapy due to the unique arterial system at doses of 54 Gy. The cochlea is susceptible to injury especially when cis-platinum is used as part of the care plan. Brachial plexus injury was described in breast cancer patients at doses of 54 Gy; however, this is an issue which identification of this dose may be inaccurate. At the time of description of the injury, radiation therapy techniques unintentionally created overlap with anterior and posterior fields under the lateral third of the clavicle where the entire nerve plexus enters the upper extremity. It is rare to see plexopathy in head and neck patients, therefore the experience with the breast cancer population and regional treatment may have related to technique rather than radiation dose. This again point to the importance of increasing the knowledge of radiation therapy in the general medical community and acute care providers [33, 44].

7.12. Endocrine

Hypothyroidism is exceptionally common in patients treated with both surgery and radiation therapy to the upper thorax and neck. This can have significant health issues and is often overlooked and underappreciated in the acute care environment. The thyroid is also highly vulnerable to injury with unintended exposure and a source of secondary malignancies due to exposure. Gonadal exposure leads to both fertility issues and endocrine dysfunction, which can affect every organ system including growth and development in children. Atrophy and dysfunction of multiple organ systems is identified in patients where limitations in estrogen and testosterone function are not identified. Pituitary dysfunction is well described in multiple disease systems especially in patients treated with high retropharyngeal adenopathy or primary disease in the nasopharynx. Modern survivorship plans need to include strategies for endocrine malfunction [33, 26].

7.13. Pediatrics

Children are a highly vulnerable population. Although treated at a young age, late effects often become more visible when these cancer survivors transfer their long-term care into adult medicine. At radiation doses of 20 Gy, limitations in musculo-skeletal development are seen and at dose of 55 Gy bone necrosis can occur, especially in patients treated with chemotherapy. Exit dose from cranio-spinal radiotherapy can impose changes in cardiovascular and pulmonary health and development. Treatment for Wilms tumor makes children vulnerable to renal health problems as adults. Because these children are treated as infants and young children, even low dose therapy affects gonadal function and other gastrointestinal injuries including maldevelopment of bowel segments. With advanced imaging techniques, structures once thought immune to radiation effects now are known to be more vulnerable to injuries. Sacral insufficiency fractures are now visible at radiation doses of 50 Gy. Stereotactic body radiosurgery is now associated with injuries once thought historical in nature including rib fractures from pulmonary therapy. Often childhood patients do not have survivorship plans that can detail what is needed when they become adult patients and adult physicians need to detail a plan when caring for these patients as they become adults to provide a comprehensive survivorship plan.

Intentional and unintentional radiation exposure can have significant impact on normal tissue, both immediate and late. In assessing acute exposure, it is essential to determine exposure and dose. Optical imaging may be a tool moving forward which can validate computational extrapolation of dose as injury can be seen within 12 hours of exposure. Appropriate support needs to be applied to victims of acute exposure and intentional therapy needs to be mitigated by strategic planning and application of therapy. Survivorship plans for those exposed to radiation including those with unintentional exposure need to be developed. An understanding of these effects is essential for modern healthcare providers in the acute care setting [19–21, 26, 33, 45].

8. Conclusions

It has been more than 100 years since the discovery of X-rays and radium. The power of radiation is significant and appropriate application of radiation has saved lives and become an extraordinary source of energy. The devastating side of radiation is equally visible. Both intentional and unintentional injury remains at significant risk in spite of a century worth of knowledge concerning radiation safety and application of safety measures. Radiation therapy and diagnostic imaging remain tools that are essential to mission for patient care, nevertheless we must remain vigilant and apply continuous process improvements in practice to ensure optimal patient care and secure safe environment. Enhanced knowledge of the impact of radiation on normal tissue is important for emergency care workers.

Conflict of interest

The authors certify that there is no conflict of interest in relation to this manuscript.

Author details

Thomas J. FitzGerald[1*], Maryann Bishop-Jodoin[1], Killian Dickson[1], Yuan-Chyuan Lo[1], Carla Bradford[1], Linda Ding[1], Jessica Hiatt[1], Harry Bushe[1], Jonathan Saleeby[1], I-lin Kuo[1], Elizabeth Bannon[1], Kenneth Ulin[1], David DeSantis[2], Sherri L. Shul[1], Bashera Nochomowitz[1], Julie Trifone[1], Thomas Quinn[1], Catherine Whelan[1], Joshua Taylor[1], Maureen Britton[1], Shannon Higgins[1], Karen Morano[1], Jean Quigley[1] and Kathleen Briggs[1]

*Address all correspondence to: tj.fitzgerald@umassmemorial.org

1 Department of Radiation Oncology, University of Massachusetts Medical School, Worcester, MA, USA

2 Department of Radiation Oncology, Steward Health Care Network, Boston, MA, USA

References

[1] Frei GA. Deleterious effects of X-rays on the human body. Electrical Review. 1896;**29**:95

[2] Stickney N. The cause of burns from X-rays. Boston Medical and Surgical Journal. 1896; **135**:719

[3] Sansare K, Khanna V, Karjodkar F. Early victims of X-rays: A tribute and current perception. Dentomaxillofacial Radiology. 2011;**40**:123-125. DOI: 101259dmfr/73488299

[4] Aronowitz JN. Ethereal fire: Antecedents of radiology and radiotherapy. AJR. American Journal of Roentgenology. 2007;**188**:904-912

[5] Wikipedia. Nuclear and Radiation Accidents and Incidents [Internet]. 2018. Available from: https://en.wikipedia.org/wiki/Nuclear_and_radiation_accidents_and_incidents {Accessed: Jan 30, 2018]

[6] Lushbagh CC, Ricks RC, Fry SA. Radiological accidents: A historical review of sealed source accidents. In: Proceedings of the International Conference on Radiation Protection in Nuclear Energy. Sydney (Australia): US Nuclear Regulatory Commission; April 18-22, 1988; IAEA-CN-51/92. 1988. p. 522

[7] International Atomic Energy Agency. Scientific and Technical Basis for the Geological Disposal of Radioactive Wastes. Technical Reports Series 413. 2003. STI/DOC/010/413. ISBN: 92-0-100103-7

[8] Kellerer AM. The Southern Urals radiation studies. A reappraisal of the current status. Radiation and Environmental Biophysics. 2002;**41**:307-316. DOI: 10.1007/s00411-002-0168

[9] Hall EJ, Giaccia AJ, editors. Radiology for the Radiologist. 7th ed. Philadelphia: Lippencott, Williams, and Wilkins; 2012. 546 p

[10] Standring WJ, Dowdall M, Strand P. Overview of dose assessment developments and the health of riverside residents close to the "Mayak" PA facilities, Russia. International Journal of Environmental Research and Public Health. 2009;**6**:174-199

[11] United States Nuclear Regulatory Commission. Information Notice No. 85-87: Lost Irridium-192 Source Resulting in the Death of 8 Persons in Morocco. [Internet]. 1985. Available from: https://www.nrc.gov/reading-rm/doc-collections/gen-comm/info-notices/1985/in85057.html [Accessed: Jan 30, 2018]

[12] Bogdanich W. Radiation offers new cures, and ways to do harm. The New York Times. Jan 23, 2010. Available from: http://www.nytimes.com/2010/01/24/health/24radiation.html[Accessed: Dec 19, 2017]

[13] Williamson JF, Dunscombe PB, Sharpe MB, Thomadsen BR, Purdy JA, Deye JA. Quality assurance needs for modern image-based radiotherapy: Recommendations from 2007 interorganizational symposium on "quality assurance of radiation therapy: challenges of advanced technology". International Journal of Radiation Oncology, Biology, Physics. 2008;**71**:S2-S12

[14] Connor MJ, Marshall DC, Moiseenko V, et al. Adverse events involving radiation oncology medical devices: Comprehensive analysis of US Food and Drug Administration data, 1991 to 2015. International Journal of Radiation Oncology, Biology, Physics. 2017; **97**:18-26

[15] Turai I, Veress K. Radiation accidents: Occurrence, types, consequences, medical management, and the lessons to be learned. Central European Journal of Occupational and Environmental Medicine. 2001;**7**:3-14

[16] Donnelly EH, Nemhauser JB, Smith JM, et al. Acute radiation syndrome: Assessment and management. Southern Medical Journal. 2010;**103**:541-546

[17] Baranov A, Gale RP, Goskova A, et al. Bone marrow transplantation after the Chernobyl nuclear accident. The New England Journal of Medicine. 1989;**321**:205-212

[18] Citrin D, Cotrim AP, Hyodo F, Krishna MC, Mitchell JB. Radioprotectors and mitigators of radiation-induced normal tissue injury. The Oncologist. 2010;**15**:360-371

[19] Bentzen SM. Preventing or reducing late side effects of radiation therapy: Radiobiology meets molecular pathology. Nature Reviews. Cancer. 2006;**6**:701-713

[20] Guo H, Seixas-Silva JA Jr, Epperly MW, et al. Prevention of radiation-induced oral cavity mucositis by plasmid/liposome delivery of human manganese superoxide dismutase (SOD2) transgene. Radiation Research. 2003;159:361-370

[21] FitzGerald TJ, Aronowitz J, Cicchetti MG, et al. The effect of radiation therapy on normal tissue function. Hematology/Oncology Clinics of North America. 2006;**20**:141-163

[22] Anscher MS, Thrasher B, Rabbani Z, Teicher B, Vujaskovic Z. Antitransforming growth factor-beta antibody 1D11 ameliorates normal tissue damage caused by high-dose radiation. International Journal of Radiation Oncology, Biology, Physics. 2006;**65**:676-881

[23] Massague J. TGFbeta in cancer. Cell. 2008;**134**:215-230

[24] Miller DL, Balter S, Cole PE, et al. Radiation doses in interventional radiology procedures: The rad-IR study: Part II: Skin dose. Journal of Vascular and Interventional Radiology. 2003;**14**:977-990

[25] Miller DL, Balter S, Wagner LK, et al. Quality improvement guidelines for recording patient radiation dose in the medical record. Journal of Vascular and Interventional Radiology. 2004;**15**:423-429

[26] Armstrong GT, Kawashima T, Leisenring W, et al. Aging and risk of severe, disabling, life-threatening, and fatal events in the childhood cancer survivor study. Journal of Clinical Oncology. 2014;**32**:1218-1227

[27] FitzGerald TJ, Jodoin MB, Tillman G, et al. Radiation therapy toxicity to the skin. Dermatologic Clinics. 2008;**26**:161-172

[28] Fajardo L, Berthrong M, Anderson R. Radiation Pathology. 1st ed. New York: Oxford University Press; 2001. 472 p

[29] Majno G, Joris I. Cells, Tissues, and Disease: Principles of General Pathology. 2nd ed. New York: Oxford University Press; 2004. 1040 p

[30] Chin MS, Freniere BB, Bonsey CF, et al. Skin perfusion and oxygenation changes in radiation fibrosis. Plastic and Reconstructive Surgery. 2013;**131**:707-716

[31] Chin MS, Freniere BB, Lo YC, et al. Hyperspectral imaging for early detection of oxygenation and perfusion changes in irradiated skin. Journal of Biomedical Optics. 2012;**17**:026010. DOI: 10.1117/1.JBO.17.2.026010

[32] Hoppe BS, Laser B, Kowalski AV, et al. Acute skin toxicity following stereotactic body radiation therapy for stage I non-small-cell carcinoma: Who's at risk? International Journal of Radiation Oncology, Biology, Physics. 2008;**72**:1283-1286

[33] Bentzen SM, Constine LS, Deasy JO, et al. Quantitative analyses of normal tissue effects in the clinic (QUANTEC): An introduction to the scientific issues. International Journal of Radiation Oncology, Biology, Physics. 2010;**76**:S3-S9

[34] Guha C, Kavanagh BD. Hepatic radiation toxicity: Avoidance and amelioration. Seminars in Radiation Oncology. 2011;**21**:256-263

[35] Sioshansi S, Rava PS, Karam AR, et al. Diaphragm injury after liver stereotactic body radiation therapy. Practical Radiation Oncology. 2014;**4**:e227-e230. DOI: 10.1016/j.prro.2014.01.001

[36] Ding L, Lo YC, Kadish S, et al. Volume modulated arc therapy (VMAT) for pulmonary stereotactic body radiotherapy (SBRT) in patients with lesions in close approximation to the chest wall. Frontiers in Oncology. 2013;**3**:12. DOI: 10.3389/fonc.2013.00012 2013

[37] Evans SB, Sioshansi S, Moran MS, et al. Prevalence of poor cardiac anatomy in carcinoma of the breast treated with whole breast radiotherapy: Reconciling modern cardiac dosimetry with cardiac mortality data. American Journal of Clinical Oncology. 2012;**35**:587-592

[38] Lenihan DJ, Cardinale DM. Late cardiac effects of cancer treatment. Journal of Clinical Oncology. 2012;**30**:3657-3664

[39] Weintraub NL, Jones WK, Manka D. Understanding radiation-induced vascular disease. Journal of the American College of Cardiology. 2010;**55**:1237-1239

[40] Lam WW, Leung SF, So NM, et al. Incidence of carotid stenosis in nasopharyngeal carcinoma patients after radiotherapy. Cancer. 2001;**92**:2357-2363

[41] Adams MJ, Hardenbergh PH, Constine LS, Lipshultz SE. Radiation-associated cardiovascular disease. Critical Reviews in Oncology/Hematology. 2003;**45**:55-75

[42] Katz NM, Hall AW, Cerqueira MD. Radiation induced valvulitis with late leaflet rupture. Heart. 2001;**86**:E20

[43] McCulloch TM, Jaffe D. Head and neck disorders affecting swallowing. In: Goyal R, Shaker R, editors. GI Motility Online. Part 1: Oral cavity, pharynx and esophagus. 1st ed. London: Nature Publishing Group; 2006. DOI:10.1038/gimo36

[44] Giese W, Kinsella T. Radiation injury to peripheral and cranial nerves. In: Gutin P, Leibel S, Sheline G, editors. Radiation Injury to the Nervous System. New York: Raven; 1991. pp. 383-403

[45] Hopewell JW. Radiation therapy effects on bone density. Medical and Pediatric Oncology. 2003;**41**:208-211

Chapter 2

Shock

Rana Jaffer Hamed Hussein

Additional information is available at the end of the chapter

http://dx.doi.org/10.5772/intechopen.76242

Abstract

This chapter targets to provide information to medical students, residents, and nurses on emergency medicine. The concept and definitions of shock have been mentioned. An overview about shock has been given at the beginning of the chapter. Different categories of shock have been elaborated with comparison. Each type of shock has been discussed with its specificities and its management. Septic shock has been extensively discussed and different definitions and terminology have been used. Latest surviving sepsis campaign guidelines have been scribbled down. Hemorrhagic shock has been widely discussed too and a table provided for the differentiation of stages of hemorrhagic shock. Finally, the chapter is concluded with all the references used for accomplishing this chapter.

Keywords: hypovolemia, sepsis, distributive shock, obstructive shock, cardiogenic shock

1. Introduction

Shock is a life-threatening condition that leads to global tissue hypoperfusion and circulatory collapse. It can be reversible if detected, treated, and resuscitated early; otherwise it can cause multi-organ failure and death. Almost one million cases of shock are seen at the emergency department, annually in the USA [1].

Septic shock causes highest rates of mortality (40–60%), compared to other types of shock.

Identification of the cause of shock can be challenging [1].

There is no one specific vital sign that is diagnostic of shock [1].

Bedside ultrasound is a useful tool for diagnosing some types of shock. It can help to evaluate the volume status and cardiac contractility. It can detect tension pneumothorax and cardiac tamponade [2].

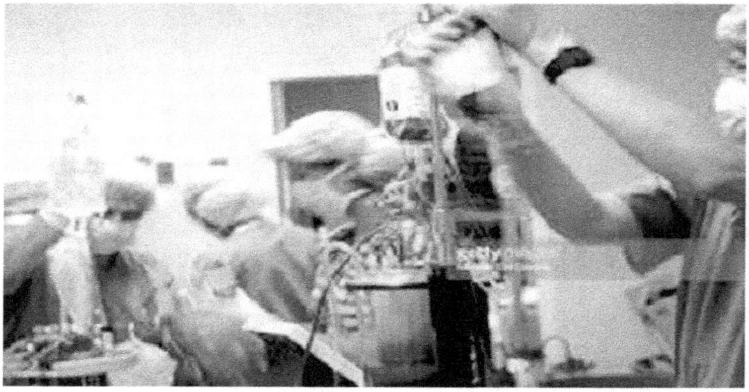

Figure 1. Management of shock [2].

Shock management requires securing airway, controlling breathing, and optimizing circulation to ensure adequate tissue perfusion [2] (**Figure 1**).

2. Pathophysiology

Shock is a state of circulatory insufficiency creating imbalance between oxygen delivery and demand to the tissues, resulting in end-organ dysfunction. At the cellular level, shock first affects the mitochondria. Majority of the aerobic energy comes from combustion of substrates (carbohydrates and fats) along with oxygen, forming carbon dioxide and water. But in shock there is cellular hypoxemia; the tissues enter in anaerobic state and accumulate lactic acid. Lactate starts building up in the blood and acidosis develops [3].

Measurement of serum lactic acid aids in detecting tissue hypoxemia. It is a reliable tool for predicting the outcome and prognosis [4] (**Figure 2**).

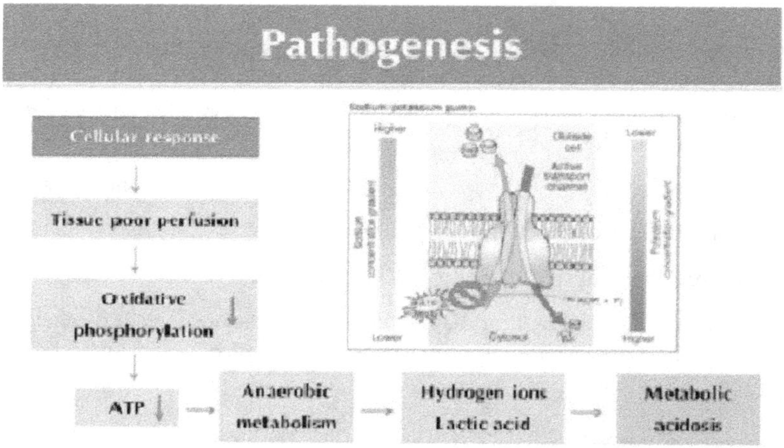

Figure 2. Pathophysiology of shock [2].

3. Stages of shock

- Pre-shock: compensated phase where patient usually has normal blood pressure.
- Shock: the compensatory mechanism of the body is overwhelmed (almost 20–25% of blood volume is lost).
- End-organ failure: there is irreversible organ damage and death [4].

4. Recognition of shock

After the airway is secured and ventilation is optimized, the circulatory status must be evaluated. Tachycardia and cutaneous vasoconstriction may be early signs of shock. Respiratory rate and pulse pressure (difference between systolic pressure and diastolic pressure) are of significance, too [2].

Hypotension develops in late stages of shock, and its absence does not exclude shock [2].

Serum lactic acid and base deficit are good parameters for detecting the presence and severity of shock [2].

The cause of shock can be determined by taking good history, detailed physical examination, and ordering for necessary investigations (e.g., imaging, bedside ultrasound) [2].

5. Classification of different categories of shock

- Hemorrhagic shock (or hypovolemic shock)
- Non-hemorrhagic shock includes:

  a. Septic shock

  b. Cardiogenic shock

  c. Obstructive shock (tension pneumothorax, pericardial tamponade)

  d. Neurogenic shock

  e. Anaphylactic shock

Sometimes there is a combination or coexistence of more than one type of shock [2].

5.1. Hemorrhagic shock (hypovolemia)

There is loss in intravascular volume which decreases preload and diminishes the cardiac output. Sometimes despite fluid or blood replacement, inotropes and vasopressors might need to be added on [1].

In hemorrhagic shock, due to rapid drop in the blood volume, there is activation of the baroreceptors causing peripheral vasoconstriction and increased cardiac contractility and heart rate. Initially, as a response to the blood loss, the body tries to compensate by increasing the pulse rate and diastolic pressure, causing the pulse pressure (difference between systolic and diastolic pressure) to narrow. As the volume deficit continues, the cardiac output drops followed by reduction in the blood pressure. Simultaneously there is renal vasoconstriction too, leading to tubular necrosis. There is impaired fuel delivery to all the vital organs including the brain, due to impaired hepatic glucose output and peripheral lipolysis. The most common cause of hemorrhage is trauma [2].

5.2. Management of hemorrhagic shock.

The main treatment is to stop bleeding and restore volume by administering fluids, including blood.

- Establish a secure patent airway and optimize breathing.
- Establish intravenous access for fluid resuscitation.
- Determine the level of conscious (by evaluating the eye, verbal, and best motor response) (Glasgow Coma score, GCS).
- Expose the patient from head to toe to look for injuries or deformities, bearing in mind to avoid hypothermia.

Patient may need to have orogastric tube in place to relieve gastric distension and urinary catheter to monitor output. Patient may need central venous access for measuring central venous pressure, fluid resuscitation, and blood sampling. Imaging studies would aid to the diagnosis of the source of hemorrhage. Initial resuscitation should start with 1–2 L of fluid bolus in adults and 20 ml/kg in pediatric patients. Blood transfusion might be needed too. Balanced resuscitation must be the target in hemorrhagic shock management, which means balancing organ perfusion with risks of rebleeding and accepting lower than normal blood pressure [2].

Target goal of resuscitation is to maintain a urinary output of 0.5 ml/kg/hr. in adults and 1 ml/kg/hr. in pediatric patients [2].

In severe bleeding, uncross-matched blood can be used. Consider O negative blood in women of childbearing age. Vasopressors would usually worsen the hypoperfusion, so it must be considered only if resuscitation by fluids and blood fails. Bedside ultrasound scanning (E-FAST) can help in detecting hemorrhage in intra-abdominal, pleural, pericardial, and pelvic cavities. Knowing the base deficit is important as it can help to distinguish trivial bleeding from significant blood loss. Base deficit is the amount of base needed to be added in 1 L of blood to normalize the pH. Normal base deficit is more positive than −2 mEq/L. It can become negative early in hemorrhage when the pH and blood pressure remain normal [2].

During hemorrhage, tissues suffer academia and accumulation of lactic acid which can be treated if resuscitated promptly and adequately. Treatment is with fluids, blood, and control of hemorrhage [2].

http://dx.doi.org/10.5772/intechopen.76242

5.2.1. Stages of hemorrhagic shock

Stage 1: Loss of approximately 750ml of blood, with no significant change in physiological parameters,

Stage 2: loss of 750-1500ml of blood, with mild changes in the vital signs,

Stage 3: loss of 1500ml- 2000ml of blood, affecting the normal body physiology, requiring urgent attention,

Stage 4: loss of >2000ml of blood resulting in severe disturbance of body functions, calling for urgent replacement of blood to restore normal functions.

See **Figure 3**.

5.3. Effects of hemorrhage

There are some factors that can alter the outcome in patients with shock. Factors like:

- Extremes of age.
- Site and severity of injury.
- Time lapse (from injury to resuscitation).
- Comorbidities and medications.

Class	I	II	III	IV
Blood loss (ml)	≤750	750-1500	1500-2000	≥ 2000
Blood loss (% blood volume)	≤15%	15-30%	30-40%	≥40%
Pulse rate	<100	>100	>120	≥ 140
Blood pressure	Normal	Normal	Decreased	Decreased
Pulse pressure (mmHg)	Normal or increased	Decreased	Decreased	Decreased
Capillary refill test	Normal	Positive	Positive	Positive
Respiratory rate	14-20	20-30	30-40	>35
Urine output (ml/hr)	≥ 30	20-30	5-15	Negligible
CNS-mental status	Slightly anxious	Mildly anxious	Anxious and confused	Confused, lethargic
Fluid replacement (3:1 rule)	Crystalloid	Crystalloid	Crystalloid + Blood	Crystalloid + Blood

Figure 3. Stages of hemorrhagic shock [2].

Hemostasis and balanced fluid therapy (including blood) should be started as soon as signs of hemorrhage are suspected [2].

As mentioned in the table above, patients in classes I and II have good compensatory mechanism to overcome the blood loss and may just need crystalloid infusion, while patients in classes III and IV have lost significant amount of blood and need to have blood transfusion [2].

Soft tissue injuries and fractures compromise the hemodynamics of patients with trauma, e.g., 1500 ml blood can be lost in femur fractures [2].

The cytokines released during tissue injury increase permeability of tissues. Fluid shifts and volume depletion in the intravascular compartment cause hypovolemia [2].

6. Septic shock

It is the most common form of distributive shock. The body's defense system is overwhelmed by infection leading to life-threatening organ dysfunction. In resuscitating septic shock, few effects should be considered: hypovolemia, cardiovascular depression, and systemic inflammation. Besides, there is capillary leak, which causes intravascular volume loss. The combined interaction of chemical mediators, inflammation, and disturbed metabolism causes heart injury during septic shock. There is also capillary leak in the lungs, presenting as acute respiratory distress syndrome (ARDS) [2].

Common causative organisms are pneumococcus, methicillin-resistant *Staphylococcus aureus* (MRSA), *Klebsiella pneumoniae, Pseudomonas aeruginosa,* etc. [4].

Thus, the early use of antibiotics is advised. Ensuring good oxygenation and ventilation, the use of fluids and vasopressors is the main pillar of treatment in septic shock [1].

The use of parenteral steroids is controversial and can only be considered in patients who are on chronic steroid therapy [1].

Definitions and criteria for septic shock:

Systemic inflammatory response syndrome (SIRS) includes (**Figure 4**):

Two or more of the following:

- Temperature > 38°C or < 36°C.
- Heart rate > 90 beats/min.
- Respiratory rate > 20 breaths/min or $paCO_2$ < 32 mmHg.
- White blood cell count >12,000 or < 4000 or > 10% band neutrophilia [5].

Severe sepsis:

SIRS with suspected infection associated with organ dysfunction [5].

http://dx.doi.org/10.5772/intechopen.76242

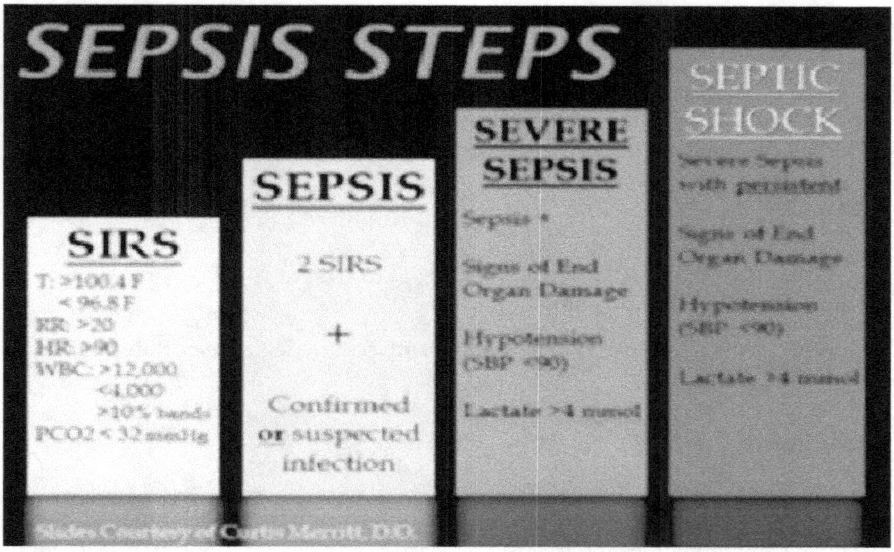

Figure 4. Steps of sepsis [6].

Septic shock:

SIRS with suspected infection and hypotension, despite adequate fluid resuscitation [5].

Surviving Sepsis Campaign has altered the approach to managing sepsis and septic shock, worldwide. It has helped to deliver early timely care to critically ill patients in as less than 6 h [5].

The latest **Surviving Sepsis Campaign Bundles** are as follows:

To be completed 3 h of time of presentation:

1. Measure lactate level.
2. Obtain blood cultures prior to administration of antibiotics.
3. Administer broad spectrum antibiotics.
4. Administer 30 ml/kg crystalloid for hypotension or lactate ≥4 mmol/L [5].

To be completed within 6 h of time of presentation:

5. Apply vasopressors (for hypotension that does not respond to initial fluid resuscitation) to maintain a mean arterial pressure (MAP) ≥65 mmHg.
6. In the event of persistent hypotension after initial fluid administration (MAP <65 mm Hg) or if initial lactate was ≥4 mmol/L, reassess volume status, tissue perfusion, and document findings.
7. Remeasure lactate if initial lactate is elevated [5].

Document reassessment of volume status and tissue perfusion with either:

- Repeat focused exam (after initial fluid resuscitation) including vital signs, cardiopulmonary examination, and skin findings.

Or any two of the following:

- Measure CVP.
- Measure $ScvO_2$.
- Bedside cardiovascular ultrasound.
- Dynamic assessment of fluid responsiveness with passive leg raise or fluid challenge [5].

7. Cardiogenic shock

Cardiogenic shock results when more than 40% of the myocardium is damaged by necrosis from ischemia, inflammation, and toxins. There is decreased cardiac output due to pump failure such as cardiomyopathy, myocardial infarction, valvular insufficiency, and arrhythmias. This shock can further persist and eventually lead to cardiac arrest. Usually patients in cardiogenic shock look ill, drowsy, sweaty, and pale and can have tachycardia with weak pulse and hypotensive. The urine output would be deceased to less than 0.5 ml/kg/h, and serum lactic acid would be as high as 4 mmol/L, indicating circulatory insufficiency. Left ventricular dysfunction can be detected by echo early in the course of cardiogenic shock. Patients with severe left ventricle dysfunction are more liable to develop shock than those with mild to moderate dysfunction. Serial cardiac markers and bedside echo for such cases are worth doing as they can aid in diagnosis and effective management. Patient needs to be monitored closely and vital signs recorded frequently. It is worth to have an arterial line in place for accurate blood pressure readings. Monitoring urine output, base deficit, and serum lactic acid is important for the assessment of resuscitation in all patients who are in shock [4] (**Figure 5**).

Management of cardiogenic shock includes:

1. Improve the work of breathing by adequate oxygenation and ventilation.
2. Initiation of vasopressors or inotropes, e.g., norepinephrine (0.5 μg/min or dobutamine (5μg/kg/min).
3. Treating arrhythmias.
4. Aspirin and heparin (if indicated).
5. Treatment of the cause, e.g., thrombolysis or angioplasty (e.g., myocardial infarction). In refractory cases of cardiogenic shock, intra-aortic balloon pump can be used.

Emergency reperfusion procedure (thrombolysis/PTCA) is not superior to medical management in cardiogenic shock, secondary to myocardial infarction. There is no reduction in the mortality rate [1].

http://dx.doi.org/10.5772/intechopen.76242

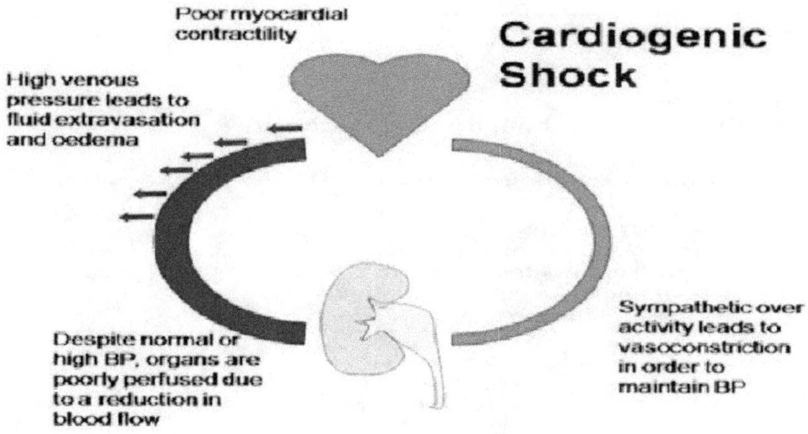

Figure 5. Pathophysiology of cardiogenic shock [7].

8. Obstructive shock

It is usually due to extra cardiac etiologies which result in poor right ventricle output. Causes are:

- Pulmonary: right ventricular failure from pulmonary embolism or severe pulmonary hypertension, as the heart cannot generate enough pressure to overcome the high pulmonary vascular resistance.
- Mechanical: there is a reduction in venous return to the right atrium and inadequate right ventricle filling. Causes: tension pneumothorax, tamponade, constrictive pericarditis, and restrictive cardiomyopathy [4].

Bedside ultrasound would be of absolute benefit in diagnosing obstructive shock [2].

9. Neurogenic shock

It is characterized by hypotension due to severe brainstem or spinal cord injury resulting in autonomic system disruption. Trauma to the cervical or upper thoracic spine leads to sympathetic chain injury resulting in vasodilation.

Good fluid resuscitation and vasopressors would help to manage this type of shock [1].

10. Anaphylactic shock

Immunoglobulin E mediated response due to insect stings, food, and drugs. Cardinal feature is circulatory collapse associated with bronchospasm and increase airway resistance. It can be associated with skin manifestations of wheals and hyperemia. There can also be vomiting and

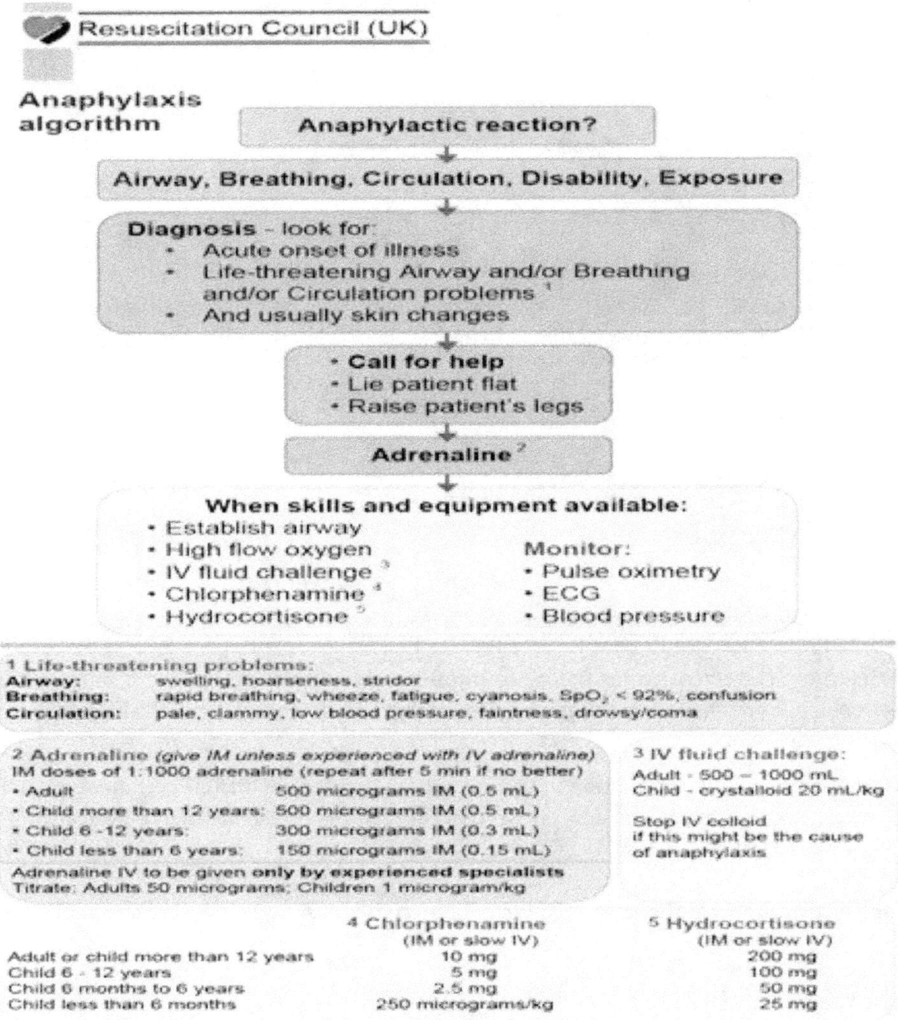

Figure 6. Anaphylaxis management algorithm [8].

diarrhea, too. Management includes stabilizing the patient; maintaining the airway patency; effective breathing; prompt use of epinephrine, fluid resuscitation, parenteral steroids, and antihistamine; and the use of bronchodilators, if necessary [3] (**Figure 6**).

11. Special considerations

11.1. Advanced age

Trauma in elderly patients needs special attention as cardiac compliance decreases with age. The heart cannot compensate for blood loss as efficiently as in youngsters. There is a decrease

http://dx.doi.org/10.5772/intechopen.76242

in catecholamine production resulting in manifestation of tachycardia, when in shock. Elderly patients are mostly on multiple medications. Beta blockers worsen hypotension caused by trauma and also mask the tachycardia, which is an early sign of shock. Volume resuscitation must be strictly monitored as most patients have decreased cardiac contractility and can easily go into volume overload [2].

11.2. Athletes

They may not manifest any signs of shock due to their unusual compensatory mechanism, despite significant amount of blood loss [2].

11.3. Pregnancy

Pregnant patients would present with signs of shock only after huge volume of blood is lost, due to their physiological maternal hypervolemia [2].

12. Conclusion

Shock is a state of global tissue hypoperfusion. After initial resuscitation, detailed physical examination is important to determine the cause of shock. Patients in shock have to be kept on monitored bed. Urine output and central venous pressure would need to be monitored in such patients [2].

In trauma patients, hypovolemia is the main reason for shock. Control of hemorrhage and blood replacement are necessary. Hypovolemia can also develop due to gastroenteritis, heat stroke, febrile illness, etc. Septic shock needs early administration of antibiotics, after drawing a full septic workup. Cardiogenic shock needs to be treated meticulously and monitored closely. Inotropes and fluids have to be administered, cautiously. Neurogenic shock needs good vasopressor support. Obstructive shock whether it is tension pneumothorax or pericardial tamponade, both, need decompression. Pulmonary embolism needs to be treated with anticoagulants. Anaphylactic shock can be managed by administration of parenteral epinephrine, crystalloids, steroids, and antihistamines [3].

Management of shock is often complicated especially in extremes of age, pregnancy, and patients with multiple comorbidities [2].

Author details

Rana Jaffer Hamed Hussein

Address all correspondence to: ranajaffer1979@yahoo.com

Hamad Medical Corporation (HMC), Doha, Qatar

References

[1] Tintinalli's Emergency Medicine. A Comprehensive Study Guide. 8th ed

[2] American College of Surgeons. Advanced Trauma Life Support, Student Course Manual. 9th ed

[3] Rosen's Emergency Medicine. Concepts and Clinical Practice. 7th ed

[4] www.uptodate.com

[5] www.survivingsepsis.org

[6] https://en.wikipedia.org/wiki/Sepsis

[7] http://nursingcrib.com/critical-care-and-emergency-nursing/cardiogenic-shock/

[8] https://www.resus.org.uk/resuscitation-guidelines/

Chapter 3

Approach to Fluid Therapy in the Acute Setting

Nor'azim Mohd Yunos

Additional information is available at the end of the chapter

http://dx.doi.org/10.5772/intechopen.74458

Abstract

In the acute medicine, fluid therapy is a common intervention. Clinicians may have different preferences in prescribing the fluids—the type, the volume and rate, and the monitoring of response—but there is a growing argument in the literature for a more consistent and evidence-based approach to these prescriptions. This coincides with the call to treat fluids as drugs and to strategize the fluid management of individual patients. A good start toward observing this call will be an appreciation of the underlying physiology. The hemodynamic, biochemical, and microcirculatory responses to fluid therapy will influence the end-organ and clinical effects. In translating these physiological insights into practice, recent studies in several acute cohorts like trauma, sepsis, and postoperative and intensive care offer valuable guides. With all this in mind, the chapter aims to review the optimal approach to fluid therapy in the acute setting, from the understanding of the relevant basic sciences to the practice at the bedside.

Keywords: intravenous infusions, crystalloid solutions, colloids, emergency medicine, critical care

1. Introduction

Majority of patients, in the early and immediate phase of their presentations to the hospital, will require fluid therapy. These fluids are given for various indications, from hemodynamic instability to the delivery of medications [1]. The clinical scenarios that demand the administration of fluids in the acute phase of these patients' stay in the hospital are often complex, yet the task in deciding the fluid regimen is often delegated to junior staff who may lack the necessary insight and experience [2]. Such attitude is compounded by the inadequate knowledge, among the doctors, on the essentials of intravenous fluids like the electrolyte components [3].

Intravenous fluids are drugs, and like other drugs, there are potential complications. In the acute setting where these fluids are commonplace, it is imperative that the practice aims at administering the right patient the right fluids, at the right volume and rate, with the right overall fluid balance.

2. Fluids and physiology

Water is the most important and abundant element of the human body, and the physiology that surrounds it is extensive. The following principles are at best, the foundations toward an informed fluid practice.

2.1. The body fluid compartments

Water, on average, makes up 60% of the total body weight. The percentage will vary depending on the gender and the fat content in the body. There is an inverse correlation between the water content of the body and the fat content as adipose tissue contains less water than lean tissue. This explains why women have lower percentages of water than men as they have a higher percentage of adipose tissue.

Water in the body is functionally distributed among the two main body fluid compartments, the intracellular fluid (ICF) and the extracellular fluid (ECF) (**Figure 1**). The ICF constitutes approximately two-thirds of the total body water or 40% of the body weight and the ECF the remaining one-third or 20% of the body weight [4]. Water crosses between the ICF and the ECF through aquaporin channels in the cell membrane to attain osmotic equilibrium. The cell

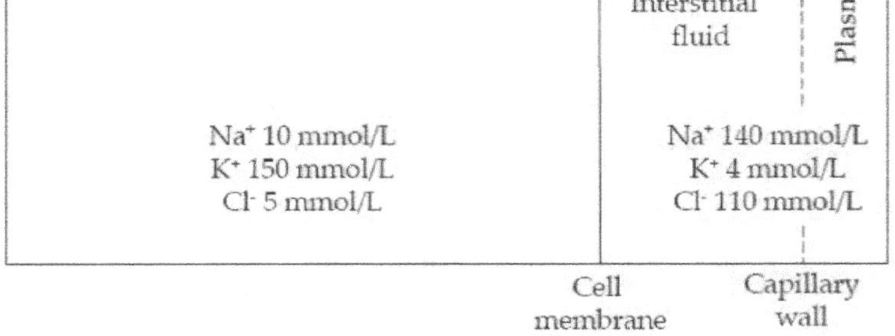

Figure 1. The distribution of total body water.

http://dx.doi.org/10.5772/intechopen.74458

membrane also contains active pumps and transporters that distribute individual solutes, including electrolytes. These electrolytes account for the effective osmolality (tonicity) that governs the water movement. The mechanisms of these electrolyte movements are further defined by the Gibbs-Donnan effect of the nondiffusible large anions like protein. The end results are an ICF compartment with potassium (K^+) as the predominant ion and an ECF compartment with sodium (Na^+) and chloride (Cl^-) as the predominant ions [5].

The ECF is further divided into the interstitial fluid and the plasma compartments, the two separated by the capillary wall. Except for plasma proteins and blood cells, the pores on the capillary wall permit the flux of water and small solutes. This contributes to the two compartments having almost similar electrolyte composition with only small differences contributed by the Gibbs-Donnan effect of the plasma proteins. By volume, these plasma proteins constitute 7% of the plasma volume with the remaining 93% plasma water. As a side note, these proteins are solids in the plasma, and the changes in their plasma load will affect the water-based measurements of plasma electrolyte concentrations [6].

2.2. The body fluid regulation

A complex interaction of regulatory mechanisms from different organs helps the body to maintain an effective fluid volume in different circumstances. The key pathway that underpins this volume regulation is the hormonally mediated renin-angiotensin II-aldosterone-system (RAAS), with the faster neutrally mediated baroreceptor reflex contributing an indirect role through its interplay of the pressure regulation. In the context of the fluid therapy scope of the chapter, the RAAS will be elaborated below.

The RAAS pathway is activated by a decrease in the renal perfusion pressure, detected by the juxtaglomerular apparatus (JGA) (**Figure 2**). In the JGA, the reduced renal perfusion stimulates the granular cells of the afferent arteriole to secrete the proteolytic enzyme renin through a direct intrarenal baroreceptor activity and detection of reduced sodium chloride concentrations by the macula densa in the wall of the ascending limb of the loop

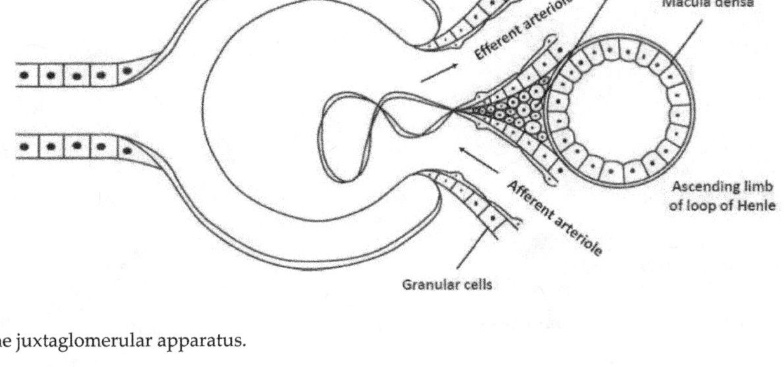

Figure 2. The juxtaglomerular apparatus.

of Henle. Besides these mechanisms, the renin release is also controlled by renal sympathetic nerves and angiotensin II.

Renin as an enzyme will then catalyze the conversion of angiotensinogen, a large protein produced in the liver, to angiotensin I, a decapeptide. This is the rate-limiting step of the RAAS pathway (**Figure 3**). Angiotensin I has little biologic activity apart from being the precursor to angiotensin II. Its conversion to angiotensin II involves the removal of two amino acid moieties by the angiotensin-converting enzyme (ACE). ACE is primarily located in the pulmonary capillaries, but it is also found in the kidney epithelial cells.

The ultimate objective of the RAAS, through the activities of angiotensin II and aldosterone as summarized in **Figure 3**, is the preservation of effective fluid volume and pressure. The RAAS demonstrates the strong interconnection between the body fluid and electrolytes in maintaining the fluid homeostasis. In the acute setting, this interconnection is very relevant given the frequent alterations of the electrolyte contents of the body in the acute phase of illness. The assessment of electrolytes in the acute patients should, therefore, be comprehensive and extend beyond the laboratory results. For example, the assessment should also consider the potential electrolyte losses from the gastrointestinal tract, a common organ affected in acute illnesses [7].

2.3. The microcirculation model

The classic microcirculation model, based on the semipermeability of the capillary and post-capillary venule walls, and the presence of hydrostatic and oncotic pressure gradients across these walls had for long described the flux of fluids and electrolytes between the plasma and the interstitial fluid [8, 9]. The identification of the endothelial glycocalyx layer, a web of membrane-bound glycoproteins and proteoglycans on the luminal side of endothelial cells, has now challenged the classic model [10, 11]. The colloid oncotic pressure from the sub-glycocalyx space is a key determinant of the trans-capillary flow. The disruption to the integrity of the glycocalyx layer, or the "leakiness," in a number of acute situations like sepsis [12], trauma, and postsurgery, has been attributed to the development of interstitial edema

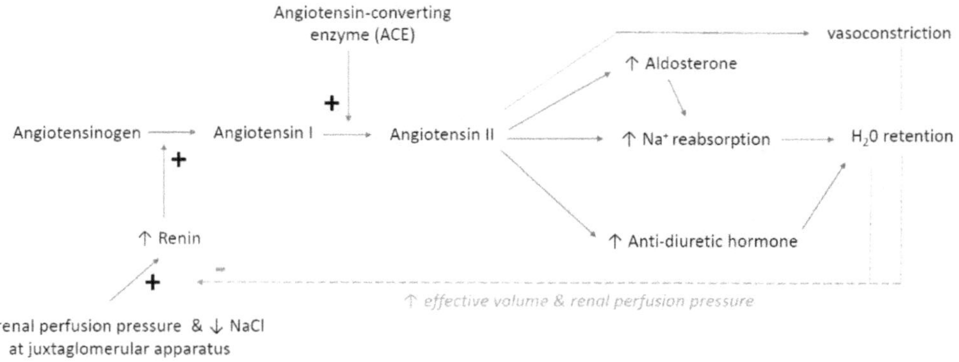

Figure 3. The renin-angiotensin II-aldosterone-system (RAAS).

http://dx.doi.org/10.5772/intechopen.74458

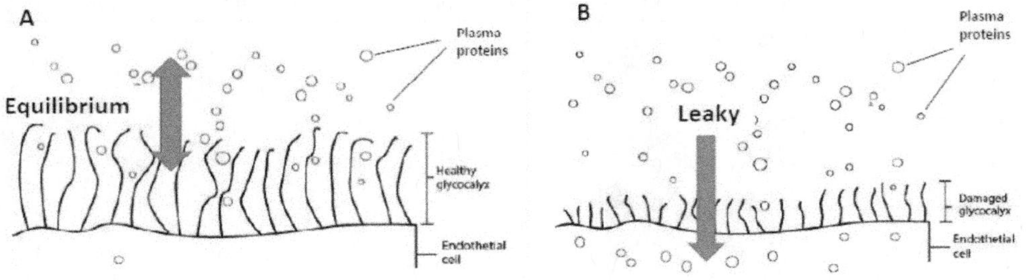

Figure 4. The endothelial glycocalyx layer in healthy, equilibrium state (A) and damaged, leaky state (B) that leads to interstitial edema.

in various organs of the body (**Figure 4**). Appreciation of the dynamics of glycocalyx in the microcirculation of the acute cohort of patients will be integral in their fluid resuscitation and in future fluid research in such population [13, 14].

3. The types of fluids

The history of intravenous fluids began during the cholera pandemic in Europe in the 1830s. The success of Thomas Latta in using a saline solution to resuscitate dying cholera patients paved the way for the widespread use of intravenous fluids and the research to refine their contents [15]. The early milestones in intravenous fluid therapy included the first experiment with albumin in 1834 [16] and the attempt by Sydney Ringer to develop a physiological solution for cardiac contractility with his Ringer's solution in 1876 [17]. Ringer's solution was modified by Alexis Hartmann in 1932 by including lactate to help overcome the acidosis in dehydrated pediatric patients [18]. The gelatins and other solutions with larger molecules only broke into the scene during the Second World War [19], although the first study in humans was performed in 1915 [20]. It is interesting that the history behind the most common type of fluids used, the 0.9% saline, is unclear. The present-day 0.9% saline, often called the "normal saline," has far higher sodium and chloride concentrations than Latta's 1832 saline solution. The only possible connection to 0.9% saline in the history was the in vitro studies of Hamburger in the 1890s that described 0.9% NaCl as an "indifferent solution" in which erythrocytes were least likely to lyse [21, 22].

From the above breakthroughs, the science of intravenous fluids has grown progressively, especially in the last couple of decades. Whether medicine will find an answer to the ideal intravenous fluid will be debatable, but more evidence has emerged in the comparison between the different types of fluids available.

3.1. Crystalloids

Crystalloids are solutions containing salts in the form of electrolytes and small molecules. The composition of commonly available crystalloids is given in **Table 1**.

	Plasma	0.9% NaCl	Hartmann's	Plasmalyte 148®	Sterofundin®
Sodium	140	150	131	140	140
Potassium	5	0	5	5	4
Chloride	100	150	111	98	127
Calcium	2.2	0	2	0	2.5
Magnesium	1	0	1	1.5	1
Bicarbonate	24	0	0	0	0
Lactate	1	0	29	0	0
Acetate	0	0	0	27	24
Gluconate	0	0	0	23	0
Maleate	0	0	0	0	5
Real osmolality	287	286	254	273	287

Plasma-Lyte 148®: Baxter International, Deerfield, IL, USA; Sterofundin®: B Braun, Melsungen, Germany. All concentrations in mmol/L; osmolality in mosmol/kg.

Table 1. The composition of commonly used crystalloids.

Based on their differing compositions, crystalloids have been divided into saline solutions and balanced solutions. Saline solutions, chiefly the 0.9% NaCl solutions, are differentiated from the rest of crystalloids by their high contents of sodium and chloride. These concentrations of 150 mmol/L, especially for chloride, are much higher than the plasma concentrations. The 0.9% saline has thus been described as supra-physiological, and the name "normal saline" has been put to question [23, 24]. Balanced solutions, on the other hand, are other solutions like Hartmann's, Plasmalyte 148®, and Sterofundin® that contains more closely resemble human plasma concentrations. These solutions achieve lower sodium and chloride concentrations through the addition of other electrolytes and buffers like lactate and acetate.

The debate is ongoing as to which will be the better choice for the acute population of patients, saline or balanced solutions. While saline is cheap and is still the most commonly used crystalloid in the world, there are significant concerns with its effect on acid-base balance and kidney function. The high chloride contents of saline contribute to the hyperchloremic or strong ion acidosis [25–27], and this has been well shown in different studies in different acute populations [28–30]. Given that acidosis is a common biochemical presentation in the acute setting, such acidosis could confuse patients' assessment. This has made a case for suggesting balanced solutions as the fluid of choice, even when saline has always been the conventional prescription like in diabetic ketoacidosis [31, 32].

On the other hand, the potential risk of acute kidney injury (AKI) from the use of saline is a main research agenda. Changing the intravenous fluid practice from chloride-rich fluids (0.9% saline, 4% succinylated gelatin, or 4% albumin) to chloride-restrictive fluids (Hartmann's solution, Plasma-Lyte 148, and 20% albumin) had been shown to reduce the incidence of AKI in the intensive care and emergency department populations in a single-center, open label sequential trial

[33–35]. Among the explanations suggested for the higher AKI incidence with the chloride-rich fluids like saline is the renal vasoconstrictive response to the high chloride delivery to the macula densa of JGA, a mechanism similar to the regulatory tubuloglomerular feedback [36, 37]. Similar trends of results implicating saline with AKI have been repeated in large retrospective trials [38, 39]. However, the only three large randomized trials comparing saline with balanced solutions to date have shown inconsistent results. These cluster randomized trials either showed no difference in renal outcomes [40] or a significant increase in major adverse kidney events within 30 days in the saline group for both the intensive care and emergency department populations [41, 42].

While large multicenter randomized controlled trials are ongoing to provide stronger evidence on the issue of saline [43, 44], there has been a notable shift in clinical practice with an increasing use of the balanced solutions [45]. 0.9% saline, nonetheless, remains the fluid of choice for patients with metabolic acidosis, hyponatremia, and traumatic brain injury, the latter attributed to its relatively high osmolality.

3.2. Colloids

Colloid solutions are characterized by the large molecules suspended in carrier solutions that would also contain electrolytes. The colloid osmotic pressure or oncotic pressure generated by these large molecules helps to retain fluid in the intravascular space longer. The composition of the commonly available colloids is in **Table 2**.

The volume effect of colloid, when compared to crystalloid, has traditionally been thought to be at a 1:3 ratio. This gives colloid a perceived advantage in reducing the volume of fluid

	Plasma	Gelofusine®	Albumex®4	Albumex®20	Voluven® (HES 6% 130/0.4)
Sodium	140	154	140	48-100	154
Potassium	5	0	0	0	0
Chloride	100	125	128	19	154
Calcium	2.2	0	0	0	0
Magnesium	1	0	0	0	0
Bicarbonate	24	0	0	0	0
Lactate	1	0	0	0	0
Acetate	0	0	0	0	0
Malate	0	0	0	0	0
Octanoate	0	0	6.4	32	0
Real osmolality	287	271	260	130	298

HES: hydroxyethyl starch. Gelofusine®: B Braun, Melsungen, Germany; Albumex®: CSL Limited, Victoria, Australia; Voluven®: Fresenius-Kabi, Bad Homburg, German. All concentrations in mmol/L; osmolality in mosmol/kg.

Table 2. The composition of commonly used colloids.

infused during resuscitation. However, data from recent large multicenter trials on the use of different types of colloids suggested a smaller colloid: crystalloid ratio, between 1:1.1 and 1:1.6 [46–49]. The finding of smaller volume effect advantage from colloid than previously thought adds to the predominant concern on the use of colloid—its effects on the kidney.

Strong evidence emerged in the last decade demonstrating a significant association between the risk of renal dysfunction, measured as AKI, and the need for renal replacement therapy, with the use of hydroxyethyl starch in the acute population of sepsis and intensive care [46, 47]. There are also doubts from observational data on the renal safety of another choice of colloid, the gelatins, in the septic population [50, 51]. The hyperoncotic albumin solutions (20–25%), on the other hand, have been associated with increased risk of renal events when used in cardiac surgery [52] and in patients in shock [53].

Besides these renal effects, colloids are more expensive than crystalloids, and there has been an absence of their clinical superiority over crystalloids in the mortality outcome of studies on different acute populations [49, 54, 55]. All these lead to the call for caution in the use of colloids. The recent Surviving Sepsis Guidelines, for example, strongly recommend against the use of hydroxyethyl starches and place albumin and gelatins as a second choice to crystalloids in sepsis fluid resuscitation [56].

4. Delivering fluid therapy

Following an evidence-informed choice of fluid, the next set of decisions will be equally crucial: how to administer the fluid, how to measure the patient's response to the fluid, and how much fluid should be given. Strategizing intravenous fluid delivery to an acute patient should include a well thought-out plan for these three important elements.

4.1. Resuscitation and the fluid challenge

A key aim of the fluid resuscitation in the acute setting is to exert a hemodynamic impact, increasing the venous return and the stroke volume. To achieve this, the concept of fluid challenge or fluid bolus was introduced almost four decades ago [57, 58]. The fluid challenge is a targeted administration approach through the delivery of a small amount of fluid over a short period of time, with an assessment of the fluid responsiveness [59].

The administration of fluid challenge has been one of the most diverse practices in fluid therapy. Recent attempts at identifying the global patterns in fluid challenge have provided valuable information. A global inception cohort study on fluid challenge involving 2213 patients across ICUs in 46 countries revealed a median amount of fluid challenge volume of 500 ml, a median time of 24 min, a median rate of fluid administration of 1000 ml/h, and a predominant choice of crystalloids [60]. Interestingly, categorizing patients as fluid responsive, non-fluid responsive, or uncertain fluid responsive did not make any difference to the receipt of further fluid administration in this study. In another study on the worldwide fluid challenge practices, involving 3138 intensive care specialists from 30 countries, more than 80% respondents defined the fluid bolus therapy as delivery of more than 250 mL of either colloid or crystalloid fluid over less than 30 minutes, with crystalloids the most acceptable [61]. These numbers only reflect the majority views on the fluid challenge and must be interpreted in the context of the other aspects of an acute fluid strategy—the fluid responsiveness and the fluid balance.

4.2. Fluid responsiveness

Clinical assessment is always an integral component of any fluid therapy approach. Identifying body volume repletion and the likelihood to respond to fluid resuscitation should begin with the background history and elicitation of signs of volume deficits, from the peripheral temperature gradient and capillary refill time [62] to the tachycardia, decreased mean arterial pressure, and oliguria. However, reliance on these clinical signs alone for assessment of volume status and responsiveness could be misleading [63–65]. For instance, an increase in the mean arterial pressure following a fluid challenge could be a result of the changes in the arterial vascular tone rather than a true increase in cardiac output.

Beyond clinical signs, the indices of fluid responsiveness—both static and dynamic—have been extensively studied. The static index of central venous pressure (CVP), arguably the most commonly used measure of fluid responsiveness, has long been shown to have no meaningful relationship to fluid volume and should be abandoned [66]. Similarly, the more invasive static index measurement of pulmonary artery occlusion pressure (PAOP) has its limitations and does not predict fluid responsiveness [67, 68].

The dynamic indices of fluid responsiveness work on the basis of inducing a change in preload and following up the effects on stroke volume and cardiac output [69]. There are different versions of these dynamic measurements with many evolving around the respiratory variation of hemodynamic indices. Examples include the pulse pressure variation (PPV), the pulse contour-derived stroke volume, the inferior vena cava (IVC) parameters assessed by ultrasonography, and the descending aortic blood flow assessed by esophageal Doppler [70–75]. There are, however, limitations to the observations of these respiratory variations. Some of these are of practical significance, like the need for tidal volumes of >7 ml/kg, the absence of spontaneous ventilatory efforts, and the absence of arrhythmia.

An approach to assessment of fluid responsiveness that is not affected by the practical ventilatory limitations above is the passive leg raising, PLR [76]. The postural change in PLR transfers around 300 mL of venous blood from the lower body to the heart. The advantage of this is it is an endogenous fluid challenge that is rapidly reversible [77]. To date, the PLR has been deemed as the most reliable measure of fluid responsiveness [78], although an increase in the intra-abdominal pressure or pain could give a false-negative result [79].

It is important to recognize that fluid responsiveness does not necessarily mean that fluid challenges must be given. It also does not mean that patients should be receiving fluid challenges until they are no longer fluid responsive. The hemodynamic benefits of the fluid boluses should be weighed against the risks of accumulating positive fluid balance, with a strong consideration of the use of vasopressors like noradrenaline to improve organ perfusion [80].

4.3. The importance of fluid balance

Fluid accumulation in the acute setting is a frequent event. While everything is geared toward early and aggressive fluid resuscitation, as it should be, less emphasis is given toward the risks associated with fluid accumulation and overload. As fluid overload is shown to contribute to poorer outcomes in different acute populations [81–84], it becomes imperative to achieve the right balance between overcoming hypovolemia and organ hypoperfusion and avoiding the dangers of fluid overload [85].

A common quantitative definition of fluid overload in the literature is a percentage fluid accumulation of >10%, determined by dividing the cumulative fluid balance in liter by the patient's baseline body weight and multiplying by 100% [86, 87]. This is, however, on the assumption that the patient is volume depleted on admission to the acute unit, which is not necessarily the case as some patients have already been accumulating fluid by then. The negative effects of the excess fluid have been shown in various organ systems. In a large RCT, higher cumulative fluid balance was associated with longer mechanical ventilation duration and length of ICU stay and without reducing the incidence of shock and the need for renal replacement therapy [88]. In managing intra-abdominal hypertension and abdominal compartment syndrome, poorer outcomes have been attributed to fluid overload [89, 90], a phenomenon linked to capillary leak and tissue edema. While fluid is often aggressively given to prevent AKI, the association between fluid overload and poorer renal outcomes has been evident [86, 91, 92], prompting questions on the cause-effect relationship between fluid overload and AKI [93].

A comprehensive fluid strategy will require a close monitoring of the fluid balance. In this context, a mindset of fluids as drugs will promote careful considerations of the indications and the doses of the fluids, recognizing that more is not always better.

5. Conclusion

In conclusion, fluid therapy in the acute setting is a challenging and complex task for the clinicians. Two areas that are beyond the scope of the chapter—the specific needs of the different subpopulations of acute patients and the different access to resources at different locations of practice—further add to the complexity. Emerging evidence on various facets of fluid therapy has helped to offer some consistency in approach in what has been a very diverse practice. The underpinning principle should be fluids are drugs that must be chosen and prescribed correctly, as wrong choice and doses lead to adverse effects.

Conflict of interest

The author declares no competing interest.

Author details

Nor'azim Mohd Yunos

Address all correspondence to: nor.azim@monash.edu

Jeffrey Cheah School of Medicine and Health Sciences, Monash University Malaysia, Johor Bahru, Malaysia

References

[1] National Institute for Health and Care Excellence. Intravenous Fluid Therapy in Adults in Hospital: Clinical Guideline. London: NICE, 2013. Available from: https://www.nice.org.uk/guidance/cg174 [Accessed: 2018-01-03]

[2] Liu B, Finfer S. Intravenous fluids in adults undergoing surgery. BMJ. 2009;**338**:b2418. DOI: 10.1136/bmj.b2418

[3] Lobo DN, Dube MG, Neal KR, Simpson JS, Rowlands BJ, Allison SP. Problems with solutions: Drowning in the brine of an inadequate knowledge base. Clinical Nutrition. 2001;**20**:125-130. DOI: 10.1054/clnu.2000.0154

[4] Costanzo LS. Physiology. 5th ed. Philadelphia, PA: Elsevier; 2014. ISBN: 9781455708475

[5] Kamel KS, Halperin ML. Fluid, Electrolyte, and Acid-Base Physiology: A Problem-Based Approach. 5th ed. Philadelphia, PA: Elsevier; 2017. ISBN 9780323355155. DOI: 10.1016/c2013-0-13529-5

[6] Story DA, Morimatsu H, Egi M, Bellomo R. The effect of albumin concentration on plasma sodium and chloride measurements in critically ill patients. Anesthesia and Analgesia. 2007;**104**(4):893-897. DOI: 10.1213/01.ane.0000258015.87381.61

[7] Macafee DA, Allison SP, Lobo DN. Some interactions between gastrointestinal function and fluid and electrolyte homeostasis. Current Opinion in Clinical Nutrition and Metabolic Care. 2005;**8**:197-203. DOI: 10.1097/00075197-200503000-00015

[8] Starling EH. On the absorption of fluids from connective tissue spaces. The Journal of Physiology. 1896;**19**:312-326. DOI: 10.1113/jphysiol.1896.sp000596

[9] Krogh A, Landis EM, Turner AH. The movement of fluid through the human capillary wall in relation to venous pressure and to the colloid osmotic pressure of the blood. The Journal of Clinical Investigation. 1932;**11**:63-95. DOI: 10.1172/JCI100408

[10] Weinbaum S, Tarbell JM, Damiano ER. The structure and function of the endothelial glycocalyx layer. Annual Review of Biomedical Engineering. 2007;**9**:121-167. DOI: 10.1146/annurev.bioeng.9.060906.151959

[11] Levick JR, Michel CC. Microvascular fluid exchange and the revised Starling principle. Cardiovascular Research. 2010;**87**:198-210. DOI: 10.1093/cvr/cvq062

[12] Lee WL, Slutsky AS. Sepsis and endothelial permeability. The New England Journal of Medicine. 2010;**363**:689-691. DOI: 10.1056/NEJMcibr1007320

[13] Myburgh JA, Mythen MG. Resuscitation fluids. The New England Journal of Medicine. 2013;**369**:1243-1251. DOI: 10.1056/NEJMra1208627

[14] Guidet B, Ait-Oufella H. Fluid resuscitation should respect the endothelial glycocalyx layer. Critical Care. 2014;**18**:707. DOI: 10.1186/s13054-014-0707-6

[15] Latta T. No. 3. Letter from DR. LATTA, of Leith, detailing three cases, of which one was successful. Lancet. 1832;**18**:370-3737. DOI: 10.1016/S0140-6736(02)94630-1

[16] Barsoum N, Kleeman C. Now and then, the history of parenteral fluid administration. American Journal of Nephrology. 2002;**22**:284-289. DOI: 10.1159/000063775

[17] Ringer S. Regarding the action of the hydrate of soda, hydrate of ammonia, and the hydrate of potash on the ventricle of the frog's heart. Journal of Physiology (London). 1880/82;**3**:195-202. PMCID: PMC1484928

[18] Hartmann AF, Senn MJ. Studies in the metabolism of sodium r-lactate. I. Response of normal human subjects to the intravenous injection of sodium r-lactate. The Journal of Clinical Investigation. 1932;**11**:327-335. DOI: 10.1172/JCI100414

[19] Hogan JJ. The intravenous use of colloidal (gelatin) solutions in shock. Journal of the American Medical Association. 1915;**LXIV**(9):721-726. DOI: 10.1001/jama.1915.02570350015004

[20] Jacobson SD, Smyth CJ. Gelatin as a substitute for plasma observations on its administration to human beings. Archives of Internal Medicine. 1944;**74**:254-257. DOI: 10.1001/archinte.1944.00210220021003

[21] Awad S, Allison SP, Lobo DN. The history of 0.9% saline. Clinical Nutrition. 2008;**27**:179-188. DOI: 10.1016/j.clnu.2008.01.008

[22] Lazarus-Barlow WS. On the initial rate of osmosis of blood-serum with reference to the composition of 'physiological saline solution' in mammals. Journal of Physiology. 1896; **20**:145-157. PMCID: PMC1512961

[23] Wakim KG. "Normal" 0.9 per cent salt solution is neither "normal" nor physiological. JAMA. 1970;**214**(9):1710. DOI: 10.1001/jama.1970.03180090074027

[24] Reid F, Lobo DN, Williams RN, Rowlands BJ, Allison SP. (Ab)normal saline and physiological Hartmann's solution: A randomized double-blind crossover study. Clinical Science. 2003;**104**:17-24. DOI: 10.1042/cs1040017

[25] Kellum JA, Bellomo R, Kramer DJ, Pinsky MR. Etiology of metabolic acidosis during saline resuscitation in endotoxaemia. Shock. 1998;**9**:364-368. DOI: 10.1097/00024382-199805000-00009

[26] Story DA, Morimatsu H, Bellomo R. Hyperchloraemic acidosis in the critically ill: One of the strong-ion acidoses? Anesthesia and Analgesia. 2006;**103**:144-148. DOI: 10.1213/01.ane.0000221449.67354.52

[27] Yunos NM, Bellomo R, Story D, Kellum J. Bench-to-bedside review: Chloride in critical illness. Critical Care. 2010;**14**(4):226. DOI: 10.1186/cc9052

[28] Scheingraber S, Rehm M, Sehmisch C, et al. Rapid saline infusion produces hyperchloremic acidosis in patients undergoing gynecologic surgery. Anesthesiology. 1999; **90**(5):1265-1270. DOI: 10.1097/00000542-199905000-00007

[29] Ho AM-H, Karmakar KM, Contardi LH, Ng SW, Hewson JR. Excessive use of normal saline in managing traumatized patients in shock: A preventable contributor to acidosis. The Journal of Trauma. 2001;**51**:173-177. DOI: 10.1097/00005373-200107000-00033

[30] Yunos NM, Kim IB, Bellomo R, Bailey M, Ho L, Story D, Gutteridge GA, Hart GK. The biochemical effects of restricting chloride-rich fluids in intensive care. Critical Care Medicine. 2011;**39**:2419-2424. DOI: 10.1097/CCM.0b013e31822571e5

[31] Mahler SA, Conrad SA, Wang H, Arnold TC. Resuscitation with balanced electrolyte solution prevents hyperchloremic metabolic acidosis in patients with diabetic ketoacidosis. The American Journal of Emergency Medicine. 2011;**29**(6):670-674. DOI: 10.1016/j.ajem.2010.02.004

[32] Chua HR, Venkatesh B, Stachowski E, et al. Plasma-Lyte 148 vs 0.9% saline for fluid resuscitation in diabetic ketoacidosis. Journal of Critical Care. 2012;**27**(2):138-145. DOI: 10.1016/j.jcrc.2012.01.007

[33] Yunos NM, Bellomo R, Hegarty C, Story D, Ho L, Bailey M. Association between a chloride-liberal vs chloride-restrictive intravenous fluid administration strategy and kidney injury in critically ill adults. JAMA. 2012;**308**:1566-1572. DOI: 10.1001/jama.2012.13356

[34] Yunos NM, Bellomo R, Glassford N, Sutcliffe H, Lam Q, Bailey M. Chloride-liberal vs. chloride-restrictive intravenous fluid administration and acute kidney injury: An extended analysis. Intensive Care Medicine. 2015;**41**(2):257-264. DOI: 10.1007/s00134-014-3593-0

[35] Yunos NM, Bellomo R, Taylor DM, Judkins S, Kerr F, Sutcliffe H, Hegarty C, Bailey M. Renal effects of an emergency department chloride-restrictive intravenous fluid strategy in patients admitted to hospital for more than 48 hours. Emergency Medicine Australasia. 2017;**29**(6):643-649. DOI: 10.1111/1742-6723.12821

[36] Wilcox CS. Regulation of renal blood flow by plasma chloride. The Journal of Clinical Investigation. 1983;**71**(3):726-735. DOI: 10.1172/JCI110820

[37] Chowdhury AH, Cox EF, Francis ST, Lobo DN. A randomized, controlled, double-blind crossover study on the effects of 2-L infusions of 0.9% saline and plasma-Lyte 148 on renal blood flow velocity and renal cortical tissue perfusion in healthy volunteers. Annals of Surgery. 2012;**256**(1):18-24. DOI: 10.1097/SLA.0b013e318256be72

[38] Shaw AD, Bagshaw SM, Goldstein SL, et al. Major complications, mortality, and resource utilization after open abdominal surgery: 0.9% saline compared to Plasma-Lyte. Annals of Surgery. 2012;**255**:821-829. DOI: 10.1097/SLA.0b013e31825074f5

[39] McCluskey SA, Karkouti K, Wijeysundera D, Minkovich L, Tait G, Beattie WS. Hyperchloremia after non-cardiac surgery is independently associated with increased morbidity and mortality: A propensity matched cohort study. Anesthesia & Analgesia. 2013;**117**:412-421. DOI: 10.1213/ANE.0b013e318293d81e

[40] Young P, Bailey M, Beasley R, et al. Effect of a buffered crystalloid solution vs. saline on acute kidney injury among patients in the Intensive Care Unit: The SPLIT randomized clinical trial. Journal of the American Medical Association. 2015;**314**(16):1701-1710. DOI: 10.1001/jama.2015.12334

[41] Semler MW, Self WH, Wanderer JP, et al. Balanced crystalloids versus saline in critically ill adults. The New England Journal of Medicine. 2018;**378**:829-839. DOI: 10.1056/NEJMoa1711584

[42] Semler MW, Self WH, Wanderer JP, et al. Balanced crystalloids versus saline in noncritically ill adults. The New England Journal of Medicine. 2018;**378**:819-828. DOI: 10.1056/NEJMoa1711586

[43] Plasma-Lyte 148® versUs Saline Study (PLUS) NCT02721654. Available from: https://clinicaltrials.gov/ct2/show/NCT02721654?term=NCT02721654&rank=1 [Accessed: 2018-01-17]

[44] Balanced Solution Versus Saline in Intensive Care Study (BaSICS) NCT02875873. Available from: https://clinicaltrials.gov/ct2/show/NCT02875873?term=NCT02875873&rank=1 [Accessed: 2018-01-17]

[45] Hammond NE, Taylor C, Saxena M, et al. Resuscitation fluid use in Australian and New Zealand Intensive Care Units between 2007 and 2013. Intensive Care Medicine. 2015; **41**(9):1611-1619. DOI: 10.1007/s00134-015-3878-y

[46] Myburgh J, Finfer S, Bellomo R, et al. Hydroxyethyl starch or saline for fluid resuscitation in intensive care. The New England Journal of Medicine. 2012;**367**:1901-1911. DOI: 10.1056/NEJMoa1209759

[47] Perner A, Nicolai H, Guttormson A, et al. Hydroxyethyl starch 130/0.42 versus Ringer's acetate in severe sepsis. The New England Journal of Medicine. 2012;**367**:124-134. DOI: 10.1056/NEJMoa1204242

[48] Annane D, Siami S, Jaber S, et al. Effects of fluid resuscitation with colloids vs crystalloids on mortality in critically ill patients presenting with hypovolaemic shock. The CRISTAL randomized trial. Journal of the American Medical Association. 2013;**310**:1809-1817. DOI: 10.1001/jama.2013.280502

[49] Guidet B, Martinet O, Boulain T, et al. Assessment of hemodynamic efficacy and safety of 6% hydroxyethyl starch 130/0.4 vs 0.9% NaCl fluid replacement in patients with severe sepsis: The CRYSTMAS study. Critical Care. 2012;**16**(3):R94. DOI: 10.1186/11358

[50] Bayer O, Reinhart K, Sakr Y, et al. Renal effects of synthetic colloids and crystalloids in patients with severe sepsis: A prospective sequential comparison. Critical Care Medicine. 2011;**39**:1335-1342. DOI: 10.1097/CCM.0b013e318212096a

[51] Pisano A, Landoni G, Bellomo R. The risk of infusing gelatin? Die-hard misconceptions and forgotten (or ignored) truths. Minerva Anestesiologica. 2016;**82**:1107-1114. PMID: 27045639

[52] Frenette AJ, Bouchard J, Bernier P, Charbonneau A, Nguyen L, Rioux J, Troyanov S, Williamson D. Albumin administration is associated with acute kidney injury in cardiac surgery: A propensity score analysis. Critical Care. 2014;**18**(6):602. DOI: 10.1186/s13054-014-0602-1

[53] Schortgen F, Girou E, Deye N, Brochard L. Cryco Study Group. The risk associated with hyperoncotic colloids in patients with shock. Intensive Care Medicine. 2008;**34**(12):2157-2168. DOI: 10.1007/s00134-008-1225-2

[54] Caironi P, Tognoni G, Masson S, et al. Albumin replacement in patients with severe sepsis or septic shock. The New England Journal of Medicine. 2014;**370**(15):1412-1421. DOI: 10.1056/NEJMoa1305727

[55] Qureshi SH, Rizvi SI, Patel NN, Murphy GJ. Meta-analysis of colloids versus crystalloids in critically ill, trauma and surgical patients. The British Journal of Surgery. 2016;**103**(1):14-26. DOI: 10.1002/bjs.9943

[56] Rhodes A, Evans LE, Alhazzani W, et al. Surviving Sepsis Campaign: International Guidelines for Management of Sepsis and Septic Shock: 2016. Intensive Care Medicine. 2017;**43**(3):304-377. DOI: 10.1007/s00134-017-4683-6

[57] Weil MH, Henning RJ. New concepts in the diagnosis and fluid treatment of circulatory shock. Thirteenth annual Becton, Dickinson and Company Oscar Schwidetsky Memorial Lecture. *Anesthesia* & Analgesia. 1979;**58**:124-132. PMID: 571235

[58] Vincent JL, Weil MH. Fluid challenge revisited. Critical Care Medicine. 2006;**34**:1333-1337. DOI: 10.1097/01.CCM.0000214677.76535.A5

[59] Cecconi M, Parsons AK, Rhodes A. What is a fluid challenge? Current Opinion in Critical Care. 2011;**17**:290-295. DOI: 10.1097/MCC.0b013e32834699cd

[60] Cecconi M, Hofer C, Teboul JL, et al. Fluid challenges in intensive care: The FENICE study: A global inception cohort study. Intensive Care Medicine. 2015;**41**:1529-1537. DOI: 10.1007/s00134-015-3850-x

[61] Glassford NJ, Mårtensson J, Eastwood GM. Defining the characteristics and expectations of fluid bolus therapy: A worldwide perspective. Journal of Critical Care. 2016;**35**:126-132. DOI: 10.1016/j.jcrc.2016.05.017

[62] Ait-Oufella H, Bakker J. Understanding clinical signs of poor tissue perfusion during septic shock. Intensive Care Medicine. 2016;**42**:2070. DOI: 10.1007/s00134-016-4250-6

[63] Saugel B, Ringmaier S, Holzapfel K, et al. Physical examination, central venous pressure, and chest radiography for the prediction of transpulmonary thermodilution-derived hemodynamic parameters in critically ill patients: A prospective trial. Journal of Critical Care. 2011;**26**:402-410. DOI: 10.1016/j.jcrc.2010.11.001

[64] Monge García MI, Guijo González P, Gracia Romero M, et al. Effects of fluid administration on arterial load in septic shock patients. Intensive Care Medicine. 2015;**41**:1247-1255. DOI: 10.1007/s00134-015-3898-7

[65] Pierrakos C, Velissaris D, Scolletta S, Heenen S, De Backer D, Vincent JL. Can changes in arterial pressure be used to detect changes in cardiac index during fluid challenge in patients with septic shock? Intensive Care Medicine. 2012;**38**:422-428. DOI: 10.1007/s00134-011-2457-0

[66] Marik PE, Cavallazzi R. Does the central venous pressure (CVP) predict fluid responsiveness: An update meta-analysis and a plea for some common sense. Critical Care Medicine. 2013;**41**:1774-1781. DOI: 10.1097/CCM.0b013e31828a25fd

[67] Michard F, Teboul JL. Predicting fluid responsiveness in ICU patients: A critical analysis of the evidence. Chest. 2002;**121**:2000-2008. DOI: 10.1378/chest.121.6.2000

[68] Osman D, Ridel C, Ray P, et al. Cardiac filling pressures are not appropriate to predict hemodynamic response to volume challenge. Critical Care Medicine. 2007;**35**:64-68. DOI: 10.1097/01.CCM.0000249851.94101.4F

[69] Marik P, Monnet X, Teboul J. Hemodynamic parameters to guide fluid therapy. Annals of Intensive Care. 2011;**1**:1-9. DOI: 10.1186/2110-5820-1-1

[70] Cannesson M, Slieker J, Desebbe O, et al. The ability of a novel algorithm for automatic estimation of the respiratory variations in arterial pulse pressure to monitor fluid responsiveness in the operating room. Anesthesia and Analgesia. 2008;**106**:1195-1200. DOI: 10.1213/01.ane.0000297291.01615.5c

[71] Cecconi M, Monti G, Hamilton M, et al. Efficacy of functional hemodynamic parameters in predicting fluid responsiveness with pulse power analysis in surgical patients. Minerva Anestesiologica. 2012;**78**:527-533. PMID: 22534733

[72] Hofer C, Müller S, Furrer L, et al. Stroke volume and pulse pressure variation for prediction of fluid responsiveness in patients undergoing off-pump coronary artery bypass grafting. Chest. 2005;**128**:848-854. DOI: 10.1378/chest.128.2.848

[73] Feissel M, Michard F, Mangin I, et al. Respiratory changes in aortic blood velocity as an indicator of fluid responsiveness in ventilated patients with septic shock. Chest. 2001; **119**:867-873. DOI: 10.1378/chest.119.3.867

[74] Vermeiren G, Malbrain M, Walpot J. Cardiac ultrasonography in the critical care setting: A practical approach to asses cardiac function and preload for the "non-cardiologist". Anaesthesiology Intensive Therapy. 2015;**47**:89-104. DOI: 10.5603/AIT.a2015.0074

[75] Feissel M, Michard F, Faller J, et al. The respiratory variation in inferior vena cava diameter as a guide to fluid therapy. Intensive Care Medicine. 2004;**30**:1834-1837. DOI: 10.1007/s00134-004-2233-5

[76] Monnet T. Passive leg raising: Five rules, not a drop of fluid! Critical Care. 2015;**19**:18. DOI: 10.1186/s13054-014-0708-5

[77] Jabot J, Teboul JL, Richard C, Monnet X. Passive leg raising for predicting fluid responsiveness: Importance of the postural change. Intensive Care Medicine. 2009;**35**:85-90. DOI: 10.1007/s00134-008-1293-3

[78] Monnet X, Marik P, Teboul JL. Passive leg raising for predicting fluid responsiveness: A systematic review and meta-analysis. Intensive Care Medicine. 2016;**42**(12):1935-1947. DOI: 10.1007/s00134-015-4134-1

[79] Malbrain M, Reuter D. Assessing fluid responsiveness with the passive leg raising maneuver in patients with increased intra-abdominal pressure: Be aware that not all blood returns! Critical Care Medicine. 2010;**38**:1912-1915. DOI: 10.1097/CCM.0b013e3181f1b6a2

[80] Marik PE. Fluid responsiveness and the six guiding principles of fluid resuscitation. Critical Care Medicine. 2016:1920-1922. DOI: 10.1097/CCM.0000000000001483

[81] Boyd JH, Forbes J, Nakada TA, Walley KR, Russell JA. Fluid resuscitation in septic shock: A positive fluid balance and elevated central venous pressure are associated with increased mortality. Critical Care Medicine. 2011;**39**(2):259-265. DOI: 10.1097/CCM.0b013e3181feeb15

[82] Kox M, Pickkers P. Less is more in critically Ill patients: Not too intensive. JAMA Internal Medicine. 2013;**173**:1369-1372. DOI: 10.1001/jamainternmed.2013.6702

[83] Acheampong A, Vincent JL. A positive fluid balance is an independent prognostic factor in patients with sepsis. Critical Care. 2015;**19**:251. DOI: 10.1186/s13054-015-0970-1

[84] Raghunathan K, McGee WT, Higgins T. Importance of intravenous fluid dose and composition in surgical ICU patients. Current Opinion in Critical Care. 2012;**18**:350-357. DOI: 10.1097/MCC.0b013e328355598c

[85] Boulain T, Cecconi M. Can one size fit all? The fine line between fluid overload and hypovolemia. Intensive Care Medicine. 2015;**41**:544-546. DOI: 10.1007/s00134-015-3683-7

[86] Bouchard J, Soroko SB, Chertow GM, et al. Fluid accumulation, survival and recovery of kidney function in critically ill patients with acute kidney injury. Kidney International. 2009;**76**:422-427. DOI: 10.1038/ki.2009.159

[87] Malbrain ML, Marik PE, Witters I, Cordemans C, Kirkpatrick AW, Roberts DJ, Van Regenmortel N. Fluid overload, de-resuscitation, and outcomes in critically ill or injured patients: A systematic review with suggestions for clinical practice. Anaesthesiology Intensive Therapy. 2014;**46**:361-380. DOI: 10.5603/AIT.2014.0060

[88] Wiedemann HP, Wheeler AP, Bernard GR, et al. Comparison of two fluid-management strategies in acute lung injury. The New England Journal of Medicine. 2006;**354**(24):2564-2575. DOI: 10.1056/NEJMoa062200

[89] Balogh Z, McKinley BA, Cocanour CS, et al. Supranormal trauma resuscitation causes more cases of abdominal compartment syndrome. Archives of Surgery. 2003;**138**:637-643. DOI: 10.1001/archsurg.138.6.637

[90] Kirkpatrick AW, Balogh Z, Ball CG, et al. The secondary abdominal compartment syndrome: Iatrogenic or unavoidable? Journal of the American College of Surgeons. 2006;**202**:668–679. DOI: 10.1016/j.jamcollsurg.2005.11.020

[91] Salahuddin N, Sammani M, Hamdan A, et al. Fluid overload is an independent risk factor for acute kidney injury in critically ill patients: Results of a cohort study. BMC Nephrology. 2017;**18**:45. DOI: 10.1186/s12882-017-0460-6

[92] Vaara ST, Korhonen AM, Kaukonen KM, et al. Fluid overload is associated with an increased risk for 90-day mortality in critically ill patients with renal replacement therapy: Data from the prospective FINNAKI study. Critical Care. 2012;**16**:R197. DOI: 10.1186/cc11682

[93] Ostermann M, Straaten HMO, Forni LG, et al. Fluid overload and acute kidney injury: Cause or consequence? Critical Care. 2015;**19**:443. DOI: 10.1186/s13054-015-1163-7

Chapter 4

Resuscitation Procedures in Emergency Setting

Aml Yousif Elemamali and Aftab Mohammad Azad

Additional information is available at the end of the chapter

http://dx.doi.org/10.5772/intechopen.76165

Abstract

The physicians of the emergency department have great mission as they have to manage these critically ill patients and stabilize them by effectively using their own skills in order to improve their patients' condition. It is very important to understand when a procedure is needed in emergency situation and to make all efforts to achieve that goal in a timely and safe manner and to follow the protocols and guidelines. There are some procedures which are lifesaving and imminent to resuscitation and considered adjuncts to resuscitation. Effective and lifesaving resuscitation cannot be completed without these procedures. This chapter will help the emergency physician (EP) to better understand and develop the required technical skills to achieve the highest level of care that will have direct impact on patients' outcome.

Keywords: resuscitation, procedures, emergency medicine

1. Introduction

The emergency department (ED) is one of the basics of any hospital, as this department is considered the gate of the hospital and its front line. Above one third of patients who present to ED are very critically ill and need urgent care and intervention [1].The physicians of the emergency department have great mission as they have to manage these critically ill patients and stabilize them by effectively using their own skills in order to improve their patients' condition. It is very important to understand when a procedure is needed in emergency situation and to make all efforts to achieve that goal in a timely and safe manner and to follow the protocols and guidelines. There are some procedures which are lifesaving and imminent to resuscitation and considered adjuncts to resuscitation. Effective and lifesaving resuscitation cannot be completed without these procedures. This chapter will help the emergency physician (EP) to better understand and develop the required technical skills to achieve the highest level of care that will have direct impact on patients' outcome.

The chapter will cover the following resuscitative procedures of emergency:

- Airway management
- Rapid sequence intubation
- Needle decompression
- Tube thoracostomy
- Central venous catheter placement
- Intraosseous line placement
- Pericardiocentesis
- ED thoracotomy
- Defibrillator
- Transcutaneous pacing

2. Airway management

2.1. Introduction

Emergency airway management is considered one of the most difficult fields of the emergency care. In order for physicians to provide proficient and effective care, they must be trained to a competent and highly efficient level of proficiency in maintaining, assessing, and managing airways using both basic airway maneuvers and advanced skills such as rapid sequence intubation (RSI). The physician's decision-making process is the core principle of highly safe and effective airway management. The decision made by the physicians should ensure the accomplishment of airway security and improvement of ventilation and oxygenation while ensuring there are none or minimal iatrogenic errors or defaults [1].

2.2. Basic airway management

The most initial part of airway management in sick patient is to assess for airway adequacy and patency and risk for compromise and take a decision for further intervention. Delivering oxygen to the lungs and ensuring a clear airway are the key principles of airway management. For this to be done, physicians must ensure the airway is guarded from foreign objects such as blood and fluids. Once breathing discontinues the body's oxygen supplies dramatically and rapidly decrease; time is the most critical part of this process of airway management which takes us back to the extreme importance of accurate decision-making when assessing adequacy of airway alongside any risks of compromise. Blood, vomit, and other foreign bodies are the main cause of the blockade to the airways; however airway injury or swelling can also be a cause. These obstructions can be treated by many lifesaving interventions such as airway maneuvers, positioning, and correct ventilations [2–5].

2.3. Airway anatomy

A complete understanding and knowledge of anatomy is important for performing any procedure. Adverse events in any procedure usually happen either due to lack of understanding of the regional anatomy or as a result of inexperience. Performing an airway procedure with a thorough understanding of airway anatomy is not exceptional. Starting by assessing the airway looking for external anatomical landmarks till the completion of intubation, an understanding of the anatomy of the airway will lead to increased success rate and reduced attempts rate and iatrogenic errors. The upper airway includes the oral and nasal cavities, the pharynx, and the larynx. The lower airway comprises the subglottic larynx, the trachea, and the bronchi. It is a complicated system that transmits filtered warm air to the lungs through the trachea and at the same time permits passage of solids and liquids to the esophagus. However, if a food particle or liquid enters the airway, a complete system of reflexes will be activated to protect its integrity [3, 4]. **Figure1** shows the anatomy of the larynx, trachea, and pharynx (graphic jump location).

2.4. Basic airway management techniques

Basic airway management is the base for advanced airway skills. Although it is easy, it can be both tricky and lifesaving. In majority of patients, a combination of patient positioning, different airway maneuvers, use of airway adjuncts, and assisted ventilation will help maintain oxygenation and can be lifesaving [3].

2.5. Positioning

The sniffing position is the preferable way to open the upper airway and it is achieved by flexion of the lower cervical spine and atlanto-occipital extension. It can be accomplished by putting a pillow or folded towel under the patient's head, and the physician then extends the head on the neck to align the three airway axes oral, pharyngeal, and laryngeal axes[2, 3, 6].If cervical spine injury is suspected, maintain the neck in a neutral position. In obese patients the sniffing position can be achieved by putting a pillow under the shoulders and another pillow under the head to raise it further. Raising the head end of the trolley or bed also improves preoxygenation in obese patients by reducing the pressure of the abdominal contents on the diaphragm, thereby increasing the functional residual capacity [2].

2.6. Head-tilt and chin-lift maneuver

After patient positioning, there are other movements that improve the airway more. Head tilt and chin lift one of them, to perform it, place the tips of index and middle fingers under the patient's chin and pull the mandible forward to elevate the tongue and open the airway. The thumb then can be used to open patient's mouth by depressing the lower lip.

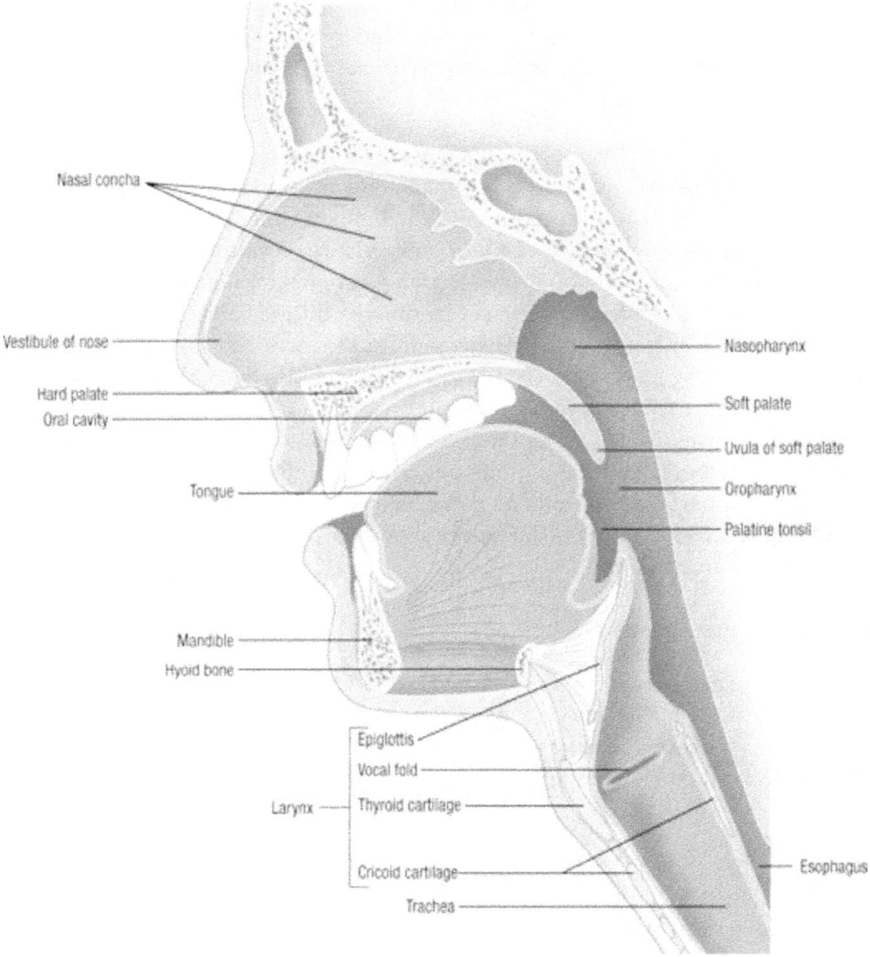

Figure 1. Airway anatomy.

2.7. The jaw-thrust maneuver

It is the favorite method for patients with possible cervical spine injury. To perform it, the tips of the middle or index fingers should be placed behind the angle of the mandible. Then lift the mandible upward to bring the lower incisors anterior to the upper incisors. Jaw thrust can be used together with the head tilt and chin lift and it is called the triple airway maneuver. The best description of this maneuver is head tilt, jaw thrust, and mouth opening [4] (**Figure 2**).

2.8. Suction

Patient positioning and airway opening maneuvers are usually insufficient to completely open the airway. Continuous vomits and bleeding usually need suctioning. The sucker should be used

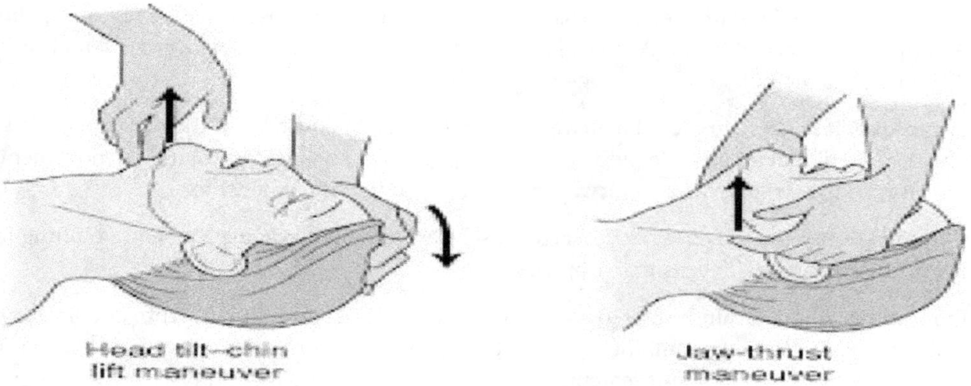

Figure 2. Head-tilt and jaw-thrust maneuver.

gently under direct vision. Using the sucker blindly might lead to airway injury, vagal stimulation, increased intracranial pressure, and vomiting. Intermediate negative pressure should be used to avoid blockage of the sucker. There are no contraindications to airway suctioning [3, 4, 6].

2.9. Airway adjuncts

2.9.1. Oropharyngeal airways

The oropharyngeal airways (OPA) are hard plastic devices with curved shape to lift the base of the tongue forward and prevent obstruction.

Indications: It is indicated for obstructed airway in an obtunded patient. Conscious patients will not tolerate an OPA.

Size: The device is sized by measuring its length from the patient's incisors to the angle of the jaw.

Technique: It is inserted inverted into the mouth after it passed the hard palate; the airway is rotated 180 degrees and advanced over the tongue. Another way is to use a tongue depressor to depress the tongue and advance the airway directly with no rotation needed.

Complications: May induce vomiting in patients with intact gag reflex, laryngospasm, raised intracranial pressure, and risk of aspiration in patients who have some airway reflexes.

Limitations: As a rule, any patient who tolerates an OPA airway should have a definitive airway. OPA is not a definitive airway. It helps with oxygenation and keep the airway open, but does not protect it.

2.9.2. Nasopharyngeal airways (NPA)

Are soft rubber tubes with a bevel at one end and a flange on the other end.

Indications: NPA is indicated when OPA cannot be used. It can be used to open the airway of conscious or semiconscious patients with intact airway reflexes who cannot tolerate OPA.

Size: The size can be estimated by measuring from the tip of the nose to the tip of the earlobe. An appropriate size of the NPA in adults is 6 mm internal diameter of an average female and 7 mm internal diameter for an average male [2, 3].

Technique: It is very simple. The airway should be lubricated first and then inserted gently into the nostril that looks wider and advanced it posteriorly with slight rotational movement. To improve the airflow, another airway can be inserted into the other side.

Complications: It may cause hemorrhage, nasal trauma, and laryngospasm and vomiting in a conscious patient with sensitive oropharynx [6].

Limitations: It is contraindicated to use NPA when there is a basal skull fracture or cribriform plate injury. These injuries might lead to intracranial placement of the airway. It is usually rare, and when there is life-threatening hypoxemia and where insertion of an OPA is not possible, careful insertion of NPA may be lifesaving [2].

The effectiveness of any airway maneuver or adjunct must always be assessed after it has been completed.

The oropharyngeal airway (OPA) and nasopharyngeal airway (NPA) are basic airway adjuncts. They are used to secure and open the airway, once it has been opened by either a head-tilt, chin-lift, or jaw-thrust maneuver and any objects or secretions have been removed by suctioning (**Figure 3**).

2.10. Oxygenation

The guidelines recommend that for most acutely ill patients, oxygen should be given to achieve a target saturation of 94–98% or 88–92% of those at risk of hypercapnic respiratory failure. Give all critically ill patients high flow oxygen 15 L/min until they are stable, and then reduce it to achieve the target saturation. These targets can be achieved by the use of nasal cannula, face mask with reservoir, or noninvasive ventilation (NIV) together with airway maneuver and adjuncts [2].

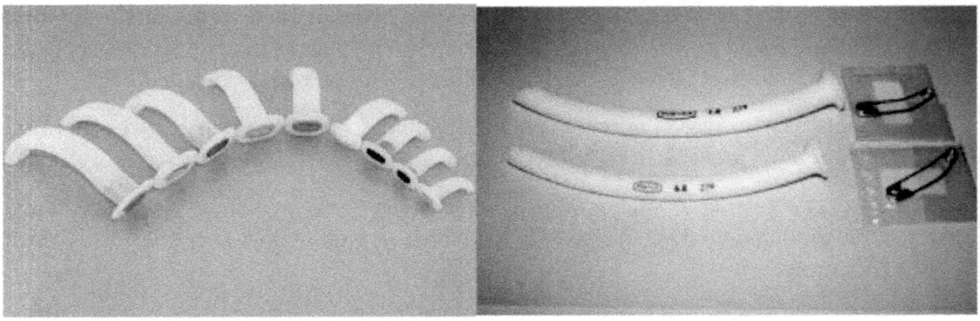

A B

Figure 3. A-oropharyngeal airway, B- nasopharyngeal airway.

http://dx.doi.org/10.5772/intechopen.76165

3. Rapid sequence induction

Rapid sequence induction (RSI) is a guided protocol of steps to reduce complications and boost success. The protocol of RSI entails the administration of anesthetic induction drug, followed by muscle-relaxing drugs (neuromuscular blockade drug) to achieve complete paralysis.

RSI is the preferred method to secure an airway on an emergent basis and where there is a risk of aspiration of gastric contents. In experienced hands, it is a relatively safe procedure with few complications. The choice of pharmacologic agents used will vary by physician experience, physician preference, the clinical condition of the patient, and the pharmacology of the agents [4].

3.1. Indication for intubation

There are four clinical situations in which intubation may be indicated:

1. Apneic patient.
2. Patient with an obstructed/partially obstructed airway where basic airway care is ineffective.
3. The patient requires invasive respiratory support for oxygenation or ventilatory failure.
4. Patient in whom basic airway care is effective, but whose predicted clinical course includes a high probability of airway obstruction, aspiration, or ventilatory failure[2].

3.2. Contraindications

RSI has just few contraindications. Firstly, inexperienced intubator should not perform RSI. Secondly, when the physician is not sure of his capability to intubate a patient with difficult airway, then he has to perform awake intubation. There are also other contraindications to RSI such as the contraindications of the muscle relaxants and absence of required equipment.

3.3. Preparation for RSI

Once the decision for intubation is taken, preparation for RSI should be started. The first attempt is always the best chance, so all efforts to make it successful should be done this by a systematic approach, maximizing the preintubation physiologic parameters of the patient and good teamwork which will all increase the success rate for intubation.

3.4. Assessment for difficult airway

Before proceeding with preparations for RSI, assessment of patient for difficult airway should be done using the LEMON mnemonic which can be done easily on any critically ill patient; this is done by:

L-looking externally for any anatomic or external characteristics that predict difficult intubation, such as facial hair, obesity, short neck, prominent upper incisors, receding mandible, edentulous, facial trauma, and airway deformity.

E-evaluate the 3-3-2 rule to evaluate the airway and predict the poor visibility of the posterior pharynx.

Starting with mouth opening should be at least 4 cm which is around three fingerbreadths. If it is less than this, it predicts difficult intubation and difficult visualization on laryngoscopy.

Thyromental distance is from the top of the thyroid cartilage to the mentum with fully extended neck. It should be 3–4 fingerbreadths, and when it is less than 3, this predicts difficult view on laryngoscopy.

The final part of the 3-3-2 rule is two fingers from the floor of the mouth to the laryngeal prominence (Adam's apple).

M-Mallampati score is used to assess oral access for laryngoscopy by viewing patients tongue, uvula, faucial pillars, and posterior pharynx (**Figure 4**).

O-obesity or obstruction obesity in addition to certain infections or swelling involving the upper airways or tumors like patients with chemical or thermal burns, infections of the larynx and pharynx, epiglottis and glottic polyps, laryngeal mass, angioedema, and neck hematoma all will affect laryngoscopy view.

N-neck mobility: any condition that limits neck mobility will impair the view on laryngoscopy, for example, patients with arthritis affecting cervical spine, e.g., ankylosing spondylitis, rheumatoid arthritis, and elderly [2, 7].

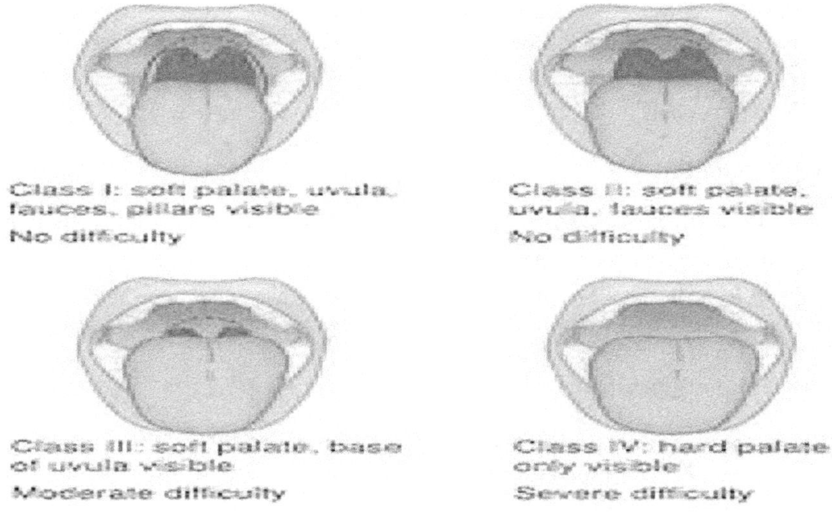

Figure 4. Mallampati score.

Once a difficult airway is predicted, EP should be prepared for it before proceeding with RSI by having other devices ready like video laryngoscopy, bougie tube, stylets, laryngeal mask airway (LMA), or a surgical airway kit, e.g., cricothyrotomy set, or awake intubation.

The most experienced EP should do the first trial and call for help early, predicting the difficulty [4, 5].

3.4.1. Equipment

- Nonrebreather face masks (different sizes) and oxygen supply and connectors.
- Nasal cannula for oxygenation.
- Bag-valve-mask devices, different sizes.
- Laryngoscope blades and handle of different sizes with extra batteries.
- Endotracheal tubes (ETT), different sizes.
- Stylet and boogie tube.
- Oropharyngeal airways, different sizes.
- Nasopharyngeal airways, different sizes.
- Alternative airway devices.
- Yankauer suction catheter.
- Syringes, 10 and 20 ml.
- Medications drawn and labeled.
- End-tidal carbon dioxide (CO_2) monitor/device.
- Crash cart.
- Resuscitation medications.
- Monitor pulse oximetry, ECG, and noninvasive blood pressure (NIBP).
- Failed intubation equipment or backup equipment should be prepared in case intubation failed. This can be a laryngeal mask airway (LMA), a cricothyroidotomy tray, and video laryngoscopy.

3.4.2. Technique

There are three major qualities of RSI; these are preoxygenation, application of cricoid pressure, and the avoidance of positive pressure ventilation before securing the airway with endotracheal tube [4, 9]. Steps for performing RSI from start to finish:

The patient is preoxygenated with 100% O_2 using a nonrebreather mask or assisted ventilation using a bag-valve-mask device. This leads to enhance oxygen reserve and prevent hypoxemia during induction [2, 4, 8].

The routine practice is to preoxygenate the patient for 5 minutes. If it is not possible, then preoxygenate for 3 minutes. However, four maximal inspirations are equally effective in the cooperative patient [4, 8]. Administering oxygen using noninvasive positive pressure ventilation has the ability to improve the process of oxygenation much faster than by using the face mask.

All the equipment should be prepared before the intubation and should be checked. The laryngoscope handles and light should be checked if they are working or not. ETT cough should be checked for any air leaks. Connect the patient at the same time to a monitor including pulse oximetry, cardiac monitor, and NIBP. The nurse at the same time should prepare the required medication and label them and get an intravenous access. Record and observe patient physiologic parameters.

The patient should be positioned in the sniffing position if no cervical spine injury is suspected. If cervical spine injury is suspected, manual in-line immobilization should be maintained during the intubation.

Premedicate the patient as indicated by the condition. Lidocaine (1.0–1.5 mg/kg) or fentanyl (2–3 μg/kg) both can be given to blunt the intracranial pressure response, transient hypertension, bronchospasm, and tachycardia associated with intubation. Phenylephrine (50 μg) can be used to lessen the hypotensive effect of intubation. Administer an appropriate induction agent as indicated by the clinical setting and patient's hemodynamic status followed by a non-depolarizing agent, if no contraindication. Flush the intravenous line after each drug to ensure delivery [10].

A cricoid pressure (the Sellick maneuver) should be applied immediately and maintained till oral endotracheal intubation is completed.

Intubate the patient after administration of succinylcholine (or rocuronium) and the patient's muscles are relaxed. Confirm the correct placement of the ETT by visualizing the tube passing through the vocal cords, monitoring continuous end-tidal CO_2 wave on the capnography, and auscultating breath sounds at the midaxillary lines and epigastric area. Release cricoid pressure. After successful intubation, secure the tube and connect to a ventilator and adjust the sitting according to patient condition. Administer additional sedative hypnotics and analgesics as indicated by clinical scenario. Obtain a chest radiograph to confirm proper placement of the endotracheal tube [2, 4, 6, 7, 9, 10].

3.4.3. Complications of RSI

- Difficult or failed intubation
- Airway injury and dental trauma
- Hypoxia
- Tachycardia and bradycardia mainly in children
- Hypertension or hypotension
- Cerebral anoxia
- Myocardial ischemia
- Death

http://dx.doi.org/10.5772/intechopen.76165

4. Needle decompression

Needle decompression is a lifesaving procedure used to decompress the chest when there is tension pneumothorax. Tension pneumothorax is the accumulation of air in the pleural cavity under pressure. Progressive buildup of pressure in the pleural space leads to mediastinum shift to the opposite side, lung collapse, and tracheal deviation to the unaffected side and obstructs venous return to the heart. This results in a hemodynamic instability and can lead to cardiac arrest [4, 11] (**Figure 5**).

4.1. Basic principle

The main idea is to insert a catheter into the pleural space, thus creating a pathway for the air to escape and release the built-up pressure. It is an emergency procedure when there is tension pneumothorax and should be followed by the chest tube insertion as a definitive management [14].

Indication for emergent needle decompression.

Traumatic cardiac arrest with chest involvement

- Tension pneumothorax

That is evident clinically in patients with tachypnea, hypoxia, tachycardia, hypotension, tracheal deviation to the unaffected side, diminished breath sound, hyperresonance chest, and increased percussion note.

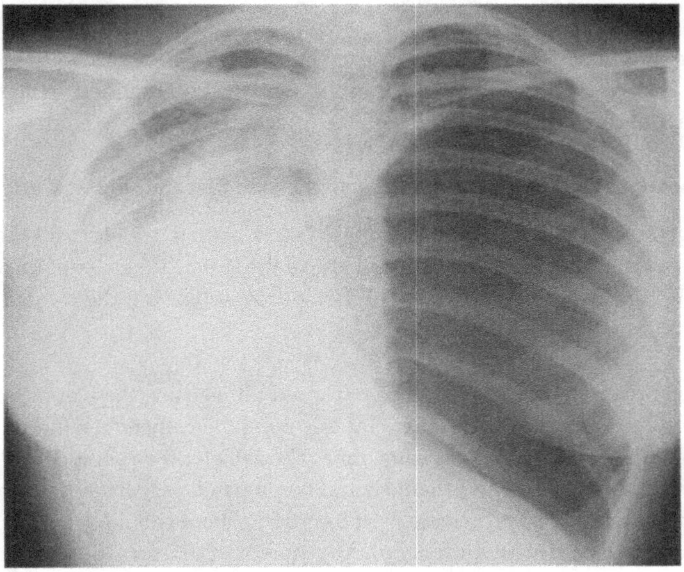

Figure 5. Radiograph of a patient with a large spontaneous tension pneumothorax.

Whenever there is deterioration in the patient's oxygenation or ventilatory status, the chest should be reexamined and tension pneumothorax should be excluded. Failure to suspect and pick it clinically will result in death.

4.2. Contraindications

There is absolute contraindication for needle decompression, but in patients with polytrauma, if the injury is not salvageable, then it should be avoided [16].

4.3. Equipment

- Povidone-iodine or chlorhexidine solution
- 12- to 16-gauge catheter-over-the-needle, 4.5 cm in length
- Syringe 5 or 10 ml
- Sterile gloves, gown, and face mask
- Ultrasound machine (optional) with sterile gel and probe

4.4. Patient preparation

The procedure should be explained to the patient or family and he should be placed in supine position. 100% oxygen through the face mask should be administered if the patient not on mechanical ventilator. Also the patient should be connected to a monitor including cardiac monitor and pulse oximetry.

4.5. Technique

The procedure should be done under aseptic technique. The EP should wear the gown, sterile gloves, mask, and cap. The anatomical landmark should be identified which is the second intercostal space at the midclavicular line on the affected side.

- Use iodine-based solution (Betadine) to clean the area that should be punctured.
- Insert a large-bore (i.e., 14 gauge or 16 gauge) needle with a catheter into the second intercostal space, perpendicular to the skin and above the superior border of the third rib at the midclavicular line, to prevent damage to the neurovascular bundle located at the second rib inferior border.

Then the catheter-over-the-needle should be advanced till reaching the pleural space. A rush of air will be heard escaping from the syringe. At this point the catheter should be advanced and the needle should be withdrawn at the same time. The catheter then should be secured in place and should be left open to air. The patient should be prepared for tube thoracostomy as needle decompression is a temporary procedure. Post insertion patient should be reevaluated and continued to be monitored, and chest X-ray should be requested. Successful placement of the catheter will be confirmed by the improvement of patient symptoms and hemodynamic status [11–14].

4.6. Tips

Failure of the procedure can be due to a short needle, especially in obese patients with a thicker chest wall, so a longer needle should be used for a successful procedure [13].Ultrasound-guided procedure can be an excellent option, and at the same time, it will confirm the presence of pneumothorax by the loss of lung's sliding movement or lung point sign which is more specific for pneumothorax. Ultrasound also can help choosing the appropriate needle length needed for the procedure.

4.7. Complications

Needle thoracostomy is not a simple procedure with no complications, and it should be done when patient scenario and clinical assessment support the clinical diagnosis of tension pneumothorax[15, 16].

Complications include

- Pneumothorax (with potential to later tension pneumothorax)
- Hemothorax
- Cardiac tamponade
- Hemorrhage (which can be life-threatening)
- Loculatedintrapleural hematoma
- Atelectasis and pneumonia
- Arterial air embolism (when needle thoracostomy is performed and no tension pneumothorax is present)
- Pain to the patient due to procedure itself
- Thoracic and abdominal organ injury
- Failure of the procedure or ineffective drainage of pneumothorax

4.8. Chest Tube

Indications

- Hemothorax
- Abscess
- Empyema
- Traumatic pneumothorax (some)
- Spontaneous pneumothorax (some)
- Indication for main theater: >1200-ml drainage immediately after insertion or continuous 150–200 mL/hr. for 2–4 hours (**Table 1**)

4.9. Relative indications

Penetrating thoracic injury and need for positive pressure ventilation.

Profound hypoxia/hypotension in patient with penetrating chest injury

- Profound hypoxia/hypotension and signs of hemothorax

4.10. Contraindications

- No absolute contraindications when performed for emergent indication

4.10.1. Relative contraindications

- Overlying skin infection
- Coagulopathy
- Multiple pleural adhesions

4.11. Equipment needed

- Chest tube
  - 14–28F for pneumothorax
  - 32–40F for hemothorax
- Scalpel
- Kelly clamp
- Sterile drapes
- Silk sutures
- Syringes and needles for anesthesia
- Lidocaine
- Betadine
- Sterile gown/gloves
- Face shield
- Pleur-evac

Procedure

1. Consider antibiotic (e.g., cefazolin) dose 1–2 gm intravenously before procedure.
2. If possible, elevate head of the bed to 30–60 degrees to lower diaphragm-decreasing risk of injury to the diaphragm/intra-abdominal organs.

3. Expose insertion site by moving the upper extremity above the head on the affected side.
    - Insertion site = mid- to ant axillary line at fourth/fifth intercostal space.
        - ~Nipple line in men and inframammary crease in women.
        - Place 1–3 intercostal spaces higher in pregnant patients (especially those in the third trimester) due to elevated diaphragm.
4. Clean with Betadine and drape.
5. Confirm rib space and anesthetize with up to 5 mg/kg of lido with or without epinephrine.
    - Must anesthetize the skin, soft tissue, muscle, periosteum, and pleural space.
6. Incise along the upper border of the lower rib of the intercostal space.
7. Use curved clamp to bluntly dissect through the muscle until you reach the rib.
8. Angle the clamp to go above and over the rib and push until enter the pleural space.
9. Open the clamp and pull it out with the clamp still open to create a larger tract.
10. Premeasure chest tube from skin incision to ipsi clavicle to avoid advancing chest tube too far.
11. Clamp the proximal end of the chest tube and pass it along the tract into the pleural cavity.
    - Ensure that inner tract/incision can fit your finger and tube.
    - It helps to have your finger in the tract and pass the tube along your finger, particularly in obese patients.
12. Once in the space, remove the clamp.
13. Feed the chest tube until all the holes are inside the thoracic cavity.
    - Aim superoanterior for pneumothorax; aim posteriorly for hemothorax.
        - Controversial as to whether this is important.
14. Rotate the tube 360 degrees.
    - Reduces likelihood of tube kinking.
    - If tube rotates easily, it can help indicate correct location inside pleural cavity.
15. Attach distal end of tube to the Pleur-evac and place on suction (20–30cmH_2O suction).
16. Secure tube with silk suture and cover with gauze and cloth tape.
17. Obtain CXR position of tube.

Chest tubesize	Type of patient	Underlying causes
Small (8–14 Fr)	• Most spontaneous pneumothorax (primary and secondary) • Most iatrogenic pneumothorax	• Alveolar-pleural fistulae (small air leak) • Iatrogenic air
Medium (20–28 Fr)	• Pneumothorax on mechanical ventilation • Non-traumatic tension pneumothorax • Malignant effusion	• Bronchial-pleural fistulae (large air leak) • Malignant fluid
Large (36–40 Fr)	• Traumatic pneumothorax • Empyema	• Bleeding (hemothorax/hemopneumothorax) • Thick pus

Table 1. Adult chest tubesizes.

4.12. Drainage system and suction

- Spontaneous pneumothorax
  - The least amount of suction (including none) needed to maintain full expansion of the lung is appropriate.
  - Starting with Heimlich valve (no suction) or − 10 cm of water and increasing only as needed
- Fluid drainage
  - −20 cm of water
  - Increased as indicated with the goal of achieving full lung expansion
- For thoracic trauma, few data are available.
  - Start −20 cm of water

Complications

- Exsanguination (secondary to removing the tamponade effect of the hemothorax)
  - Clamp tube immediately; take patient to the OR for emergent thoracostomy.
- Air leak
  - Reason why you never clamp the tube once it is in place (could cause tension pneumothorax)
- Failure
- Infection

  - Give prophylactic antibiotics (e.g., Ancef) to decrease rate of empyema.
- Re-expansion pulmonary edema
- Damage to nerves/vessels/heart/lung/diaphragm/abdomen
- Improper positioning of the tube
- Tension pneumothorax

Failure to drain

- Improper connections or leaks in the external tubing/water seal system
- Improper positioning of the tube
- Occlusion of bronchi or bronchioles by secretions or foreign body
- Tear of one of the large bronchi
- Large tear of the lung parenchyma
- Clotting of a smaller diameter chest tube or pigtail catheter by blood (may require low-dose TPA to declot pigtails)
- If pneumothorax persists or large air leak despite well-placed tube, there is a need for emergent bronchoscopy [17].

5. Central venous catheter placement

Central venous catheterization is one of the fundamental requirements for resuscitating critically ill patient in ED and intensive care unit (ICU).

5.1. Indications

Rapid venous access in emergency situation, e.g., cardiac arrest.

- Hemodynamic monitoring such as central venous pressure measurement (CVP) and central venous oxygen saturation.
- Rapid fluid and drug infusion.
- Parenteral nutrition.
- Central venous access can be used for hemodialysis and transvenous pacemaker placement.

5.2. Contraindications

Local infection in the area to be punctured.

Distorted anatomy-bleeding disorder.

- -Anticoagulant therapy-IV drug abuse through the access.
- -Pneumothorax on the contralateral side.

5.3. Equipment

-Lidocaine 1%–Needles and swabs and antiseptic solution.

Gloves, gown, cap, and mask.

- 10-ml syringe for catheter placement.
- Catheter kits–drapes and gauze pads.
- Needle holder and suture material and scissors.
- Ultrasound and sterile probe.

5.4. Technique

Seldinger (guidewire) technique is the most commonly used and it should be done under aseptic technique. The procedure should be explained to the patient if possible or his family and consent should be taken. All the equipment should be prepared. Patient should be placed in supine position and connected to a monitor. The selected area for puncture should be cleaned using the antiseptic solution and alcohol swabs. Locate the vein selected for puncture by anatomical landmark. It can also be done with ultrasound guidance as well.

Local anesthetic lidocaine 1% can be used at the site of puncture and sedation for patient comfort. A large-caliber needle connected to 10-ml syringe with 1-ml saline is used for the venipuncture and should be advanced slowly under negative pressure till a free flow of blood is seen in the syringe; at this point the syringe should be removed, and at the same time occlude needle and stabilize it carefully to avoid air embolism and displacement. Then thread the guidewire through the needle and remove the needle. After that insert the catheter over the guidewire. A dilator can be used before passage of the catheter over the guidewire and tight control of the guidewire at the skin should be kept during placement. Once the catheter is inserted, then guidewire should be removed, and connect the catheter to intravenous tubing after checking blood backflow and flush with saline and secure it with suture. Confirm the position by ultrasound and obtain X-ray of the chest and abdomen.

5.5. Complications

Arterial puncture

Air embolism and catheter embolus

Local hematoma

Pericardial tamponade

Arteriovenous fistula

Pneumothorax and hemothorax

Hemomediastinum

Neck hematoma

Tracheal obstruction or perforation

Bowel or bladder perforation

Local cellulitis and sepsis

Neurologic injury

Venous thrombosis[11].

5.6. Intraosseous access

- Provides a rapid and reliable method of getting access to the systemic circulation
- Recommended by the American Heart Association if venous access cannot be quickly and reliably established[18]
- Still a widely underutilized modality[19, 20]
- Can be used to give drugs (all the drugs given through an IV line can be given through an IO line) and infuse fluids, blood, as well as contrast for imaging [21]

5.7. Indications

In any situation where peripheral access is not easily available.

- During life-threatening situations such as CPR or trauma
- Burns
- Seizures
- Edema

5.8. Equipment

- Intraosseous needles: All are 15 G and vary in length, 15, 25, and 45 mm.
- Manual needle and trochar devices or automated EZ IO drill. Several devices like Jamshidi needle, Sur-Fast intraosseous needle, Sussmane-Raszynski needle, FAST1 Intraosseous Infusion System, new intraosseous device(NIO), and bone injection gun(BIG) are available.
- Lidocaine or lignocaine for local anesthesia and for use before starting any infusion (running infusions is more painful than insertion due to the expansion of the medullary plexus).
- 5–10-ml syringes for aspiration and flushing.
- EZ connect IV tubing if using EZ IO set.
- Dressing.

5.9. Sites and technique

Take universal precautions and prepare the insertion site with an antiseptic. Use the needle size 15 mm for <40 kg, 25 mm for>40 kg, and 45 mm for proximal humerus or excessive body tissue.

Proximal tibia: Position the patient supine with the knee flexed, and identify the tibial tuberosity. Insert the needle two fingerbreadths distal and 1–2 cm medial to it. In a conscious patient, instill local anesthetic first. Tilt the needle caudally, away from the epiphysis. Manually insert in a screw-like motion or drill till you feel a give, remove trochar (very sharp, dispose in the sharp box), fix a syringe, and aspirate. The bone marrow is not always aspirated; flush and note for any extravasation. A needle that stands upright without support indicates correct placement. Secure with tape or dressing.

Distal tibia: Palpate the medial malleolus and identify the anterior and posterior borders as well as the most prominent part of the malleolus; insert the needle 2–3 cm proximal to the most prominent part in between the anterior and posterior borders of the tibia.

Proximal humerus: With the elbow adducted and the arm internally rotated, place the hand palm down on the abdomen, palpate the anterior shaft of the humerus till you palpate the greater tuberosity, and insert the needle about a cm above that, i.e., 1 cm above the surgical neck of the humerus.

Other sites: Femur, sternum, and anterior superior iliac spine (**Figure 6**).

Complications

- Failure
- Extravasation
- Compartment syndrome
- Fracture
- Osteomyelitis
- Necrosis of the epiphyseal plate

6. ED thoracotomy

- Lifesaving procedure
- Reported survival rates of 2% in blunt trauma and 16% in penetrating trauma[22] to as great as 60% in a selected group of patients

6.1. Indications

6.1.1. Penetrating chest trauma

- Previously witnessed cardiac activity (prehospital or in-hospital) or signs of life (pulse, BP, pupil reactivity, purposeful movement, and respiratory effort)

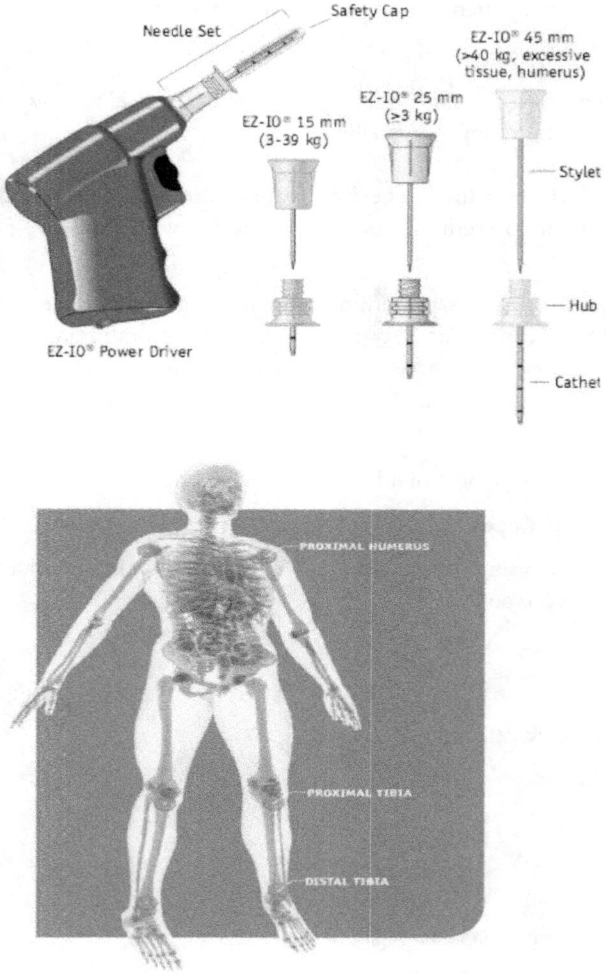

Figure 6. Intraosseous device and sites.

- Unresponsive hypotension [systolic blood pressure (SBP) <70 mm Hg] despite vigorous resuscitation [23]

6.1.2. Blunt chest trauma

- Previously witnessed cardiac activity (prehospital or in-hospital)
- Rapid exsanguination from the chest tube (>1500 mL)
- Unresponsive hypotension (SBP <70 mm Hg) despite vigorous resuscitation

The American College of Surgeons Committee on Trauma indications for EDT are as follows [24]:

- Precordial wound in a patient with prehospital cardiac arrest
- Trauma patient with cardiac arrest after arrival to ED
- Profound hypotension (<70 mm Hg) in a patient with a truncal wound who is either unconscious or an operating room is unavailable

The Eastern Association for the Surgery of Trauma strongly recommends resuscitative ED thoracotomy in patients presenting pulseless to the ED with signs of life after penetrating thoracic injury [25].

Can be considered for patients presenting with penetrating thoracic trauma without witnessed signs of life or cardiac activity and in penetrating abdominal trauma in traumatic arrest with prior witnessed cardiac activity and signs of life.

6.2. Equipment

- Sterile gloves, gown, and face shield
- Betadine and sterile drapes
- Thoracotomy set including scalpel 10 blade, Mayo scissors, rib spreaders, Gigli saw, vascular clamps, and needle holders
- Suture material
- Aortic clamp
- Chest tubes and Foley catheter
- Internal defibrillator
- Skin stapler

6.3. Technique

- Intubate the patient and pass the nasogastric tube.
- Initiate the mass transfusion and commence with the blood products.
- Wear your personal protective equipment.
- **Anterolateral approach:** Make an incision in the left fourth intercostal space extending from the sternum to the posterior axillary line cutting the skin, subcutaneous tissue, and intercostal muscles in one go. Apply the rib spreaders.
- **Clamshell approach:** Start as the left anterolateral approach, extend to the right in the space intercostal space, cut the sternum with the Gigli saw, and apply the rib spreader on the cut ends of the sternum.
- **Pericardiotomy:** Move the lung out of the way and incise the pericardium anterior to the phrenic nerve from the apex to the root of the aorta.
- Inspect the myocardium for injury, which can then be occluded digitally, by skin stapler, occluding it with a Foley catheter or sutures.

- Cardiac massage and internal defibrillation can be done.
- Hilar clamping can be done in case of extensive lung laceration.
- Cross-clamping of the aorta can be done in case of persistent hypotension.

6.4. Contraindications

- Non-traumatic cardiac arrest
- Blunt injury without witnessed cardiac activity (prehospital) or penetrating abdominal trauma without cardiac activity (prehospital).
- Severe head injury
- Severe multisystem injury
- Improperly trained team or insufficient equipment

7. Pericardiocentesis

Pericardiocentesis is the aspiration of fluid from the pericardial space that surrounds the heart. This procedure can be lifesaving in patients with cardiac tamponade, even when it complicates acute type A aortic dissection and when cardiothoracic surgery is not available.

7.1. Indications

7.1.1. Emergent pericardiocentesis

Life-threatening hemodynamic compromise due to suspected cardiac tamponade. Cardiac arrest secondary to cardiac tamponade.

7.1.2. Nonemergent pericardiocentesis

Diagnostic pericardiocentesis for pericardial effusions (due to infectious, hemorrhagic, or malignant etiology).

7.1.3. Contraindications

There is no absolute contraindication to pericardiocentesis in hemodynamically unstable patient.

7.1.3.1. Relative contraindications

- Uncorrected bleeding disorders in stable patients
- Dialysis available for uremic patients
- Immediate surgery or thoracotomy available for trauma patients

Equipment needed: Essential equipment includes the following:

- Antiseptic solution Three-way stopcock scalpel
- Ultrasound machine with sterile probe
- Pericardiocentesis kit
- Needles, 18 ga, 1.5 in and 25 ga, 5/8 inand • Spinal needle, 18 ga, 7.5–12 cm
- Continuous cardiac or ECG monitoring
- Sterile drapes, gown, and mask
- Local anesthetic (e.g., lidocaine 1%)
- Alligator clip connector for connection to V_1 lead of ECG machine

7.1.4. Technique

Ideally, patient should be in a semirecumbent position at 30–45 degrees so as to bring the pericardium close to the anterior chest wall; however, supine position is an acceptable alternative.

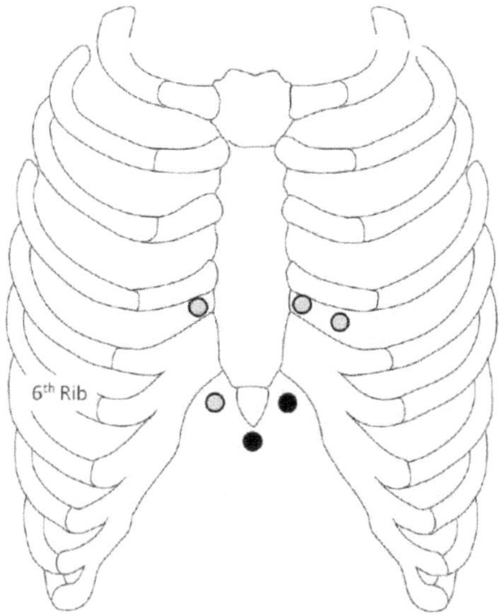

Figure 7. Various anatomical approaches for pericardiocentesis. Pericardiocentesis needle insertion sites. The subxiphoid and left sternocostal margins are the most commonly used sites (black dots).(Source: Medscape).

http://dx.doi.org/10.5772/intechopen.76165

If time and situation allow, the procedure should be explained to the patient and local anesthesia should be administered at the site of procedure. Ensure IV access, with patient connected to the monitor, and supplemental oxygen. Ideally the procedure should be done under ultrasound guidance; however, if the patient is in cardiac arrest, then the procedure should be initiated as soon as possible for pericardial fluid aspiration.

There are various anatomical approaches for pericardiocentesis, as shown in the **Figure 7**, with subxiphoid approach and left parasternal margin being the most common sites (**Figure 8**).

In subxiphoid approach, mark the area between the xiphoid process and left sternocostal margin, ideally 1 cm inferolaterally to the xiphoid process on the left side. Clean the area using an antiseptic solution and insert the needle (spinal needle) at 30–45degrees, aiming toward the left shoulder, as shown in the picture.

If time permits, connect an alligator clip from the base of the spinal needle to the V_1 lead of an ECG machine, and use bedside ultrasound to visualize the needle tip in the pericardial as depicted in **Figure 9**.

Apply constant negative pressure on the syringe until a return of fluid or blood is visualized, cardiac pulsations are felt, or abrupt change in ECG waveform is noted (**Figure 10**).

Stabilize the needle and withdraw as much fluid as possible. If a catheter-over-the-needle has been used, then the needle can be removed and catheter can be stabilized to the chest wall, with a three-way stopcock attached to allow continuous drainage of pericardial fluid.

The needle may move closer to the myocardium, and an injury pattern may appear on the ECG, in which case the needle should be withdrawn slightly to avoid myocardial injury.

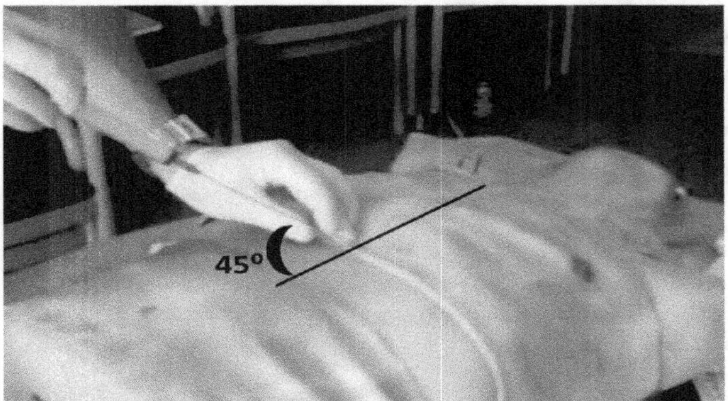

Figure 8. Needle insertion: Insert the spinal needle through the skin incision directed toward the left shoulder at a 45-degree angle to the abdominal wall and 45 degrees off the midline sagittal plane.

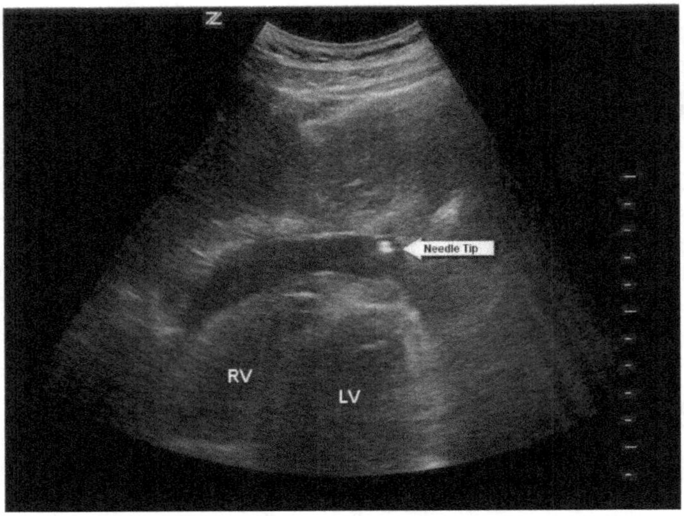

Figure 9. Subxiphoid view of the heart demonstrating the needle tip within the pericardial space.

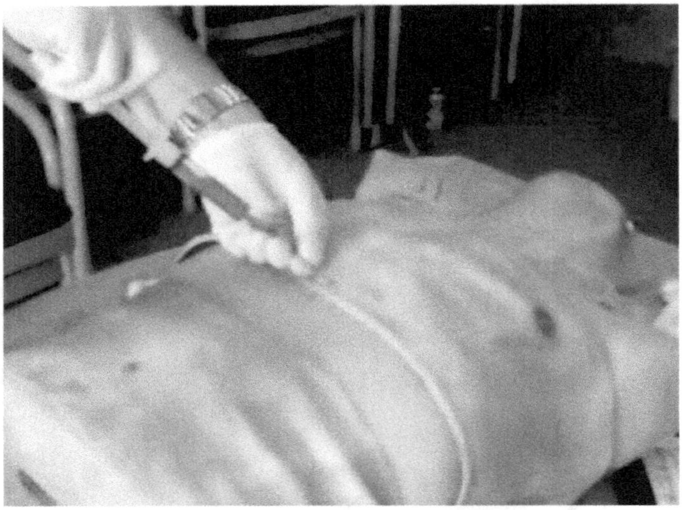

Figure 10. Needle insertion: slowly advance the spinal needle up to a depth of 5 cm while applying negative pressure on the syringe until a return of fluid is visualized.

7.2. Complications

- Dysrhythmias
- Coronary artery puncture or aneurysm
- Dry tap (failure to yield fluid)

- Pneumothorax
- Hemopericardium
- Venous air embolism
- Hepatic injury
- False-positive aspiration–intracardiac aspiration
- False-negative aspiration—clotted blood in the pericardial cavity
- Reaccumulation of pericardial fluid defibrillation

"Defibrillation" or "unsynchronized cardioversion" is the transthoracic application of unsynchronized electric current during a cardiac cycle, causing the heart muscle to contract simultaneously and, thus, terminating the abnormal electrical rhythm. This enables the sinus node to resume its normal cardiac cycle.

7.3. Indications

Indications for defibrillation include the following:

- Pulseless ventricular tachycardia (VT)
- Ventricular fibrillation (VF)
- Cardiac arrest due to or resulting in VF

7.4. Contraindications

Contraindications include the following:

- Dysrhythmias due to enhanced automaticity, such as in digitalis toxicity and catecholamine-induced arrhythmia
- Multifocal atrial tachycardia

7.5. Equipment needed

- Defibrillators [automated external defibrillators (AEDs), semiautomated AEDs, standard defibrillators with monitors]
- Paddle or adhesive patch
- Conductive gel or paste
- ECG monitor with recorder
- Oxygen equipment
- Airway management equipment
- Emergency pacing equipment

- Blood pressure cuff (automatic or manual)
- Pulse recorder
- Oxygen saturation monitor
- Intravenous access
- Suction device
- Code cart with advanced cardiovascular life support (ACLS) medications
- Sedation medications

7.6. Technique

Defibrillation is performed during a cardiac arrest while the CPR is going on simultaneously. So, it is important to carry out the CPR, along with proper administration of defibrillation technique for maximum benefit. Defibrillators can deliver either in monophasic (delivers a charge in only one direction) or biphasic (delivers a charge in one direction for half of the shock and in the electrically opposite direction for the second half) waveforms. Newer defibrillators deliver energy in biphasic waveforms as they tend to successfully terminate arrhythmias at lower energies than monophasic waveform defibrillators. The defibrillation process is done in three important steps, which are as follows:

7.6.1. Paddle placement

Apply conductive material to the entirety of the chest.

Conductive gel or paste is most commonly used, but waxy conductive pads are also available. Generous use of conductive gel on the underside and especially along the edges of the electrode paddles is essential, both to reduce transthoracic impedance and to prevent skin burns. Paste should be applied liberally but must not run onto the skin between the paddles, because the paste may divert current over the skin surface and away from the heart.

Paddle placement on the chest wall has two conventional positions:

- Anterolateral and anteroposterior.
- In the anterolateral position, a single paddle is placed on the left fourth or fifth intercostal space on the midaxillary line. The second paddle is placed just to the right of the sternal edge on the second or third intercostal space.

In the anteroposterior position, which is preferred in patients with implantable devices, to avoid shunting current to the implantable device and damaging its system, a single paddle is placed to the right of the sternum, as above, and the other paddle is placed between the tip of the left scapula and the spine (**Figure 11**).

7.6.2. Defibrillator and Charging

Turn on the defibrillator, and turn the dial to defibrillation mode on the defibrillator (**Figure12**).

Identify that the rhythm is a shockable rhythm. Select the energy of 360J for monophasic defibrillators or 120–200J for biphasic defibrillators, and select charge to start charging the defibrillator, which is indicated by beginning of a beep sound (**Figure 13**).

7.6.3. Shock delivery

As soon as the defibrillator is charged, which is indicated when the beep stops, press the shock button to deliver the shock (**Figure 14**).

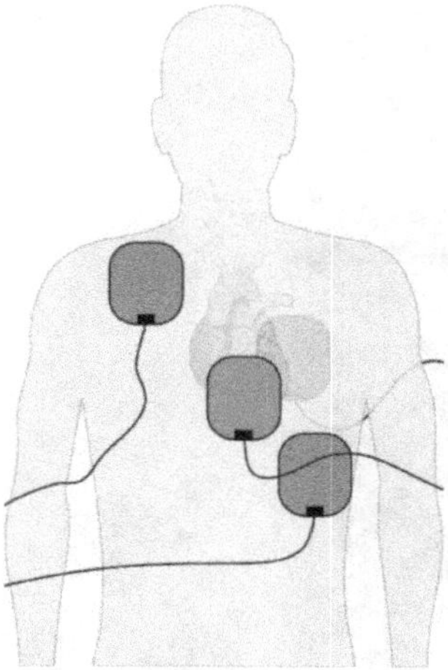

Figure 11. Paddle placement on the chest wall.

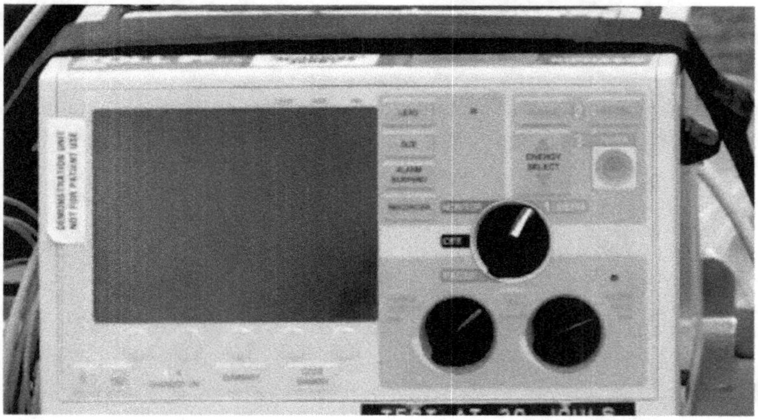

Figure 12. Defibrillation and cardioversion.

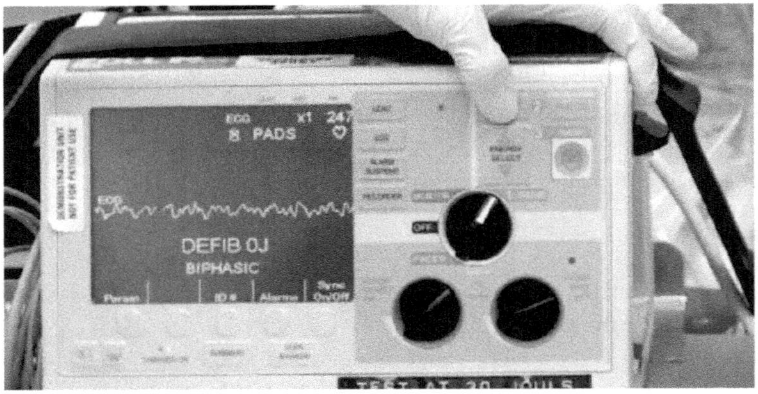

Figure 13. Defibrillation and cardioversion.

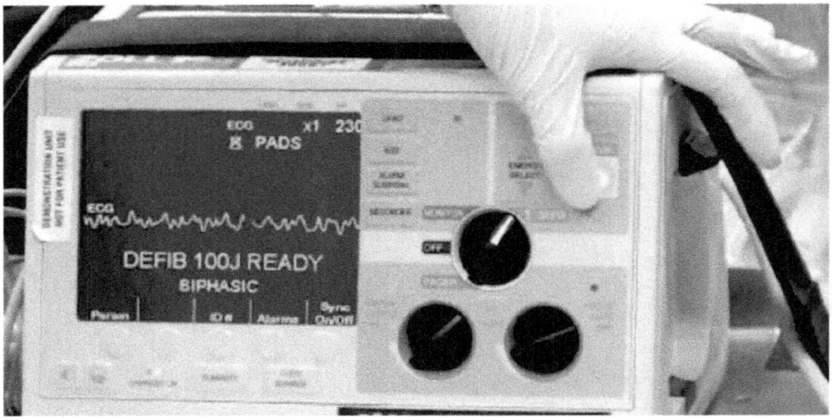

Figure 14. Defibrillation and cardioversion.

Safety is a key concern in the performance of defibrillation. Any staff member acting as a ground for the electrical discharge can be seriously injured. The operator must announce "all clear" and give staff a chance to move away from the bed before discharging the paddles.

Care must be taken to clean up spills of saline or water, because they may create a conductive path to a staff person at the bedside.

After the shock is delivered, continue the CPR.

7.7. Complications

- Harmless arrhythmias, such as atrial, ventricular, and junctional premature beats (commonest)

- Ventricular fibrillation (VF) resulting from high amounts of electrical energy, especially in patients with digitalis toxicity, severe heart disease, or improper synchronization of the shock with the R wave
- Thromboembolization
- Myocardial necrosis
- Hypoxia due to excessive sedation
- Chest wall skin burns (most likely are due to improper technique or electrode placement and inadequate conductive gel)
- Injuries to healthcare personnel (shock and burns)

8. Transcutaneous pacing

Transcutaneous pacing is a temporary means of pacing a patient's heart in an abnormally slow heart rate. It is accomplished by delivering pulses of electric current through the patient's chest, which stimulates the heart to contract in a minimally effective manner.

8.1. Indications

Indications for TCP can be grouped in bradyarrhythmias and tachyarrhythmias as follows:

8.1.1. Bradyarrythmias

- Symptomatic sinus node dysfunction (sinus arrest, tachybrady [sick sinus] syndrome, sinus bradycardia)
- Second- and third-degree heart block
- A-fib with slow ventricular response
- Malfunction of implanted pacemaker
- New left bundle-branch block (LBBB), right bundle-branch block (RBBB) with left axis deviation, bifascicular block, or alternating bundle-branch block
- Trauma patient with hypotension and unresponsive bradycardia
- Prophylaxis—cardiac catheterization, after open heart surgery, threatened bradycardia during drug trials for tachydysrhythmias

8.1.2. Tachyarrythmias

- Supraventricular dysrhythmias (e.g., postoperative atrial flutter)
- Ventricular dysrhythmias (monomorphic ventricular tachycardia)

- Prophylactically in cardiac catheterization, after open heart surgery and in cases of bradycardia-dependent tachycardias (e.g., torsades de pointes)

8.1.3. Contraindications

There are no absolute contraindications; however, it is advisable to avoid pacing in the following conditions:

- First-degree AV block
- Mobitz type I block
- Stable escape rhythm
- Bradyarrhythmias secondary to profound hypothermia

8.1.4. Equipment needed

Equipment used in transcutaneous cardiac pacing includes the following (**Figure 15**):

- Pacing unit
- Cardiac monitor
- Defibrillator (see the image below)
- Pacing electrodes (pads)
- Procedural sedation/analgesia medications
- Airway equipment

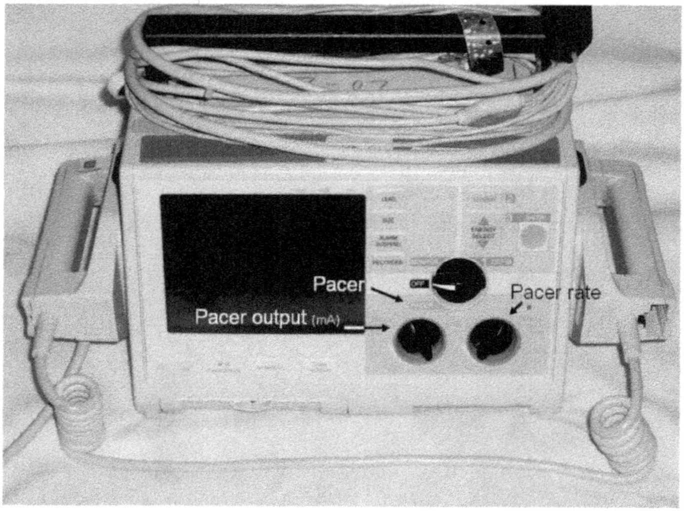

Figure 15. Defibrillator with pacing capability.

PreparationThe process of electrical pacing can be of significant discomfort to the patient if not prepared adequately.

It is, therefore, advised to consider analgesia or sedation to ease patient's discomfort.

Also, patient's skin should be wiped with alcohol and dried, any foreign body should be removed, and careful shaving of the excessive hair should be done, taking care to avoidabrading the skin as it can elevate the pacing threshold and increase burning and discomfort.

8.2. Technique

The electric pads can be placed either in anterolateral position or anteroposterior position.

The anterior electrode should have negative polarity and should be placed at the cardiac apex or at lead V3 position.

The positive or posterior electrode should be placed inferior to the scapula or between the right or left scapula and the spine; it should not be placed over the scapula or the spine. Alternatively, the positive electrode can be placed anteriorly on the right upper part of the chest (see the image below) (**Figure 16**).

To initiate TCP, after application of pads and activating the device, turn the selection knob to the "pacer" mode, and select pacer rate of 60–80; as shown in **Figure1**.

Select the current, and look for one QRS complex after each pacing spike. This is called "electrical capture." Look for corresponding pulse by checking patient's pulse (**Figure 17**). If the pulse corresponds with the electrical capture along with improved BP and clinical status of the patient, "mechanical capture" is attained as shown in **Figure 3**.

The electrical output should be started from maximum output if the patient is in cardiac arrest, and then decrease to keep 10–15 mA above the threshold to maintain adequate mechanical capture.

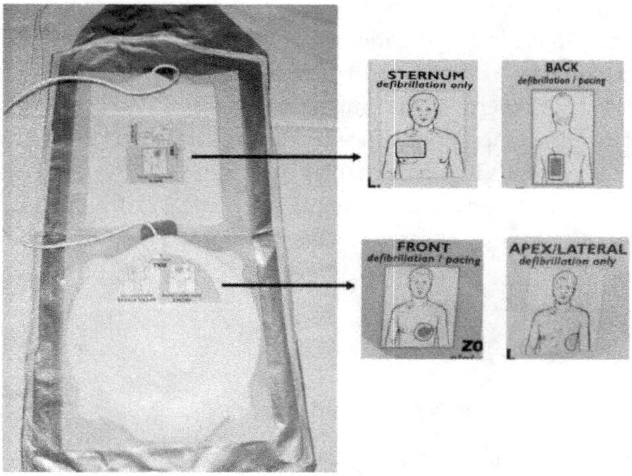

Figure 16. Pacing electrode pads of external pacing unit and locations in which each pad should be placed.

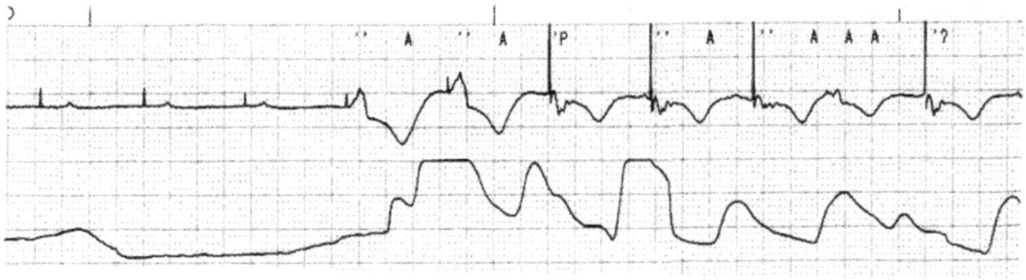

Figure 17. Rhythm strip showing failure to capture in the first four pacing stimuli that did not produce any pulse. When capture occurred, each pacing artifact is followed by QRS complex (albeit bizarrely shaped) and pulse.

However, in a patient who has a hemodynamically compromising bradycardia but is not in cardiac arrest, the operator should start from a low current output to get an electrical capture and slowly increase the output from the minimal setting until mechanical capture is achieved.

8.3. Complications

- Induction of dysrhythmias (VF)
- Burns (rarely)
- Pain/discomfort

9. Conclusion

The physicians of the emergency department have great mission as they have to manage critically ill patients and stabilize them by effectively using their own skills in order to improve their patients' condition. The emergency physicians should provide the best when providing lifesaving treatment to a critically ill patients either doing RSI to secure airway or inserting a central venous catheter for vasopressors and intravenous fluid administration or any other resuscitative procedure in emergency setting. In this chapter we focused on the fundamental knowledge for performing emergency procedures and what steps EP should know to deliver best cars and save the patient's life. This chapter was a guide to help the emergency physician (EP) to better understand and develop the required technical skills and have the basis needed to achieve the highest level of care that will have direct impact on patients' outcome.

Author details

Aml Yousif Elemamali* and Aftab Mohammad Azad

*Address all correspondence to: aftab.azad@me.com

Department of Emergency Medicine, Hamad Medical Corporation, Doha, Qatar

References

[1] http://www.lww.co.uk/emergency-medicine-toxicology/decision-making-in-emergency-critical-care;2015

[2] https://www.cambridge.org/core/books/emergency-airway-management/65F6E8117405BA92AD27281939DB1EB8

[3] https://www.scribd.com/document/353543024/Roberts-Hedges-Clinical-Procedures-in-Emergency-Medicine-6th-Ed-PDF-Tahir99-VRG

[4] http://accessemergencymedicine.mhmedical.com/book.aspx?bookID=683

[5] http://bookstore.acep.org/emergency-department-resuscitation-of-the-critically-ill-1st-ed-560000

[6] https://www.amazon.com/Emergency-Medicine-National-Medical-Independent/dp/0781788846

[7] https://www.elsevier.com/books/rosens-emergency-medicine-concepts-and-clinical-practice-2-volume-set/marx/978-1-4557-0605-1

[8] Gambee MA, Hertzka RE, Fisher DM. Preoxygenation techniques: Comparison of three minutes and four breaths. Anesthesia and Analgesia. 1987;**66**:468-470. [PubMed: 3578856]

[9] Smith CE. Rapid sequence intubation in trauma. The 10th Annual Trauma Anesthesia and Critical Care Society Symposium, May 1997 (poster)

[10] Schneider RE, Caro DA. Pretreatment agents (Chapter 16). In: Walls RM, Murphy MF, editors. Manual of Emergency Airway Management, 2nd ed. Philadelphia: Lippincott, Williams & Wilkins; 2004:183-188

[11] American College of Surgeons. Advanced Trauma Life Support Instructor Manual. 6th ed. Chicago: American College of Surgeons; 1997. p. 150

[12] Taylor RW, Civetta JM, Kirby RR: Techniques and Procedures in Critical Care. Philadelphia: Lippincott; 1990. 306

[13] Britten S, Palmer SH, Snow TM. Needle thoracentesis in tension pneumothorax: Insufficient cannula length and potential failure. Injury. 1996;**27**(5):321-322. [PubMed: 8763284]

[14] http://www.trauma.org/thoracic/CHESTtension.htmlPreparepatient

[15] https://www.ncbi.nlm.nih.gov/pmc/articles/PMC4613415/complications

[16] http://www.emedicine.com/med/topic2793.htm#section~relevant_anatomy_and_contraindications

[17] Chest tube Life in the fast lane/Wikem.org/BTS guidelines/American chest society

[18] Intraosseous [Guideline]. Kleinman ME, Chameides L, Schexnayder SM, Samson RA, Hazinski MF, Atkins DL, et al. Part 14: Pediatric advanced life support: 2010 American

Heart Association Guidelines for Cardiopulmonary Resuscitation and Emergency Cardiovascular Care. Circulation. 2010 Nov 2;**122**(18 Suppl 3):S876-S908. [Medline]. [Full Text]

[19] Bloch SA, Bloch AJ, Silva P. Adult intraosseous use in academic EDs and simulated comparison of emergent vascular access techniques. The American Journal of Emergency Medicine. 2013;**31**(3):622-624. DOI: 10.1016/j.ajem.2012.11.021

[20] Hallas P, Brabrand M, Folkestad L. Reasons for not using intraosseous access in critical illness. Emergency Medicine Journal. 2012;**29**(6):506-507. DOI: 10.1136/emj.2010.094011

[21] Winkler M, Talley C, Woodward C, Kingsbury A, Appiah F, Elbelasi H, et al. The use of intraosseous needles for injection of contrast media for computed tomographic angiography of the thoracic aorta. Journal of Cardiovascular Computed Tomography. 2017 Mar 16. [Medline]

[22] Ed thoracotomy Hopson LR et al. Guidelines for withholding or termination of resuscitation in prehospital traumatic cardiopulmonary arrest: Joint Position Statement of the National Association of EMS Physicians and the American College of Surgeons Committee on Trauma. Journal of the American College of Surgeons. 2003;**196**:106

[23] Iwata T, Inoue K, Hige M, Yamazaki K, Kawata Y, Suehiro S. Multiple thoracoabdominal gunshot wounds with complicated trajectories. Japanese Journal of Thoracic and Cardiovascular Surgery. 2006 Oct;**54**(10):444-447

[24] American College of Surgeons Committee on Trauma. Advanced Trauma Life Support. 7th ed. Chicago, Ill: American College of Surgeons Committee on Trauma; 2004

[25] Seamon, Mark J, Haut, Elliott R, et al. Emergency Department Thoracotomy. Journal of Trauma.July 2015;**79**(1):159-173

Chapter 5

Disasters and Disaster Medicine

Abdulnasir F. Al-Jazairi

Additional information is available at the end of the chapter

http://dx.doi.org/10.5772/intechopen.72947

Abstract

The rate of disaster occurrence has increased greatly in the recent decades in both natural and man-made ones. There are more hurricanes and other natural disasters occurring now than a century ago. In addition, there is marked increase in the terrorist attacks on cities and civilians in both conventional weapons and in chemical and biological ones. The increase in the rate of disasters obliges medical society to pay more and more attention to the disaster response. There are attempts to make the subject of disaster as an independent specialty of medicine because it has unique focus in managing cases and it involves dealing with several issues other than direct medical treatment of patients.

Keywords: natural disasters, man-made disasters, hazard, risks, vulnerability, incident command system, triage

1. Introduction

The frequency of disasters has increased markedly over the last 30 years [1, 2]. This increases the probability that an emergency physician may face a disaster, and he/she needs to be well trained in order to decrease the losses. Moreover, the consequences of the disasters are increased to reach billions of dollars according to **Margareta Wahlström** *(United Nations Special Representative of the Secretary-General for Disaster Risk Reduction).* In her forward to the Atlas of natural disasters in 2015, she stated that "Economic losses as a result of disasters continue to escalate. In each of the past 3 years direct economic losses from disasters have surpassed $100 billion in the world" [3]. Such threats will lead us to the conclusion that we need to study disaster as a unique phenomenon and have preplanning to manage risks, trying to prevent them or decrease their effects on the community, instead of reaction to the disaster itself. As a matter of fact, education and training in disaster medicine are mandatory [4].

2. Definitions and classifications

2.1. Why we need to define and classify disasters?

We need to define and classify disasters to have better knowledge and understanding of the problem. This will enable concerned specialists and leaders to discuss the conditions and responses needed in more detail. The response may include shifting of resources and manpower or preparing alternative places to shift victims. Analysis of disasters shows that all disasters share common characteristics; they include temporal and geographic footprints, triggering hazard (or hazards), and vulnerabilities [5, 6].

Disaster: The word *disaster* is derived from Middle French *désastre* and that from Old Italian *disastro*, which in turn comes from the Ancient Greek pejorative prefix δυσ-, (*dus*-) "bad" and ἀστήρ (*aster*), "star." The root of the word *disaster* ("bad star" in Greek) comes from an astrological sense of a calamity blamed on the position of planets and ἀστήρ (aster), "star" [7].

The **linguistic definition** of the world disaster is "a sudden calamitous event bringing great damage, loss, or destruction" [8].

World Health Organization (WHO) definition of disaster: "A **disaster** is an occurrence disrupting the normal conditions of existence and causing a level of suffering that exceeds the capacity of adjustment of the affected community" [9].

United Nation Office for Disaster Risk Reduction (UNISDR) defines disasters as "A serious disruption of the functioning of a community or a society at any scale due to hazardous events interacting with conditions of exposure, vulnerability and capacity, leading to one or more of the following: human, material, economic and environmental losses and impacts" [10].

Federal Emergency Management Agency (FEMA) defines disaster as "An occurrence that has resulted in property damage, deaths, and/or injuries to a community. FEMA 1990" [11].

International Federation of Red Cross (IFRC) added another factor to the definition: "A disaster is a sudden, calamitous event that seriously disrupts the functioning of a community or society and causes human, material, and economic or environmental losses that exceed the community's or society's ability to cope using its own resources." Though often caused by nature, disasters can have human origins [11].

3. Social definition of disaster

The difference between this definition and others is that the previous ones concentrate on the event while this one concentrates on the social phenomena accompanying the event. David Alexander in 2005 reported that disasters are not defined by fixed events, but by social constructs, and these are liable to change [12]. There is large debate and discussions between sociologists regarding the definition of disasters. There are more than 36 definitions of disasters from sociology perspective. Many scientists are involved in the evolution of the definition. E. L. Quarantelli in 2000 identified disasters in terms of a variety of defining features. They are as follows:

1. Of sudden-onset occasions,
2. Seriously disrupt the routines of collective units,
3. Cause the adoption of unplanned courses of action to adjust to the disruption,
4. Have unexpected life histories designated in social space and time, and
5. Pose danger to valued social objects [12].

4. Quantitative definition of disasters

There are trials to define disasters on the quantitative basis. This has huge variations because disasters, as noticed in the previous definitions, depend on the balance between needs and resources. Depending on that, if there are low resources, then a disaster can occur in a lower scale. On the contrary, if there are many resources then it requires larger-scale events to create a disaster. In the USA, FEMA put the following quantitative descriptions for disaster depending on Lesley Sheehan & Kenneth Hewitt's work in 1969:

"A major disaster was defined as an incident that includes one of the following events:

- At least 100 human deaths, or
- At least 100 human injuries, or
- At least US $1 million economic damages" [13].

If we look at the previous definitions by well-known organizations, we will find that they all agree about the serious effects on community and that community cannot respond to the incident depending on its own resources. The social explanation of the disaster encourages us to make changes in our social system and make improvement on the disaster outcome. Also, it confirms that there is no one definition for disaster.

5. When we consider an incident as a disaster?

The news all over the world provides a substantial number of incidents occurring every day, but not all of them are described as a disaster! Moreover, the same incidents occurring in one area are considered disaster, but if it occurred in another area, it is not.

The outcome of the triggering event by its effects on human and environment decides whether this is a disaster or not. The factors affecting the disaster outcome are (1) scope of the impact, (2) speed of the impact, (3) duration of the impact, and (4) social preparedness of the community [12].

From this perspective, we can realize the importance of studying disasters, study the disaster response plan, and train the communities on how to respond. With this, we can get a better result in case there is a disaster.

Hazard: "A hazard is an agent which has the potential to cause harm to a vulnerable target" [14]. In disaster medicine, it is: "A Hazard is a potential source of harm or adverse health effect on a person or persons" [15].

Risk: "someone or something that creates or suggests a hazard" [16]. In disaster medicine, it is: "risk is the likelihood that a person may be harmed or suffers adverse health effects if exposed to a hazard" [15].

Vulnerable: "capable of or susceptible to being wounded or hurt" [17]. IFRC defines it as "the diminished capacity of an individual or group to anticipate, cope with, resist and recover from the impact of a natural or man-made hazard" [18].

For more definitions, please see the links at the end of the chapter.

6. Reasons for increase in disasters

The disasters increased for many reasons are multifactorial: overpopulation, urbanization, expanding industrialization, increased traffic, climate change, ongoing threat of terrorism, and armed conflicts

1. The world population shows an increase from 1.6 billion in 1900 to 7.8 billion in 2017, with disproportionate growth in developing countries [19, 20].

2. A rapid-expanding industrialization especially in the chemical industry involving production, storage, and transportation of rapidly ever-increasing amounts of toxic and explosive agents, often in and through densely populated areas and with insufficient safety measures [21].

3. An increased traffic density of people and goods in more rapid and higher capacity modes of transport [22, 23]. Increasing international trade and travel provides myriad opportunities for the emergence or re-emergence of infectious disease threats and other public health risks [21].

4. Global climate change makes people susceptible to severe weather events, especially the coastal communities around the world [24, 25].

5. A continuous threat of terroristic acts [26, 27].

6. Armed conflicts with a high vulnerability of the civilian population to forced migration or displacement heightening the risk of infectious disease epidemics. A collateral impact of armed conflicts is often the destruction or malfunctioning of health systems [21, 27].

Considering the reasons for increased disasters in the world, we can notice that many of those are related to human behavior. Wrong decisions made by human lead to the occurrence of disasters like deforestation leading to landslides and global warming leading to increase in floods and cyclones. Sometimes, it leads to an increase in the effects of them, for example, badly distributed population with little safety precautions in houses, bad health systems, or increase in transportation all escalated the negative effects of infections and faster and wider distribution.

7. Disasters are social phenomena

Building upon the notes in the previous paragraph, several experts changed the concepts of disaster from a natural phenomenon for which nothing can be done to a social act which can be changed and manipulated to prevent it or decrease its effect.

The focus of studying disasters shifted from the causative agent-centered approach to the vulnerable population approach by researchers like David Alexander, Dennis Mileti, and Allen Barton. This concept leads to a change in the results and outcomes of disasters [28].

E. L. Quarantelli, 1992, stated in his article "The Importance of Thinking of Disasters as Social Phenomena" that it is not causative agent or the triggering event that makes the disaster. It is argued, *disasters are, one way or another, primarily the results of human actions*. A disaster is not a physical happening, it is a social event. There is a conjuncture of certain physical happenings and certain social happenings. Therefore, if there is no human injury or loss and/or no environmental effect, then there is no disaster [29].

8. Why we study disasters

There are several reasons for studying disasters as follows:

1. Although disasters are of diverse types and effects, their medical responses have common features. The needs are always more than the resources in disasters which need changes in our focus from individual benefit to community benefit. Also change in the way of delivering the care.
2. Majority of hazards have return periods on a human time scale. Examples include a 5-, 50-, and a 100-year flood. This reflects a statistical measure of how often a hazard event of a given magnitude and intensity will occur. The frequency is measured in terms of a hazard's recurrence interval [30].
3. Studying will help planners to make better plans and preparation to avoid needless life losses and decrease the effects of the disasters expected in any area.

9. Consequences of disasters

Hazardous process of all types can have primary, secondary, and tertiary effects:

1. ***Primary effects*** occur because of the process itself. For example, water damage during a flood or collapse of buildings during an earthquake, a landslide, or a hurricane.

2. ***Secondary effects*** occur only because a primary effect has caused them. For example, fires ignited because of earthquakes, disruption of electrical power and water service because of an earthquake, a flood, or a hurricane, or flooding caused by a landslide into a lake or a river.

3. ***Tertiary effects*** are long-term effects that are set off because of a primary event. These include things like loss of habitat caused by a flood, permanent changes in the position of a river channel caused by flood, crop failure caused by a volcanic eruption, and so on [31].

10. Classification of disasters.

Classification of disasters has several benefits:

1. It helps in better understanding of the disasters and helps interchange information regarding disasters in some detail.
2. It helps in the planning process and the types and amounts of resources devoted for response to each category.
3. It facilitates the response to a disaster by better knowledge and training on similar disasters.

Disasters are classified in a variety of ways:

1. Classification according to the triggering event: A common system divides incidents into natural and technological (human-made) disasters. There is a crossover between the two types, for example, a building collapse due to a hurricane or an earthquake [32].

   1.1. Natural hazards: They are naturally occurring physical phenomena caused by either rapid- or slow-onset events [33]. They are caused by nature, and men have no control over them. Earthquakes, tsunamis, floods, landslides, hurricanes, wildfires, droughts, and volcanic eruptions are some examples of natural disasters. Such disasters cause massive loss of life, property, and many other miseries. **Table 1** shows the different subgroups of the natural disasters [34].

Natural Disasters				
Biological	**Geophysical**	**Hydrological**	**Meteorological**	**Climatological**
Epidemics of • Viral, • Bacterial, • Parasitic, • Fungal, • Prion **Insect infestation**	**Earthquake,** **Volcano,** **Mass Movement (Dry)** • Rock fall, • Landslide, • Avalanche, • Subsidence,	**Flood:** • General flood, • Flash flood, • Storm surge/coastal flood **Mass Movement (Wet)** • Rock fall, • Landslide, • Avalanche, • Subsidence	**Storm:** • Tropical cyclone, • Extra-tropical cyclone. • Local storm.	**Extreme temp.** • Heat wave, • Cold wave, • Extreme winter condition. **Drought** **Wild fire** • Forest fire, • Land fire.

Table 1. Classification of natural disasters.

http://dx.doi.org/10.5772/intechopen.72947

1.2. Technological (or man-made) hazards are events that are caused by humans and occur in or close to human settlements [33]. Man-made disasters are less complicated and occupy smaller areas making them easier to control [35]. **Table 2** shows the man-made disasters with its subgroups and examples [36].

2. Classification based on the speed of onset

2.1. Rapid-onset disasters

Hazards that arise suddenly, or whose occurrence cannot be predicted far in advance, trigger rapid-onset disasters. Earthquakes, cyclones and other windstorms, landslides and avalanches, wildfires, floods, and volcanic eruptions are usually categorized as rapid-onset events. The warning time ranges from seconds or at best a few minutes in the case of earthquakes and many landslides, to several days in the case of most storms and floods. Some volcanic eruptions may be preceded by weeks or months of activity, but predicting volcanoes' behavior remains very difficult and the warning time for the eruption itself may be only days or hours. Most disasters are rapid-onset events [37].

2.2. Slow-onset disasters

Most discussion of slow-onset disasters concentrates on one hazard: drought. It can take months or sometimes years for the results of drought to become disastrous, in the form of severe water and food shortages and, ultimately, famine. Other examples are pollution of the environment, and human activities that degrade the environment and damage ecosystems (deforestation for instance) also contribute to disasters. Their cumulative impact may not be felt for decades, although the hazards that they make more likely, such as flash floods and landslides, may be sudden-onset events [37].

Man-Made (Human-Induced) Hazards		
Hazard Sub-Family	**Hazard Type**	**Hazard Sub-Type**
Technological Hazard	Structural Collapse	Standing Structure
		Underground Structure
	Utility Failure	
	Fire	
	Explosion	
	Contamination[23]	Chemical Contamination
		Hydrocarbon Contamination
		Radiation Contamination
Transport Hazard	Crash/Collision	Road
		Rail
		Water
		Air
		Space
Social Hazard	Social	Riot
		Stampede
	Economic	Currency Devaluation
		Mass Bank/Corporate Failures

Table 2. Classification of technological (man-made) disasters.

3. Classification according to **severity and who provide the resources**:

3.1. Level I disaster is one in which local emergency response personnel and organizations can contain and effectively deal with the disaster and its aftermath.

3.2. Level II disaster requires regional efforts and mutual aid from surrounding communities.

3.3. Level III disaster is of such a magnitude that local and regional assets are overwhelmed, requiring statewide or federal assistance and may even need international help.

This classification reflects a tiered response, which is a fundamental principle of the National Response Framework, a component of national disaster response planning in the United States [30].

4. **Simple and compound disasters:**

4.1. Simple disasters: the location's infrastructure remains intact and effective. Communication is possible. Health system and other emergency services work [38].

4.2. Compound disasters: all or most of the infrastructures are disrupted. Communication is difficult; roads, electricity, and water supply are unavailable. Hospitals may be affected, and there is no place to treat the victims [38].

5. **Complex disasters:**

This is a special kind of disasters in which there is a combination of both man-made and natural causes threatening the livelihood of people. It can be caused by wars and civil disturbance. Rescue operation may be done which is critical and risky to the environment [39].

Such "complex emergencies" are typically characterized by

- extensive violence and loss of life;
- displacements of populations;
- widespread damage to societies and economies;
- the need for large-scale, multifaceted humanitarian assistance;
- the hindrance or prevention of humanitarian assistance by political and military constraints;
- significant security risks for humanitarian relief workers in some areas [40].

6. **Compensated and uncompensated major incidents**:

Countries using this classification differentiate between major incidents and disaster:

6.1. Compensated major incidents are incidents in which there are sufficient local resources to deal with the consequences [38, 41].

6.2. Uncompensated major incidents occur where the medical and other responding emergency services are totally inadequate. This is a disaster condition [38, 41].

7. **Possibilities for further casualties**:

This classification depends on the possibilities of continuous injuries and victims or no:

7.1. Static: no more casualties are expected after evacuating the scene, for example, motor vehicle collision [42].

7.2. Dynamic: more casualties are expected as long as the disaster is active, for example, continuing wildfires [42].

11. Disaster severity

The severity index is used to assess the severity of any disaster. It depends on seven factors [43]:

1. Effect of the disaster on the surrounding community: if the effect is simple, it scores 1 and becomes 2 if the effect is compound.
2. Man-made versus natural: man-made disasters score 0 while natural disasters score 1.
3. Duration of the disaster:

Duration	Severity
Less than 1 h	0
1–24 h	1
More than 24 h	2

4. The radius of the area in which the casualties are fallen:

Area radius	Severity
Less than 1 km	0
1–10 km	1
More than 10 km	2

5. Number of casualties:

Number of casualties	Severity
Less than 100	0
100–1000	1
More than 1000	2

6. Average severity of the injuries sustained:

   Average $(S) = T1 + T2/T3$.

No. of severe cases	Severity
$T1 + T2 << T3$	0
$T1 + T2$ nearly equal $T3$	1
$T1 + T2 >> T3$	2

7. Medical rescue time: rescue, primary treatment, and transportation.

Time	Severity
Less than 6 h	0
6–24 h	1
More than 24 h	2

From the above mentioned factors, we can see that the severity index of disasters can lead to a score which make the basis upon which disasters can be compared with confidence and can be used for further study of disasters. **Figure 1** shows the relation of severity index (*S*) and disaster severity scale (DSS) with examples [44].

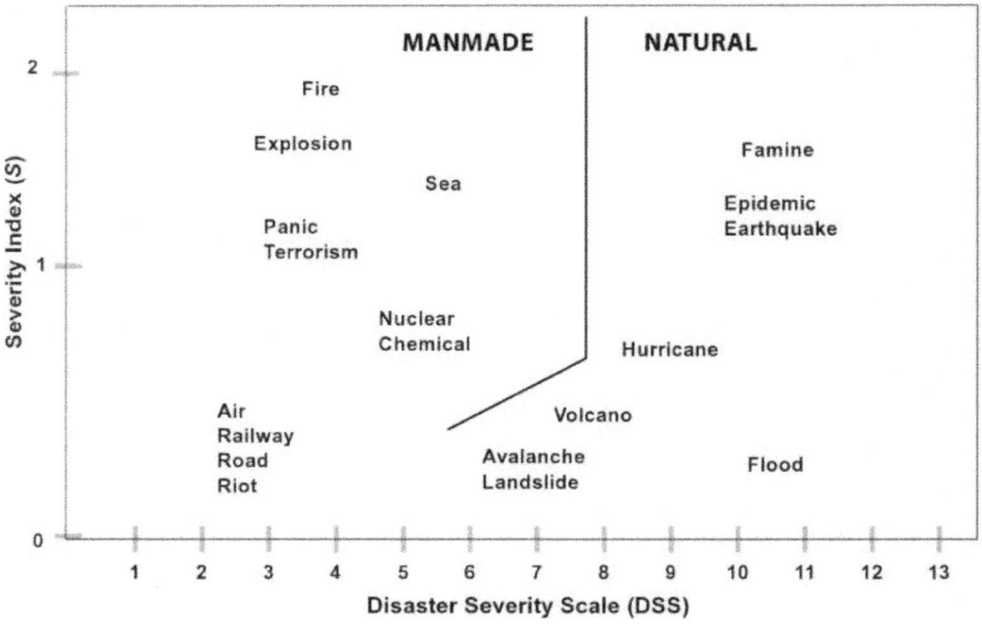

Figure 1. Disaster severity scale (DSS) versus severity index (*S*) for man-made and natural disasters. Adapted from de Boer and van Remmen (2003).

12. Disaster stages

The time frame for a disaster is a principal factor in innovating methods for management of the disaster. Quarantelli in 1980 divided the time factor into three phases [45, 46]:

1. **Pre-impact phase**: In this phase, there is enough time for investigating choices, inventing ways to prevent or mitigate the disasters, and training communities on the methods. Strategic planners and leaders are involved in this phase. They will make the needed large-scale decisions and policy shifts intended to change people's perception of risk.
2. **Trans-impact phase**: This phase includes the period that is immediately before, during, and after event. Policymakers and operation leaders are involved and are under strong time pressure to deal with the effects of disasters.
3. **Post-impact phase:** This phase includes two subphases, the early and late phases. In the early one, there is a need to restore pre-impact norm. In the late phase, there is a need to set new norms to prevent or mitigate future disasters.

13. Disaster management life cycle

Definition: It is the discipline dealing with and avoiding risks. It is a discipline that involves preparing, supporting, and rebuilding society when natural or human-made disasters occur [47].

To reach the best expected response during the impact of a disaster, a community should perform several steps long before the disaster had occurred. There should be a study of the area and expected hazards, know the available resources, then make a plan and train people on the plan. In such circumstances, we expect the best response in case there is a disaster. In other words, we need to have a planned response instead of reflex reactions [3].

The process of disaster management involves four phases: mitigation, preparedness, response, and recovery. Those stages can be divided according to the disaster phase as shown in **Figure 2**.

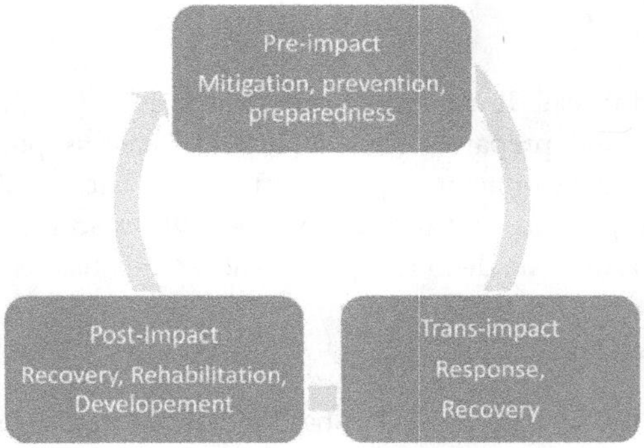

Figure 2. Disaster management components in relation to disaster phases.

All our responses follow models consciously or subconsciously. The benefits of incorporating a model for disaster management are as follows [48]:

1. Using a model simplifies complex events by helping leaders to distinguish important issues which need actions and set priorities.
2. It helps in better understanding of the current disaster situation and expected evolvement of the disaster.
3. It is important in quantifying disaster events.
4. It helps in establishing a common base for understanding the disaster management cycle by all involved personnel.
5. It helps disaster management to explain the course of the disaster and its future evolvement to nonspecialists.

There are important points we need to consider before studying models. First, rapid change may be considered the single principal factor in changing an event into a disaster. Second, chaos may look like a random behavior, but its behavior remains unstable over time that stays within boundaries. Chaos is good and is required to accommodate and adapt to changes. Finally, dividing the disaster into stages is important for theory only; otherwise, the actions are more important and there is no benefit of knowing the stage if a leader cannot make the right decisions [48].

An overview of the models is listed subsequently and will be briefly explained hereafter [47]:

1. The traditional model.
2. The circular model.
3. The expand contract models.
4. The disaster crunch and release models.
5. Manitoba model.
6. Comprehensive model.

13.1. Traditional model

This is the mostly used model. It consists of two phases only: pre-disaster that contains the mitigation, prevention, and preparedness; the second phase is post-impact in which the response, recovery, and development is present. The drawback of this model is the sharp separation between the pre-and post-disaster phases [49]. In addition, data integration and decision making are not easily made in it. **Figure 3** shows the phases of this model [50].

13.2. The circular model

This model was proposed by Richard Kelly; he divided the disaster management cycle into eight phases to reduce the complexity of disasters and handle the nonlinear nature of disaster events. The main advantage of this model is the ability to learn from the actual disaster. It requires a database with training and a high technological infrastructure to obtain reasonable results [50]. **Figure 4** shows the model [48].

13.3. The expand contract model

This model presents the phases of disaster-risk reduction as a parallel series of activities. All the stages of the cycle are continuously present. The concentration on each stage depends on

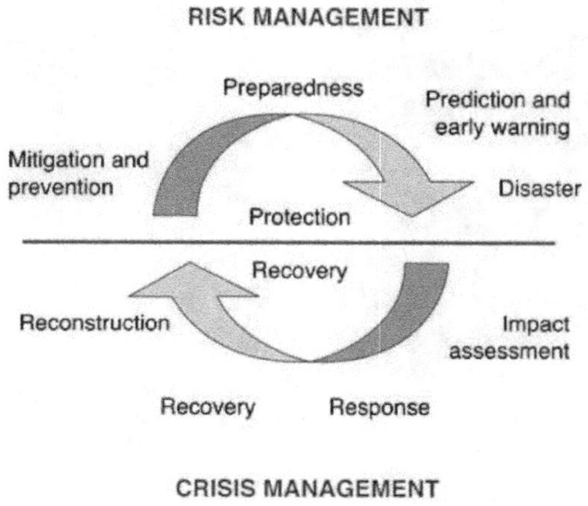

Figure 3. Traditional model.

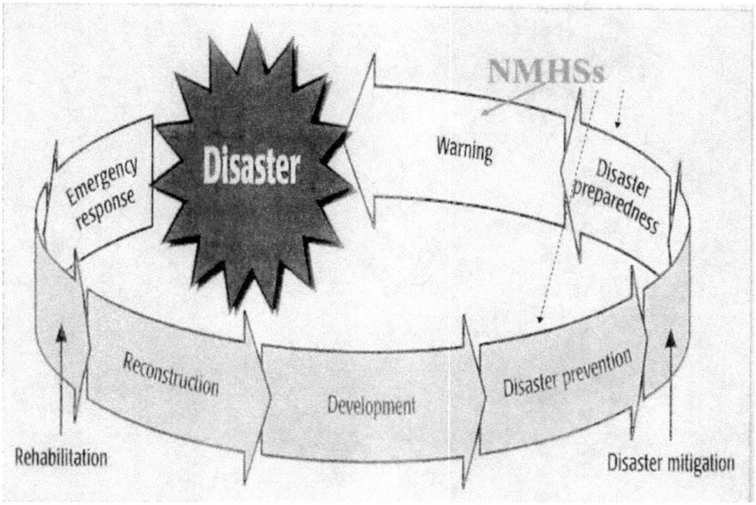

Figure 4. Kelly circular model.

the phase of the disaster. Before the disaster impact, there is concentration on mitigation and preparedness, while during the trans-impact phase the response part of the cycle gets more attention and highest weight [47]. This model overcomes the major weakness of the disaster traditional model, which regards disasters as managed in a phased sequence [5, 47, 50] (**Figure 5**).

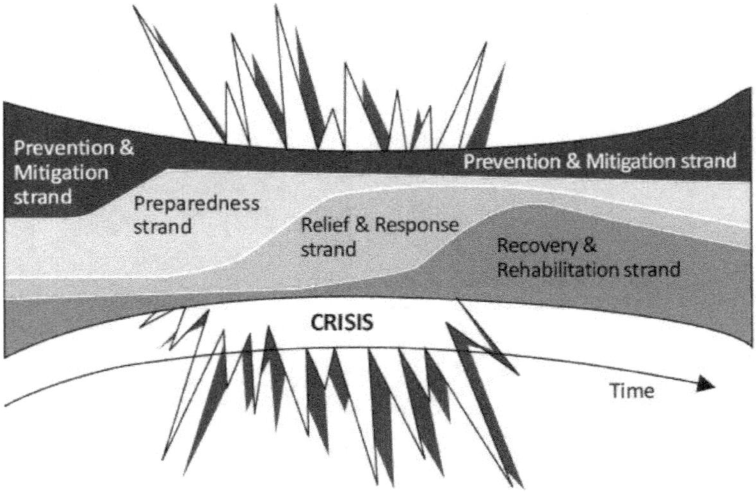

Figure 5. The expand contract model [50].

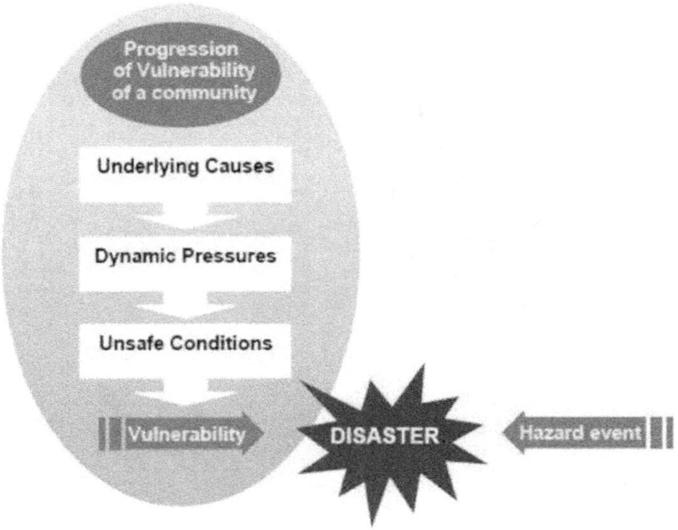

Figure 6. The crunch model.

http://dx.doi.org/10.5772/intechopen.72947

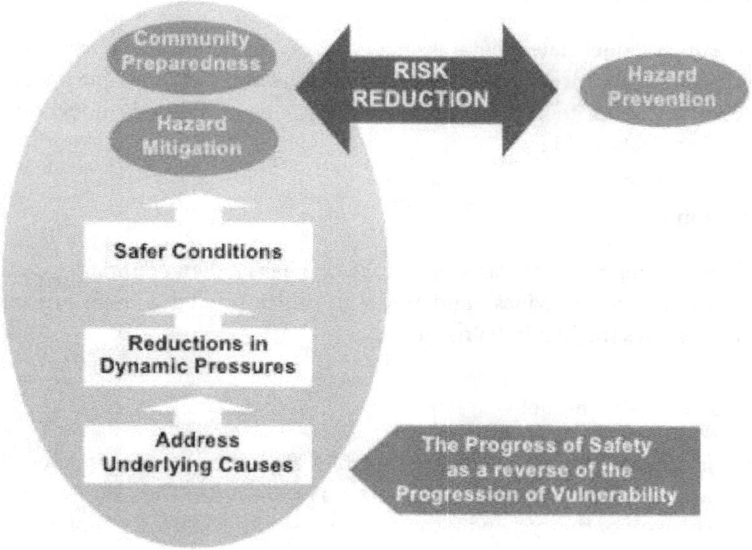

Figure 7. The release model [47].

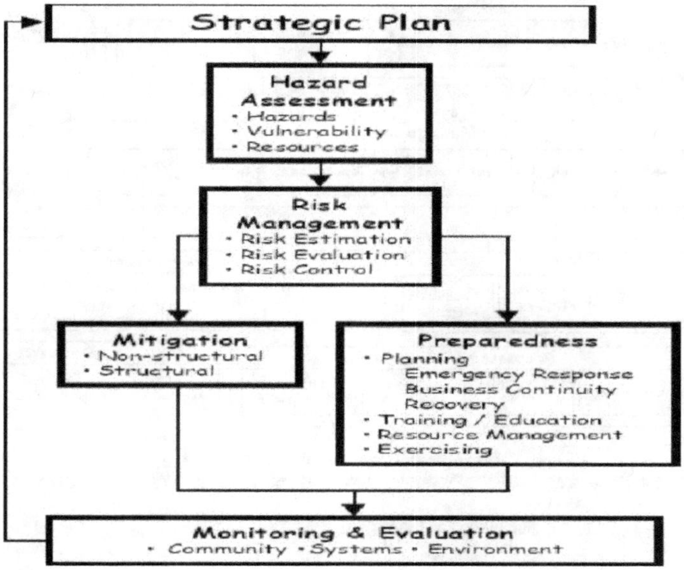

Figure 8. The Manitoba model.

13.4. The disaster crunch and release models

The disaster crunch model states that a disaster occurs only when a hazard affects vulnerable people [51] (**Figure 6**). It concentrates on the causes of disasters and how the impact can lead to them. On the other hand, the release model concentrates on the risk reduction and hazard prevention and mitigation (**Figure 7**).

13.5. Manitoba model

It separates the disaster cycle into six stages; each one has its own boundaries and limitations. The balance between preparedness and flexibility is considered a main advantage of this model. **Figure 8** shows the Manitoba model [52].

13.6. The comprehensive model

The previous models are meant to deal with certain aspects of the management cycle; therefore, they do not help decision makers in all phases of the cycle. The comprehensive model is built to link all aspects of the cycle with the disaster response acts in each phase [53]. **Figure 9** shows the comprehensive model.

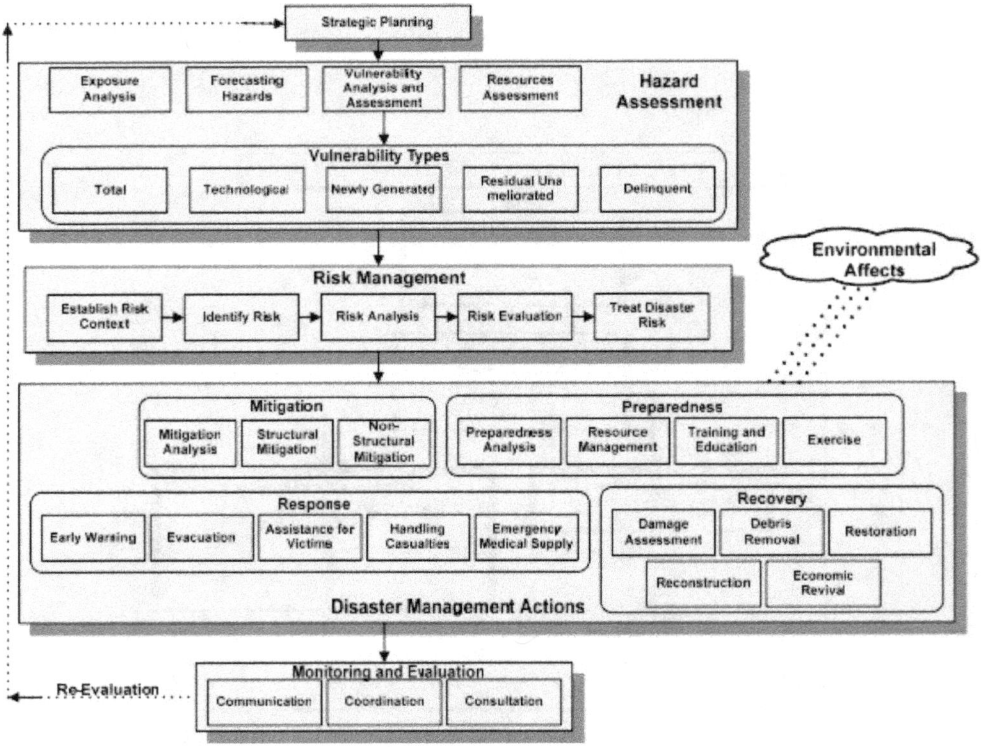

Figure 9. The comprehensive model.

14. Disaster planning

Having good knowledge on the disaster management cycle and the models, it is time to advance for discussing the disaster planning.

- Prerequisites for planning [54]:
    - recognition that hazards and vulnerability exist and that emergencies can occur;
    - awareness among the community, government, and decision;
    - makers of the need to plan and of the benefits of planning;
    - appropriate legislation to guarantee implementation of the plan;
    - a designated organization responsible for coordinating both planning and response recovery in the event of a disaster.
- Concepts of disaster management [54]:
    - All hazards approach: This means that the set of actions put in the plan should be flexible to accommodate several types of hazards. Even if there are counteract measures for some hazards, it is desirable to make this type of response.
    - Comprehensive approach: This means all phases of the disaster cycle which include mitigation, preparedness, response, and recovery.
- **Mitigation:**

Mitigation is defined as: "The act of making a condition or consequence less severe" [55].

In the medical field, it is defined as "the effort to reduce loss of life and property by lessening the impact of disasters. It is most effective when implemented under a comprehensiv, long-term mitigation plan" [56]. The mitigation deals with the identification of the risks and trying to prevent them or decrease their effects. The fundamental steps in risk management are as follows:

1. Risk identification,
2. Risk impact assessment,
3. Risk prioritization analysis,
4. Risk mitigation analysis.

These steps are better described with their relation and interaction as shown in **Figure 10** [57].

Cost-effective mitigation measures on long term are the key for reducing disaster losses on long term and **Table 3** lists the examples of measures that are not exhaustive [57].

- **Preparedness:**

Merriam Webster dictionary defined preparedness as: "the quality or state of being prepared; *especially*: a state of adequate preparation in case of war" [58].

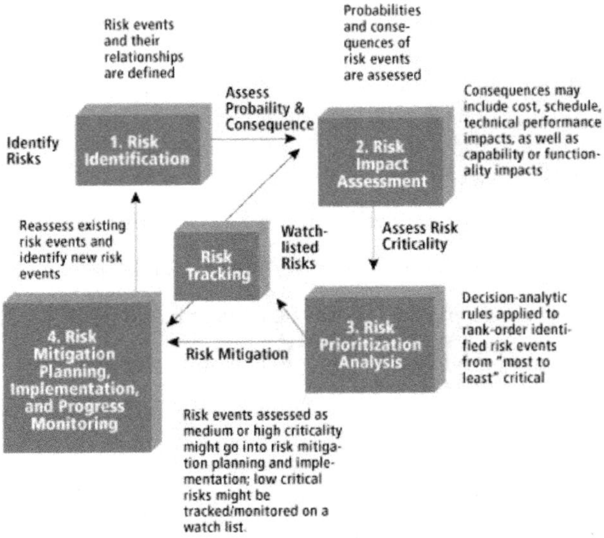

Figure 10. Fundamental steps in risk analysis [57].

• Zoning/land-use management	• Building codes and building use regulations
• Relocation of people living in vulnerable and risky areas.	• Safety improvements, for example, annual technical care checking.
• Legislations to put disaster response plan.	• Public information
• Community awareness and education	• Tax, insurance incentives or disincentives

Table 3. Examples of cost-effective mitigation measures.

IFRC defines preparedness as: "Disaster preparedness refers to measures taken to prepare for and reduce the effects of disasters; that is, to predict and, where possible, prevent disasters, mitigate their impact on vulnerable populations, and respond to and effectively cope with their consequences" [59]. It takes the results of mitigation and uses it to prepare the community on how to deal with them.

The goal of preparedness is to raise the ability and readiness of a community, an organization, or a country to respond timely and efficiently to any disaster that may occur. The basic components of disaster preparedness involve the following [60]:

1. Identifying organizational resources,
2. Determining roles and responsibilities,
3. Developing policies and procedures and planning activities.

- **Response:**

Response in biology means: "Any behavior of a living organism that result from an external or internal stimulus" [61].

http://dx.doi.org/10.5772/intechopen.72947

In disaster perspective, response encompasses the decisions and actions taken to deal with the immediate effects of an emergency [62]. Usually, it is for a short period of hours or days starting from the time of the impact or shortly before that if there are predicting signs like hurricanes. Response plan is the best put with the preparedness and whole plan to make a complete coordinated plan rather than making a fragmented plan and there is difficulty in incorporating the different fragments together [54].

Medical response during disaster can be summarized in the CO-S-TR Model framework [63]. This framework can be expressed by 4Cs, 4Ss, and 4Ts as shown in **Table 4**.

The first column (C4) in **Table 4** deals with the higher-management level and reaching the frontline staff in direct response to the disaster.

The second column (S4) looks on the surges of the resources to accommodate the increase in demands because of the disaster.

The third one (T4) deals with victims, how to define and follow them in different places, and how to deliver treatment to them in different places.

- **Recovery:**

It is the restoration or return to any former and better state or condition [64]. In disaster medicine, recovery for hospitals is defined as: "The process by which a hospital minimizes the impact an emergency has made on its operations in an effort to resume normal operations or establish new norms for operations" [65]. The concept of recovery has changes over years from regaining normality in four added-on steps proposed by Hass et al. in 1977 [66] to a more long and complex process that incorporates all other phases of the disaster [67]. To get best results and rapid regain of normality, recovery planning should be incorporated with mitigation process [68]. In disasters with a short response time, recovery starts after ending the acute phase. However, if the disaster took a long time, then review the situation every 12-h period and assess the possibility of starting the recovery processes. Sometimes, in long-lasting disasters, both response and recovery processes go side by side. We can divide recovery into three stages:

1. **Early recovery**: in this stage, regaining the basic services and trying to work as normal as possible or having a new normal. For example, working in an alternative place and this becomes the new normal place.

CO-S-TR framework		
C4	**S4**	**T4**
Command	Staff	Tracking
Control	Stuff	Triage
Communication	Space	Treatment
Coordination	Special	Transportation

Table 4. An outline of CO-S-TR framework.

2. **Rehabilitation**: in this stage, save the undamaged issues, restore the restorable, and try to go back to pre-disaster condition. In the example in the first point, work to fix and rebuild the health-care facility is done in this stage.

3. **Development**: this will be a long-lasting stage (maybe to the next disaster impact); it will intermingle with the mitigation plan, and in it, new standards are set in the building codes or electricity sources to decrease the harmful effects of disasters and go back to normality more rapidly with less damage or work with better efficiency. In the same example as discussed earlier, building or making modifications in other buildings to use them as alternative places will serve patients in time of disaster.

15. International efforts to deal with disasters

There are disasters, mostly natural ones, with scale beyond the ability of the country. Such disasters need the cooperation of the international community to deal with them. The earthquake in Pakistan in 2004, tsunami in 2005, and the earthquake in Haiti in 2011 are just recent examples of such disasters. One of the problems faced during such huge efforts is the duplication of some aspects of the humanitarian acts and missing of some other aspects. This leads to the foundation of the Sphere project under the care of the UN. It was launched in 1997 to develop a set of minimum standards in core areas of humanitarian assistance [69]. For better arrangements and coordination of the various organizations involved in the response, the cluster approach was developed to coordinate the efforts. **Figure 11** shows the cluster approach with the organizations' responsibilities [70].

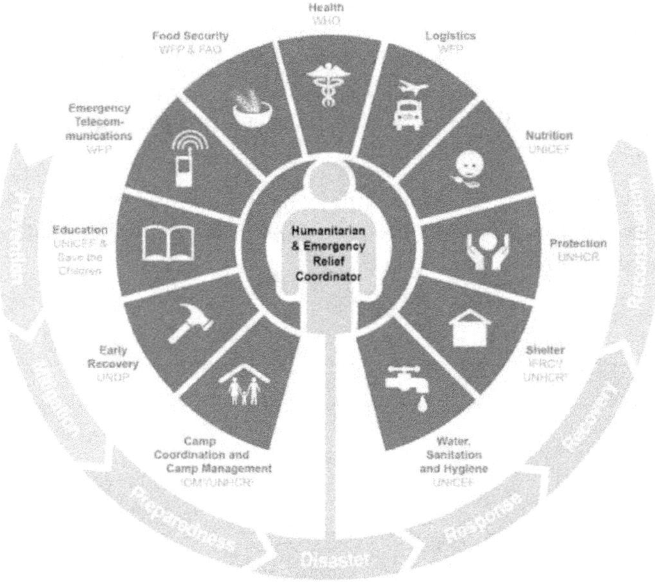

Figure 11. The cluster approach.

http://dx.doi.org/10.5772/intechopen.72947

16. CBRNE

This abbreviation denotes the use of abnormal or unusual agents which are as follows:

- C: chemical,
- B: biological,
- R: radiological,
- N: nuclear, and
- E: high-yield explosives.

These weapons can create large disruption in terms of the number and level of wellness of the community. Details are beyond the scope of this book.

17. Conclusion

Disaster is a special situation requiring different management styles and techniques. It is mainly the difference in number which exceeds the resources, and for its proper management there is a desperate need for planning to recall staff and surge space and stuff. There are situations which require the utilization of the entire country's resources, while others may even necessitate international aid. The recent examples of Haiti earthquakes, Iraq and Syrian mass immigration due to internal wars, and anti-terrorism war are still going on.

Acknowledgements

I would like to acknowledge my mentors in the European Masters in Disaster Medicine who taught me a lot and allowed me to refer to their valuable lectures and articles on disaster medicine. I would also specially wish to thank my department and chairman who provided me with the needed time to finish the chapter.

Conflict of interest

I have no conflict of interest of any sort.

Author details

Abdulnasir F. Al-Jazairi

Address all correspondence to: ahuaidi@hamad.qa

Emergency Department, Adult Urgent Care Centers, Hamad General Hospital, Doha, Qatar

References

[1] Emanuel K. Increasing destructiveness of tropical cyclones over the past 30 years. Nature. Aug 4, 2005;**436**(7051):686-688. Accessed November 1, 2017

[2] FEMA (Federal Emergency Management Agency). (2011). Declared Disasters by Year. Available from http://www.fema.gov/news/disaster_totals_annual.fema. Accessed November 1, 2017

[3] Shi P, Kasperson R, editors. IHDP/Future Earth-Integrated Risk Governance Project Series. World Atlas of Natural Disaster Risk. ISBN 978-3-662-45430-5 (eBook)

[4] Lennquist S. Education and training in disaster medicine. Scandinavian Journal of Surgery. 2005;**94**:300-310

[5] McEntire DA. Triggering agents, vulnerabilities and disaster reduction: Towards a holistic paradigm. Disaster Prevention and Management. 2001;**10**:189-196

[6] Koenig KL, Dinerman N, Kuel AE. Disaster nomenclature: A functional impact approach: The PICE system. Academic Emergency Medicine. 1996;**3**(7):723

[7] Wikipedia, the Free Encyclopedia. https://en.wikipedia.org/wiki/Disaster. Accessed November 2, 2017

[8] https://www.merriam-webster.com/dictionary/disaster. Accessed on October 28, 2017 at 14:09

[9] training.fema.gov/hiedu/docs/hazdem/session%206–defining%20disaster%20slides.ppt. Accessed October 28, 2017

[10] https://www.unisdr.org/we/inform/terminology. Accessed October 29, 2017

[11] http://www.ifrc.org/en/what-we-do/disaster-management/about-disasters/what-is-a-disaster/. Accessed October 29, 2017

[12] Rodriguez H, Quarantelli EL, Dynes RR. Handbook of Disaster Research. Springer; 2007. e-ISBN: 978-0-387-32353-4

[13] Lesley S, Kenneth H. A pilot survey of global natural disasters of the past twenty years. University of Toronto, 1969. Accessed 29/10/2017. https://hazdoc.colorado.edu/bitstream/handle/10590/779/NHC-A-WP-1969-11.pdf?sequence=1

[14] https://en.wikipedia.org/wiki/Hazard. Accessed on November 22, 2017

[15] Health and Safety Authority. http://www.hsa.ie/eng/Topics/Hazards/. Accessed on November 22, 2017

[16] https://www.merriam-webster.com/dictionary/risk. Accessed at November 22, 2017

[17] http://www.dictionary.com/browse/vulnerable. Accessed November 22, 2017

[18] http://www.ifrc.org/en/what-we-do/disaster-management/about-disasters/what-is-a-disaster/what-is-vulnerability/. Accessed on November 22, 2017

[19] United Nations, Department of Economic and Social Affairs, Population Division. World Population Prospects: The 2008 Revision, Highlights, Working Paper No ESA/P/WP. 210; 2009

[20] World Population, Wikipedia. https://en.wikipedia.org/wiki/World_population. Accessed November 1, 2017

[21] World Health Organization. The World Health Report 2007: A Safer Future: Global Public Health Security in the 21st Century. Geneva: Switzerland; 2007. www.who.int/whr/2007/whr07_en.pdf

[22] Quarantelli EL. Disaster Planning: Small and Large – Past, Present and Future. Disaster Research Center: University of Delaware; 1981

[23] Kreps G. Disaster and the social order. Sociological Theory. 1985;**3**:49-65

[24] Noji EK. Public health issues in disasters. Critical Care Medicine. 2005;**33**(Suppl):S29-S33

[25] Intergovernmental Panel on Climate Change. Climate Change 2007: Synthesis Report. Summary for Policymakers. www.ipcc.ch/pdf/assessment-report/ar4/syr/ar4_syr_spm.pdf

[26] James JJ, Subbarao I, Lanier WL. Improving the art and science of disaster medicine and public health preparedness. Mayo Clinic Proceedings. 2008;**83**:559-562

[27] Burkle FM Jr, Greenough PG. Impact of public health emergencies on modern disaster taxonomy, planning, and response. Disaster Medicine and Public Health Preparedness. 2008;**2**:192-199

[28] Rodriguez R, Quarantelli EL, Dynes R. Handbook of Disaster Research. https://books.google.com.qa/books?id=_LjS_lS2hQEC&pg=PA10&lpg=PA10&dq=disasters+as+a+social+phenomenon&source=bl&ots=ozzSp-Rjy&sig=_2WRkKgH_5KJ4n0U3z9BsDvtJSE&hl=en&sa=X&ved=0ahUKEwiTkN6F1J3XAhXBcRQKHXfeAp4Q6AEIWjAJ#v=onepage&q&f=false. Accessed 01/11/17

[29] Quarantelli EL. The Importance of Thinking of Disasters as Social Phenomena. 1992. University of Delaware Disaster Research Center PRELIMINARY PAPER f184. http://udspace.udel.edu/bitstream/handle/19716/572/PP184.pdf. Accessed 29/10/2017

[30] Capacity Building in Asia using Information Technology Applications. http://www.adpc.net/casita/course-materials/Mod-2-Hazards.pdf. Accessed 30/10/2017

[31] Nelson SA. Natural Disasters & Assessing Hazards and Risk. http://www.tulane.edu/~sanelson/Natural_Disasters/introduction.htm. Accessed on 30/10/2017

[32] Furin MA. Disaster Planning. Brenner BE. https://emedicine.medscape.com/article/765495-overview#a2. Accessed on 29/10/2017

[33] http://www.ifrc.org/en/what-we-do/disaster-management/about-disasters/definition-of-hazard/. Accessed 29/10/2017

[34] Akinci H, Dogan S, Kiliçoglu C, Temiz MS. Production of landslide susceptibility map of Samsun (Turkey) City Center by using frequency ratio method. International Journal of

the Physical Sciences. 4 March 2011 Available online at http://www.academicjournals.org/IJPS;**6**(5):1015-1025. Accessed on 30/10/2017

[35] De Boer J. Order in chaos: Modelling medical management in disaster. European Journal of Emergency Medicine. 1999;**6**(2):141-148. P 51

[36] Michael Lerner and Inter-Agency Group members. Alternative Classification Schemes for Man-Made Hazards in the Context of the Implementation of the Sendai Framework. 5 June 2016. Accessed on 30/10/2017

[37] http://www.bvsde.paho.org/bvsacd/cd46/disaster/cap15.pdf. Accessed on 30/10/2017

[38] Greaves I, Porter K. Oxford Handbook of Pre-Hospital Care. Chapter 10

[39] Environmental health in emergencies and disasters: a practical guide (WHO). 2002 http://www.who.int/environmental_health_emergencies/complex_emergencies/en/. Accessed 03 /11/2017

[40] Website of the IFRC. www.ifrc.org/en/what-we-do/disaster-management/about-disasters/-definition-of-hazard/complex-emergencies/. Accessed on 30/10/2017

[41] Greaves I, Porter K, Hodgetts TJ, Woollard M. Emergency Care: A Textbook for Paramedics. Chapter 58

[42] Robert AP, Lawrence P, David M. Oxford American Handbook of Disaster Medicine. Oxford University Press. 2012

[43] De Boer J. Order in chaos: Modelling medical management in disaster. European Journal of Emergency Medicine. 1999;**6**(2):141-148. P 49–55

[44] Gad-el-Hak M. Large-scale disasters: Prediction, control, and mitigation. Cambridge University press. 2008

[45] Rodriguez H, Quarantelli EL, Dynes RR. Handbook of Disaster Research. Springer; 2007 e-ISBN: 978-0-387-32353-4

[46] FAO website. A handbook for trainers on participatory local development. http://www.fao.org/docrep/006/ad346e/ad346e0d.htm. Accessed November 4, 2017

[47] Debacker M. Modelling medical disaster management. Lecture in the EMDM. 2014

[48] Kelly C. Simplifying disasters: Developing a model for complex non-linear events. Australian Journal of Emergency Management. 1999;**14**(1):25-27. Accessed November 7, 2017

[49] Blaikie P, Cannon T, Davis I, Wisner B. At Risk: National Hazards, People's Vulnerability and Disasters, Rouledge, London. 1994

[50] Dube E. Improving disaster risk reduction capacity of District Civil Protection Units in managing veld fires: A case of Mangwe District in Matabeleland South Province, Zimbabwe. Jamba. 2015;**7**(1) http://jamba.org.za/index.php/jamba/article/view/143/319. 11/11/2017

[51] Hai VM, Smyth I. The Disaster Crunch Model for a Gendered approach. Oxfam. https://www.scribd.com/document/342337736/The-Disaster-Crunch-Model-Guidelines-for-a-Gendered-Approach#fullscreen&from_embed. Accessed November 11, 2017

[52] https://www.researchgate.net/figure/265151071_fig2_Fig-4-The-Manitoba-model. Accessed November 12, 2017

[53] Asghar S, Alahakoon D, Churilov L. A Comprehensive Conceptual Model for Disaster Management. Monash University, Australia: Clayton School of Information Technology; file:///F:/My%20Folders/OneDrive/Disaster%20Medicine%20books/A%20Comprehensive%20Conceptual%20Model%20for%20Disaster%20Management.pdf. Accessed November 12, 2017

[54] Debacker M. General and medical disaster planning. EMDM lecture. 2014

[55] Dictionary.com. http://www.dictionary.com/browse/mitigation. Accessed November 13, 2017

[56] Hazards mitigation plan. FEMA. https://www.fema.gov/hazard-mitigation-planning. Accessed November 13, 2017

[57] Garvey PR. Probability Methods for Cost Uncertainty Analysis: A Systems Engineering Perspective. Taylor & Francis Group (UK), Boca Raton, London, New York, ISBN: 0824789660. https://www.mitre.org/publications/systems-engineering-guide/acquisition-systems-engineering/risk-management/risk-management-tools: Chapman-Hall/CRC Press; January 2000 Accessed November 13, 2017

[58] https://www.merriam-webster.com/dictionary/preparedness. Accessed November 13, 2017

[59] International Federation of Red Cross and Red Crescent Societies. Preparing for disasters. http://www.ifrc.org/en/what-we-do/disaster-management/preparing-for-disaster/. Accessed November 13, 2017

[60] International Federation of Red Cross and Red Crescent Societies. Preparedness Planning. http://www.ifrc.org/Global/Preplan.pdf. Accessed November 13, 2017

[61] Dictionary.com. http://www.dictionary.com/browse/responses. Accessed November 14, 2017

[62] Disaster Response. Wikipedia. https://en.wikipedia.org/wiki/Disaster_response. Accessed November 14, 2017

[63] Hick JL, Koenig KL, Barbisch D, Bey TA. Surge capacity concepts for health care facilities: The CO-S-TR model for initial incident assessment. Disaster Medicine and Public Health Preparedness. 2008 Sep;**2**(Suppl 1):S51-S57. DOI: 10.1097/DMP.0b013e31817fffe8

[64] Dictionary.com. http://www.dictionary.com/browse/recovery. Accessed November 14, 2017

[65] Essential Functions and Considerations for Hospital Recovery. Harvard School of Public Health Emergency Preparedness and Response Exercise Program September 2013. Accessed November 15, 2017

[66] Haas JE, Kates RW, Bowden MJ. Reconstruction Following Disaster. Cambridge, MA: MIT Press; 1977

[67] Rachel LF. In: Robert AP, Lawrence P, David M, editors. Oxford American Handbook of Disaster Medicine. Chap 7

[68] National Disaster Recovery Framework. https://www.fema.gov/pdf/recoveryframework/ndrf.pdf. Accessed November 15, 2017

[69] https://en.wikipedia.org/wiki/Sphere_Project. Accessed November 19, 2017

[70] Humanitarian response. https://www.humanitarianresponse.info/en/about-clusters/what-is-the-cluster-approach. Accessed November 19, 2017

Section 2

Focused Topics

Chapter 6

Point-of-Care Ultrasound in the Emergency Department

Irma Faruqi, Maryam Siddiqi and Rasha Buhumaid

Additional information is available at the end of the chapter

http://dx.doi.org/10.5772/intechopen.74123

Abstract

Point-of-care ultrasound (POCUS) is a useful diagnostic tool and has become an integral part of the care provided in the Emergency Department. It has evolved over the past two decades to include diagnostic and therapeutic skills. POCUS helps emergency physicians improve their diagnostic accuracy and provide better overall patient care. This chapter will summarize 13 core POCUS applications that are considered within the diagnostic armamentarium of all emergency physicians.

Keywords: ultrasound, bedside ultrasound, point-of-care ultrasound, POCUS, emergency medicine

1. Introduction

The use of point-of-care ultrasound (POCUS) in the Emergency Department (ED) has come a long way, from 1994 when the first Emergency Medicine (EM) Ultrasound Curriculum was published by Mateer et al. to current times, when it has become a core competency in EM training [1]. In a specialty, that is synonymous with quick decision-making in the presence of limited resources, ultrasound is, arguably, the most powerful and often underutilized tool [2].

POCUS is a quick, focused, bedside ultrasound examination performed by one of the primary caregivers, and aimed at guiding the evaluation and management of the patient. As such, it works hand-in-hand with the history and physical examination of a patient in order to identify the presence or absence of certain pathology and evaluates the change in patient's condition in real time. At times, it assists in the treatment by guiding certain procedures that may be performed as part of the patient's management [3].

An emergency physician (EP) skilled in the use of this technology can optimize patient management by providing timely care, improving diagnostic accuracy, and increasing procedural safety. Moreover, in this day and age, when the cost of healthcare is under critique, ultrasound is also an effective means of cost reduction [4].

2. Emergency ultrasound core applications

The American College of Emergency Physicians (ACEP) classifies emergency POCUS into five functional clinical categories: **resuscitative**—POCUS use directly related to an acute resuscitation, **diagnostic**—POCUS utilized in an emergent diagnostic imaging capacity, **symptom or sign-based**—POCUS used in a clinical pathway based upon the patient's symptom or sign, **procedure guidance**—POCUS used as an aid to guide a procedure, and **therapeutic and monitoring**—POCUS use in therapeutics or physiological monitoring [4].

Included within the 5 categories are 13 core applications for emergency POCUS, which will be discussed in this chapter.

2.1. Ultrasound in trauma

Trauma is seen frequently in the ED. The latest National Center for Health (NCH) statistics revealed that trauma comprised almost 30% of all ED visits in the United States in 2014 [5]. Of these, chest and abdominal trauma pose unique challenges for the EPs, particularly in the case of blunt trauma. This is because injuries in blunt trauma are often concealed and imaging modalities like CT are not always feasible either due to limited resources or patient instability. In the past, these patients were evaluated by diagnostic peritoneal aspiration (DPA) or lavage (DPL). However, this modality has largely been replaced by focused assessment with sonography for trauma (FAST) due to its ability to provide expedient care [6], noninvasive nature, cost-effectiveness [7], and ease-of-learning [8] with similar accuracy [9–11]. Now, with the advent of extended focused assessment with sonography for trauma (EFAST), thoracic views are included as part of the exam, helping physicians quickly diagnose and treat pneumothorax and hemothorax, as well [12, 13].

EFAST in a trauma patient identifies hemoperitoneum (**Figure 1**), pericardial effusion (**Figure 2**), hemothorax (**Figure 3**) and pneumothorax (**Figure 4**)/(Video* 1). EFAST has been studied extensively in the setting of blunt trauma and to some extent, stable penetrating trauma. It has been shown to accurately diagnose hemoperitoneum in blunt abdominal trauma (BAT) non-invasively, decrease time-to-diagnosis in BAT, and lead to decreased need for DPA/DPL and fewer CTs [14–17]. Nonetheless, all applications of ultrasound are both operator- and patient-dependent, and the results vary from provider-to-provider and patient-to-patient. It is prudent to remember that while ultrasound has often been shown to be more sensitive than radiography at ruling out a pneumothorax/hemothorax [18–22], this is not the case with all injuries. All healthcare providers performing an EFAST must always be cognizant of its limitations in

*All videos are availble in the online version.

http://dx.doi.org/10.5772/intechopen.74123

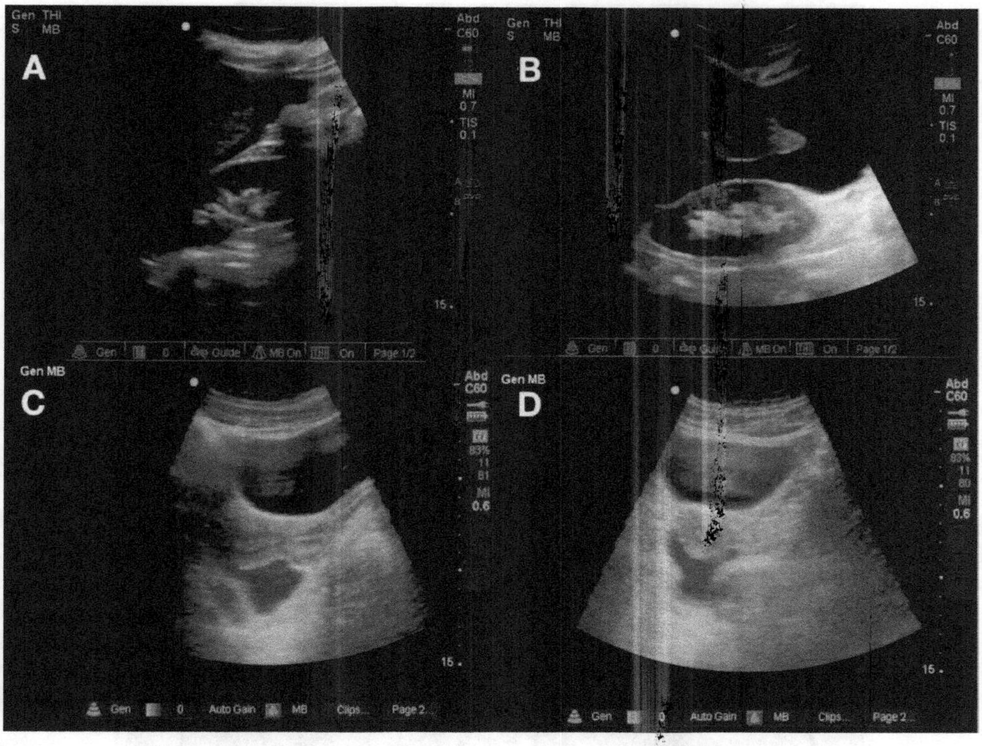

Figure 1. Positive intraperitoneal free fluid. In trauma setting, it is presumed to be hemoperitoneum. (A) Free fluid in the right upper quadrant view, hepatorenal space (Morison's pouch). (B) Free fluid in the left upper quadrant view, evident at the tip of the spleen extending to the space between the spleen and the kidney. (C) Free fluid in rectouterine pouch (pouch of Douglas) in a longitudinal view. (D) Free fluid in pouch of Douglas in a transverse view.

children, in penetrating trauma, diaphragmatic, hollow viscus and retroperitoneal injuries, pelvic trauma and obstetric patients, among others [23]. The bottom line is that a negative EFAST in a stable patient does not rule out significant injury and must frequently be followed by serial EFAST exams and/or CT according to the level of clinical suspicion.

2.2. First trimester pregnancy ultrasound

All emergency physicians are familiar with the diagnostic challenge posed by a female patient of reproductive age with acute abdominal pain and/or vaginal bleeding. This is particularly true when the patient's vital signs are on the verge of instability and some difficult, yet quick, decisions need to be made.

Obstetricians utilize ultrasound for a rather detailed examination of the pregnant patient, including gestational age and anomaly scans. In the ED, however, there is predominantly one all-important question that needs to be answered in the patient with a first-trimester pregnancy complicated by abdominal pain and/or vaginal bleeding—is there an intrauterine pregnancy

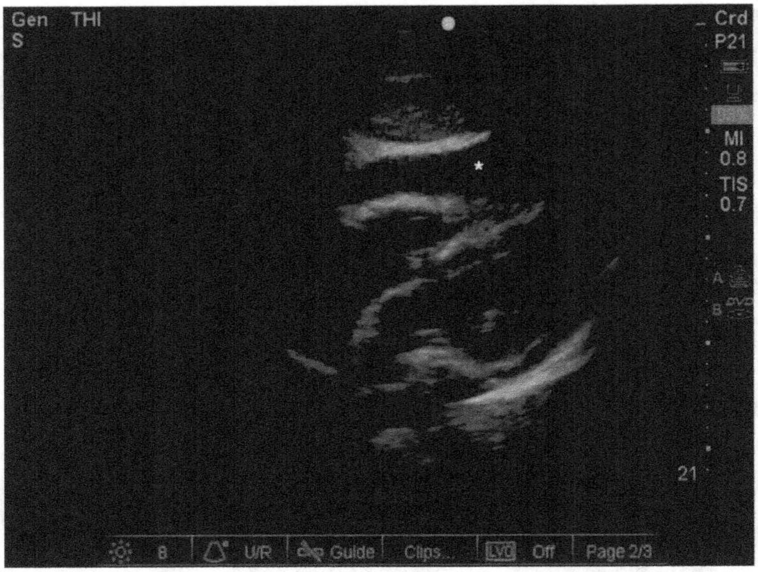

Figure 2. Pericardial effusion evident by the anechoic fluid in the pericardial space (marked by the *).

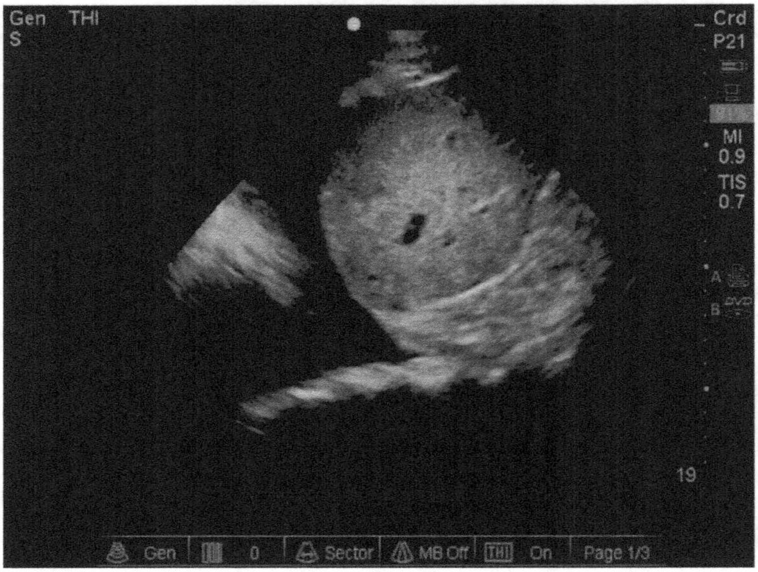

Figure 3. Anechoic fluid collection above the diaphragm. In trauma setting, it is presumed to be hemothorax; while in a non-traumatic setting, it is an undifferentiated pleural effusion.

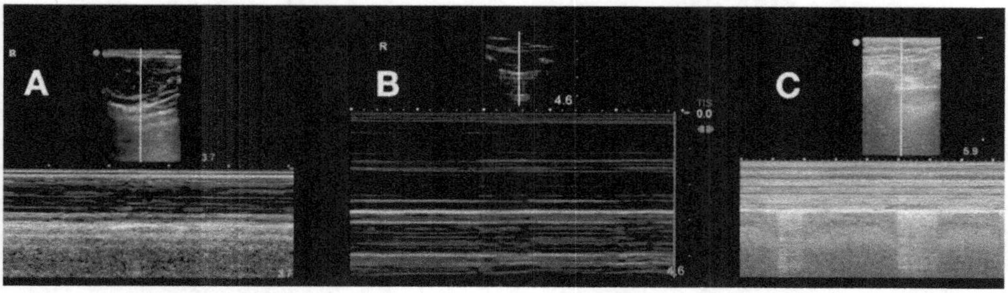

Figure 4. (A) Motion mode demonstrating pleural sliding (sea shore sign), ruling out pneumothorax in the area that is imaged; (B) demonstrates absent lung sliding (bar code sign), which in trauma setting suggests pneumothorax; (C) demonstrates a lung point, the area where half part of the pleura is sliding and the other half is not. Lung point is close to 100% specific for pneumothorax.

(IUP)? The identification of this condition effectively confirms that the patient is pregnant and decreases the chances of an undiagnosed ectopic pregnancy [24].

Pelvic POCUS can be used to rule out ectopic pregnancy in patients where a definitive sign of IUP (**Figure 5**) is identified. This cannot be applied to patients at risk of heterotopic pregnancy

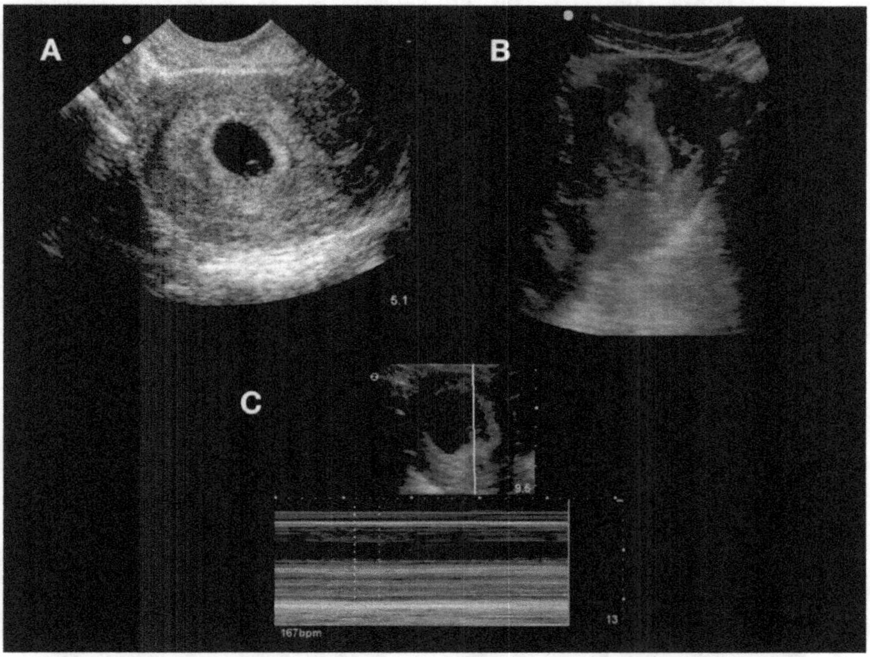

Figure 5. Pelvic ultrasound demonstrating signs of definitive intrauterine pregnancy. (A) Yolk sac within the gestational sac. (B) Fetal pole. (C) M-mode demonstrating the measurement of fetal heart rate.

(when extra-uterine and intrauterine pregnancies occur simultaneously) [25]. It is important to note that a transvaginal ultrasound can identify an IUP at lower beta-HCG levels 1000–2000 vs. 6000 mIU/mL for transabdominal ultrasound [26]. Discussion of algorithms for the diagnosis of ectopic pregnancy and the use of discriminatory zones in order to rule out an ectopic pregnancy is beyond the scope of this chapter. It is, however, imperative to note that heavy reliance on discriminatory zones to explain the presence or absence of certain ultrasound findings has been called into question, with recent guidelines highlighting close follow-up of equivocal cases instead of a rushed diagnosis of non-viable pregnancy with the consequent termination of pregnancy [27]. The use of POCUS in first-trimester pregnant patients has demonstrated decreased ED length-of-stay and time-to-ultrasound in the radiology department with a documented increase in patient satisfaction [28].

2.3. Basic cardiac ultrasound

Like other applications of POCUS, cardiac ultrasound, too, aims to answer specific questions in ED patients presenting with hypotension, dyspnea, possible pericardial effusion, cardiac arrest, cardiac trauma, chest pain, and patients after cardiac surgery [29]. These questions are [30]: (1) *Is there cardiac activity*? (Video* 2). Identifying the presence or absence of cardiac activity may help guide the resuscitation in cardiac arrest. Patients with asystole and absent cardiac activity on ultrasound have a very low survival rate [31]. (2) *Is there pericardial effusion or signs of tamponade*? Emergency physicians can rapidly and accurately identify pericardial effusion and recognize sonographic signs of tamponade. This is crucial especially in patients presenting with signs of undifferentiated shock as the management of tamponade with pericardiocentesis may be lifesaving (**Figure 6**)/(Video* 03).

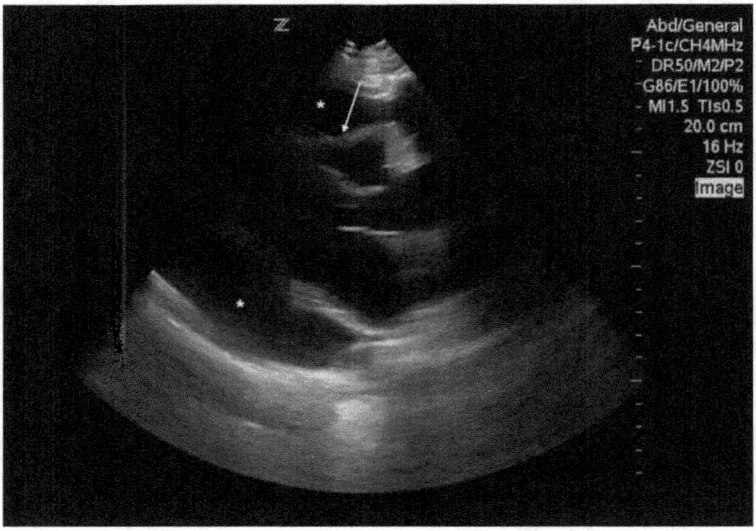

Figure 6. Cardiac ultrasound in parasternal long view demonstrating circumferential pericardial effusion (*) and collapse of the right ventricular wall during diastole (arrow) which is a sonographic sign of tamponade.

(3) *How is the global left ventricular systolic function*? EPs use visual estimation to quantify the systolic LV function as normal, decreased or hyper-dynamic (Video* 04). (4) *Is there right ventricle (RV) strain*? Signs of RV strain in the right clinical setting, although not specific, may be an indirect sign of massive pulmonary embolism [29] (**Figure 7**)/(Video* 05)

(5) *What is the status of the inferior vena cava (IVC)*? (**Figure 8**). Evaluation of the IVC along with the cardiac status can be used as an additional diagnostic tool to assess volume status and guide fluid resuscitation in patients with hypovolemic and septic shock.

EPs, with adequate training, have been shown to be as adept as cardiologists at the performance and interpretation of cardiac ultrasound [32, 33]. Its use in appropriate patients (as mentioned above) has consistently been shown to help narrow down differential diagnoses [34], diagnose and treat more accurately [35–38], and improve outcomes [39]. The use of POCUS to guide resuscitation in pulseless electrical activity (PEA) arrest has been proposed to help identify possible reversible causes such as cardiac tamponade and massive pulmonary embolism, and therefore, expedite management and improve survival [40].

2.4. Abdominal vascular US

In patients presenting to ED with abdominal, flank or back pain, an abdominal aortic aneurysm (AAA) is a diagnosis that no EP would want to miss. In spite of advances in modern medicine, mortality from ruptured aneurysms remains between 50 and 95% [41, 42] and increases by 1% each minute without appropriate intervention [43]. To make matters worse, palpation on physical exam misses roughly one out of every three patients with an AAA [44]. A ruptured AAA must also be considered in patients with unexplained hypotension, particularly in the elderly [45].

POCUS diagnoses an AAA when the identified abdominal aorta measures more than 3 cm (**Figure 9**). A significant percentage of patients do not have clinically evident aortic aneurysms,

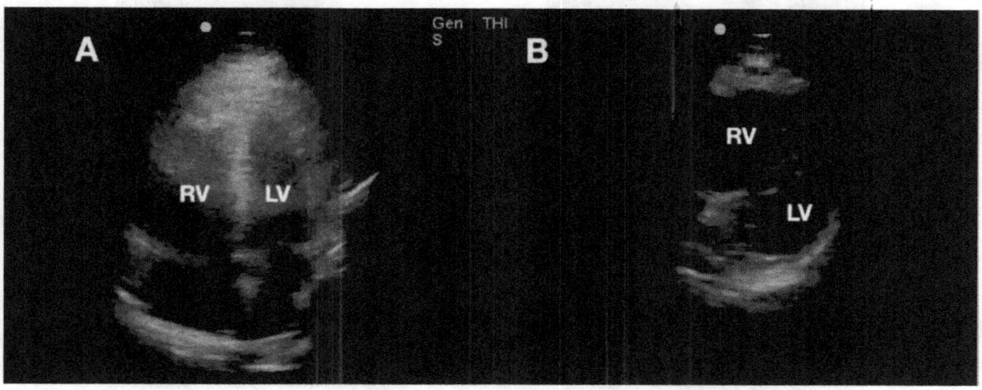

Figure 7. A case of pulmonary embolism with signs of right ventricular strain. (A) Apical four chamber view illustrating right ventricular (RV) enlargement. (B) Parasternal short view illustrating D sign; D-shaped left ventricular (LV) due to flattening of the interventricular septum from the raised RV pressure.

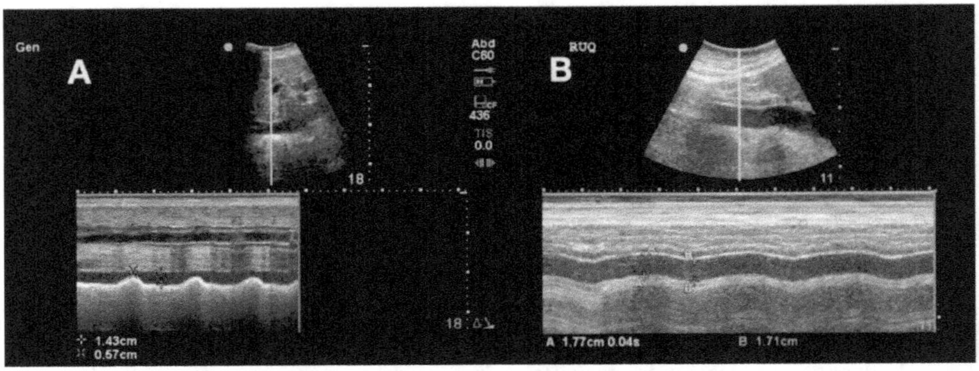

Figure 8. IVC imaged in M-mode. (A) Demonstrates small and collapsible IVC with respiratory variation. (B) Demonstrates plethoric IVC with minimal respiratory variation, which, in the right clinical setting, could suggest that the patient is volume overloaded.

and due to the time-dependent prognosis of the condition, ultrasound performed by the EP helps improve chances of survival [46]. Studies have consistently revealed that EPs are adept in the diagnosis of AAA [47, 48].

In spite of these supportive statistics, it must be mentioned that bedside ultrasound is neither the gold standard nor the imaging modality of choice in ruptured aneurysms. A CT must be performed to rule out AAA in stable patients with suspected AAA [49].

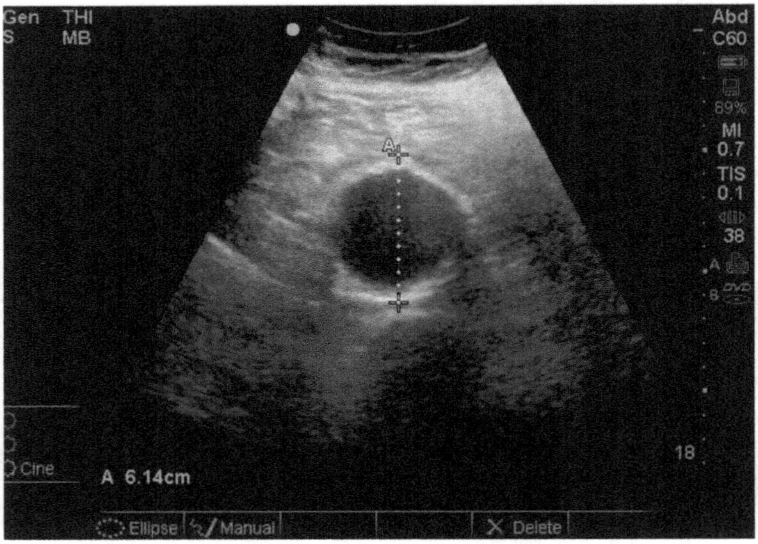

Figure 9. POCUS demonstrating an abdominal aortic aneurysm measuring 6 cm.

http://dx.doi.org/10.5772/intechopen.74123

2.5. Biliary ultrasound

The differential diagnosis in patients presenting with epigastric or right upper quadrant pain, jaundice or even undifferentiated sepsis is broad, and POCUS can easily recognize gallstones and acute cholecystitis (**Figure 10**). A sonographic Murphy's sign, defined as abdominal tenderness from the pressure of the ultrasound probe, may be elicited during biliary imaging [50]. EPs have been shown to be as adept as trained sonographers in the identification of these conditions [51, 52]. Bedside biliary ultrasound can avoid misdiagnosing patients with acute cholecystitis or biliary colic [53], decrease ED length-of-stay [54], and expedite further management [55].

2.6. Urinary tract ultrasound

ED visits for complaints secondary to urolithiasis are exceedingly common [56, 57], and ultrasound is a highly useful and often underutilized tool in the evaluation of these patients [58]. In addition to the detection of hydronephrosis (**Figure 11**), urinary tract ultrasound can also be used to measure bladder volume, an element of particular importance in those with urinary retention. Ultrasound can also be used in patients in whom urinary tract pathology may be on the list of differential diagnoses, such as those with abdominal pain, hematuria, back pain or groin pain [59]. Multiple studies have consistently demonstrated that in patients with suspected nephrolithiasis, there is a decreased need for subsequent CT scans with the use of ultrasound in the ED, resulting in decreased exposure to ionizing radiation. Although CT is superior to ultrasound in terms of sensitivity for nephrolithiasis [60], an 'ultrasound-first' approach has not revealed any significant differences in terms of serious adverse events, return ED visits or hospital admissions [61–66].

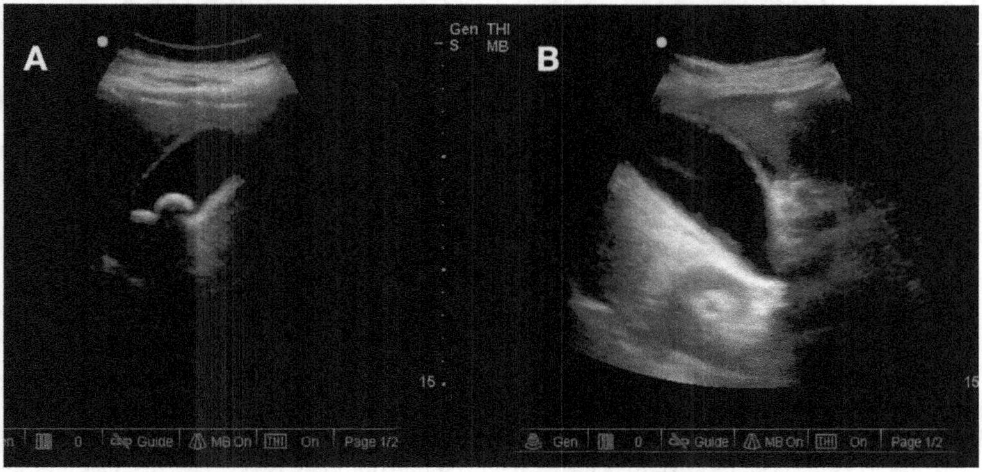

Figure 10. Biliary ultrasound demonstrating gallstones in (A) and cholecystitis in (B) suggested by the thickened gallbladder wall and pericholecystic fluid.

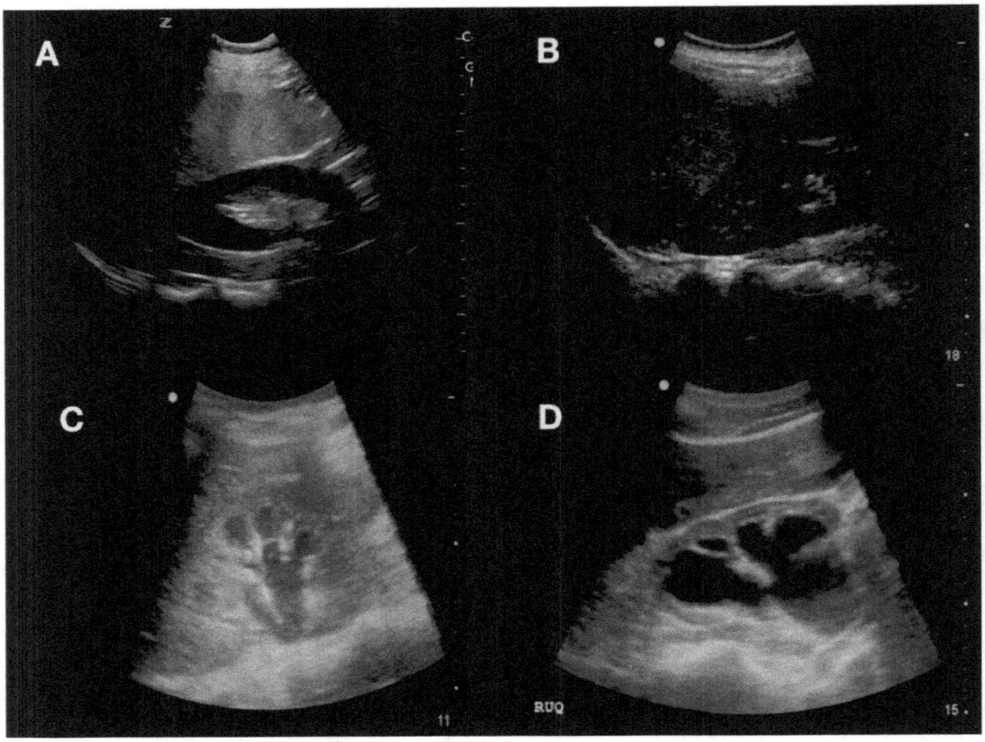

Figure 11. (A) Normal renal ultrasound, (B) mild hydronephrosis (only the renal pelvis is filled with fluid), (C) moderate hydronephrosis (fluid-filled renal pelvis extending to the renal calyces), (D) severe hydronephrosis (entire renal collecting system is dilated).

2.7. Ultrasound for deep vein thrombosis

The most common ED presentations for venous thromboembolism are deep venous thrombosis (DVT) and pulmonary embolism (PE). DVT is suspected in patients presenting with leg swelling, pain, warmth, and erythema. A study has shown that the sensitivity and specificity of these clinical symptoms and signs ranges from 72 to 97% and 19–48%, respectively [67]. In patients with suspected DVT, accurate diagnosis is essential to decrease the risk of propagation and development of PE that could lead to significant morbidity and mortality. With short training, EPs can use focused ultrasound protocol to accurately diagnose a proximal DVT in the highest probability areas (**Figure 12**) in symptomatic outpatients [68]. Several studies have suggested that incorporating POCUS along with pretest probability scoring systems (e.g. Wells Score) and/or D-Dimer improves the diagnostic accuracy of POCUS [69, 70, 72]. Using POCUS to diagnose DVT has been shown to decrease the need for comprehensive scans, decreased time-to-diagnosis, ED length of stay, and the need for return visits [71, 72]. All of these advantages make bedside ultrasound for DVT especially useful; however, it is important to understand its limitations. Most of the POCUS research was conducted on outpatients with suspected DVTs using a focused and specific protocol to diagnose only proximal (not distal or calf) DVTs [73].

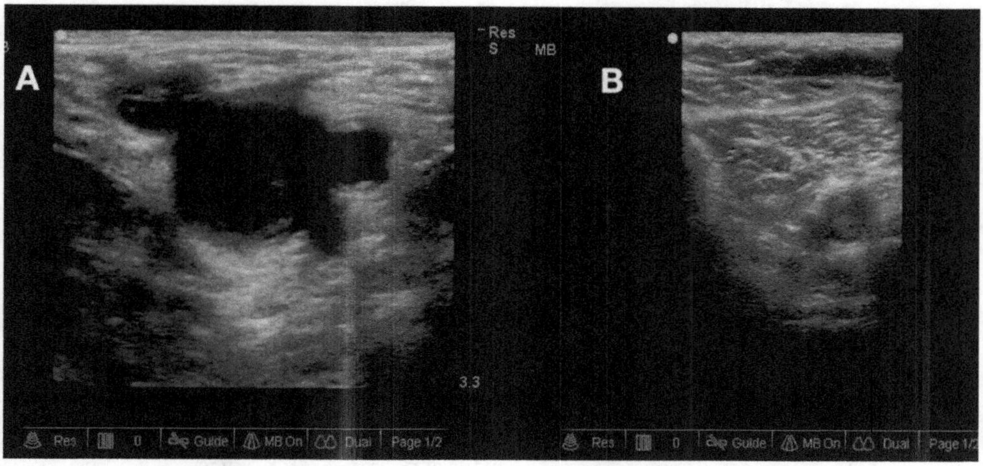

Figure 12. POCUS ultrasound demonstrates DVT of the left common femoral vein (A) and left popliteal vein (B) evident by the echogenic material within the lumen and non-compressible veins with graded compression.

2.8. Lung ultrasound

Lung POCUS may help in the evaluation of patients presenting to the ED with undifferentiated chest pain, shortness of breath (SOB) or respiratory distress. Lung POCUS can help diagnose pneumothorax (Video* 01), pleural effusion (**Figure 3**) and pulmonary edema (**Figure 13**). Ultrasound has a higher sensitivity than the traditional upright anteroposterior chest radiography for the detection of a pneumothorax [74]. Lung ultrasonography has been shown to be

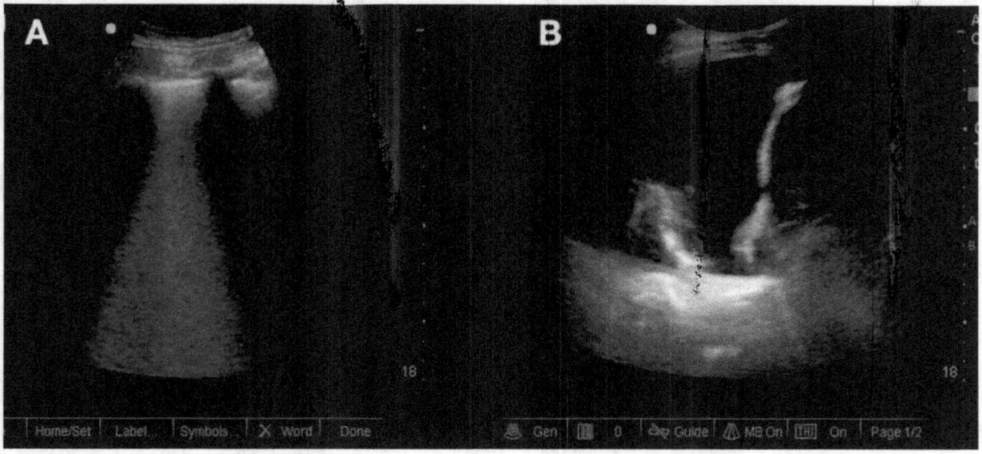

Figure 13. Case of acute cardiogenic pulmonary edema. Evident by B lines (A), which are the vertical narrow-based lines arising from the pleural line to the edge of the ultrasound screen, which was present in both hemithoraces, and bilateral pleural effusion (B). In addition, cardiac ultrasound showed decreased left ventricular systolic function (not included in the figure) which supports the diagnosis of acute cardiogenic pulmonary edema.

superior to chest radiography in the detection of pleural effusions with a sensitivity and specificity of 92 and 93%, respectively [75]. Studies have shown that POCUS is a good diagnostic tool to diagnose acute cardiogenic pulmonary edema [76, 77].

2.9. Soft tissue ultrasound

Skin and soft tissue infections are common in the ED. Physical examination findings may be insufficient to differentiate cellulitis from an abscess. Soft tissue ultrasound is one of the easiest ultrasound examinations to perform. It can be used as an adjunct to clinical evaluation of patients presenting to the ED with suspected soft tissue infections. Studies have shown that POCUS helps differentiate cellulitis, abscess and necrotizing fasciitis (**Figure 14**), and therefore, improves the diagnostic accuracy and management [78–80].

2.10. Musculoskeletal ultrasound

Musculoskeletal complaints are very common in the ED. The use of POCUS can help EPs diagnose joint effusion, long bone fractures, tendon injury and retained foreign body (FB) (**Figure 15**).

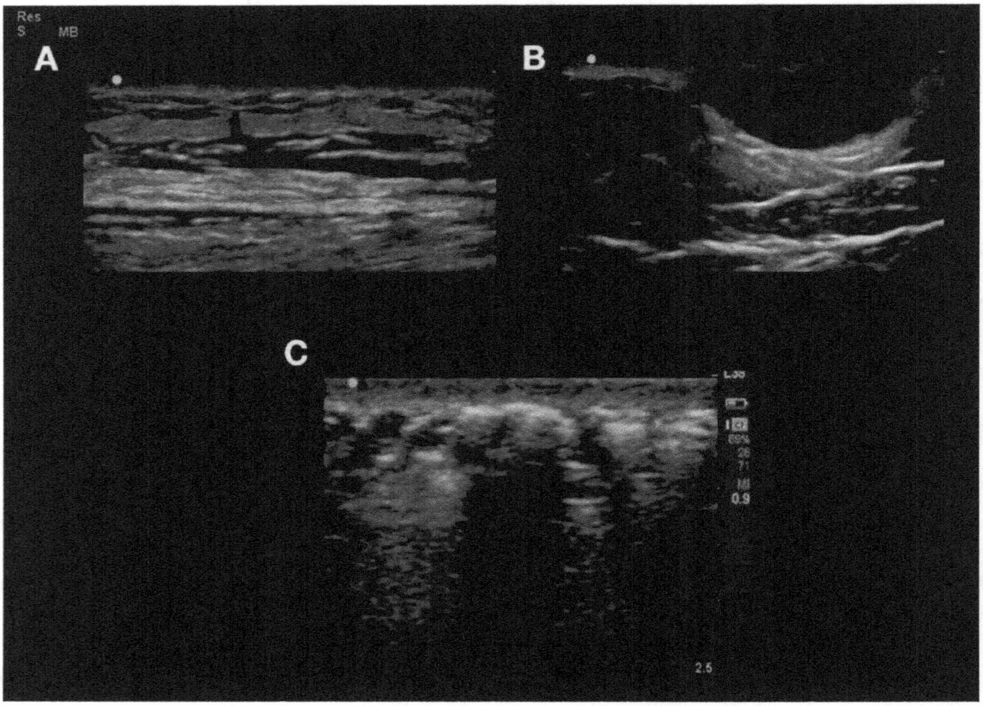

Figure 14. Soft tissue ultrasound demonstrating evidence of cellulitis (A), evident by increased echogenicity of the subcutaneous tissue separated by anechoic fluid appearing like cobble-stone. Case of abscess (B), evident by complex fluid collection mixed with debris. Case of necrotizing fasciitis (C) evident by subcutaneous thickening, fluid in the facial planes and air and shadowing.

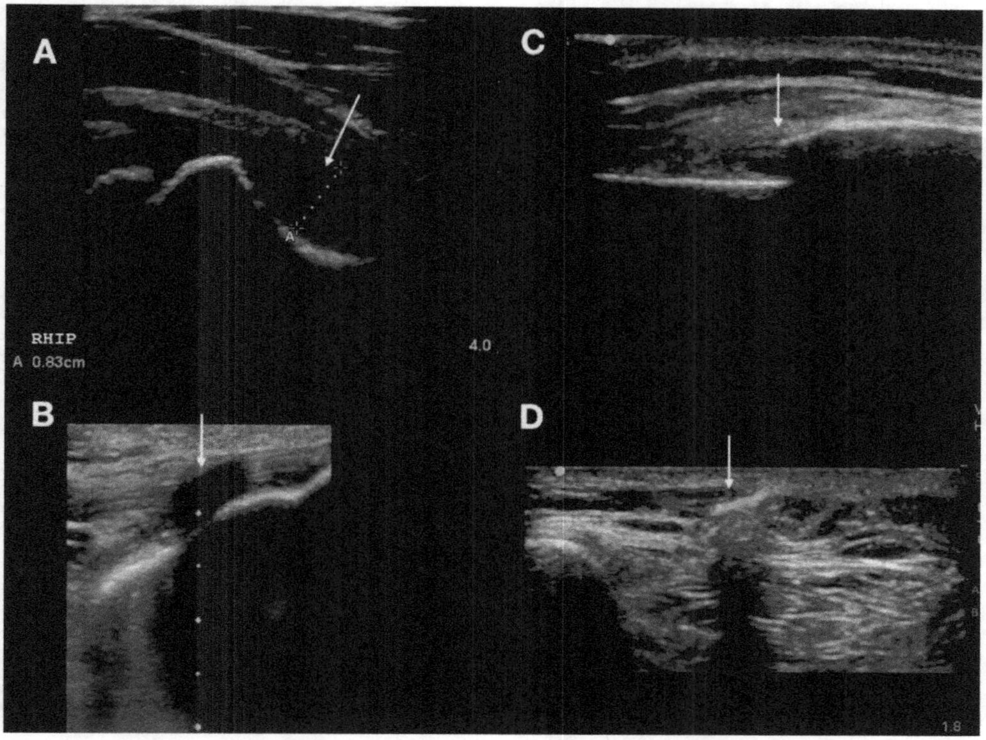

Figure 15. (A) POCUS showing hip effusion evident by the anechoic fluid in the joint space measuring 8.3 mm (arrow). (B) Case of patellar tendon tear evident by disruption of the fibular echo texture of the tendon (arrow). (C) Case of sternal fracture, evident by cortical disruption of the bone with step-off (arrow). (D) Case of retained glass in the leg that was identified as a hyperechoic structure (arrow) with posterior shadowing. FB was removed with the assistance of POCUS.

In a study of patients with joint pain, erythema, and swelling, POCUS changed the management in 65% of cases and reduced the rate of joint aspiration from 72.2 to 37% [81]. POCUS has been shown to be a good diagnostic tool to diagnose hip effusion in children [82]. It can be used to guide arthrocentesis in a safer manner via the shortest route, thus improving success rates and reducing complications [83].

POCUS has been shown to accurately diagnose long bone fractures [84, 85], assist in fracture reduction, determine realignment, and perform hematoma block [85–87]. In shorter bones and areas close to joints, POCUS is found to be inaccurate in identifying a fracture but might identify indirect signs such as soft tissue swelling and joint effusion [88].

EPs can use POCUS to help identify major tendon injuries such as achilles, quadriceps and patellar tendons [89–91].

The evaluation of retained FB can be challenging. Traditional radiography can be used to identify radiopaque FB in soft tissues and muscles. In cases of suspected radiolucent retained FB, POCUS can be used to accurately identify the location and size of FB and assist with its removal [92–94].

2.11. Bowel ultrasound

Small bowel obstruction (SBO) is a common cause of acute abdomen. It accounts for about 2% of patients presenting to ED with abdominal pain [95]. CT with contrast is considered to be the gold standard for the diagnosis of SBO as it has high sensitivity and specificity for the diagnosis [96–98]. It can often determine the location, cause, and complications related to bowel obstruction [99]. However, due to its cost and radiation, it is not the ideal initial imaging modality of choice in all suspected cases. Abdominal X-ray (AXR) is typically considered the initial imaging modality of choice in all suspected cases of SBO presenting to the ED. In recent years, POCUS has been utilized as a screening imaging modality for suspected cases of SBO (**Figure 16**). POCUS is more accurate, more sensitive, and more specific than AXR [95, 100, 101].

2.12. Ocular ultrasound

Patients present to the ED with a variety of ocular emergencies, ranging from simple conjunctivitis to sight-threatening diseases. The challenge lies in the assessment of such emergencies due to limited equipment availability and physician training; moreover, ophthalmology consultation is not available in all settings. This may place considerable burden on the EP to make a rapid decision [102].

Ocular ultrasound can non-invasively diagnose retinal detachment with high sensitivity (**Figure 17**) [103], vitreous hemorrhage/detachment [104], globe rupture, and lens dislocation [105]. Measurement of optic nerve sheet diameter has been shown to correlate with increased intracranial pressure [106].

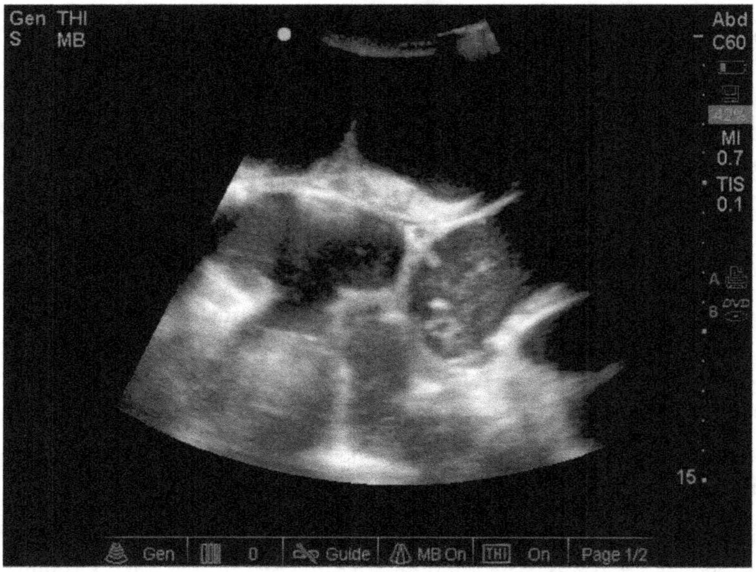

Figure 16. Case of small bowel obstruction evident by dilated (> 2.5–3 cm) fluid-filled small bowel loops and increased peristalsis of the dilated segment, as evidenced by the to-and-fro or whirling motion of the bowel contents (Video* 06).

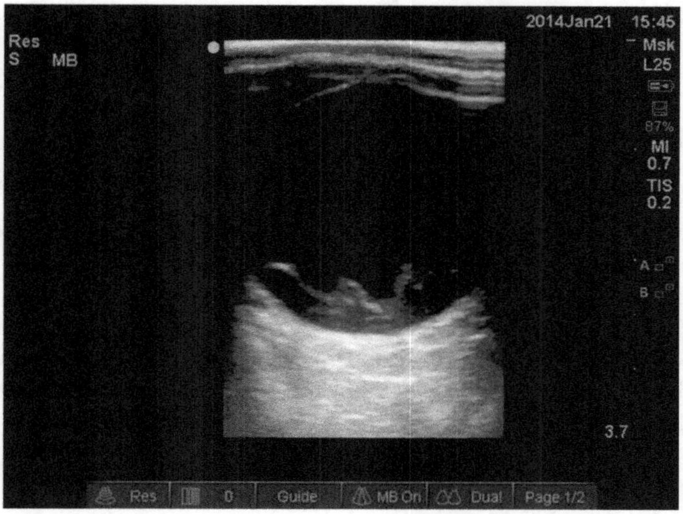

Figure 17. (A) Case of retinal detachment, evident by sharply defined, highly reflective linear membrane that is anchored to the optic disc.

2.13. Ultrasound for procedure guidance

POCUS is used to guide various ED procedures such as central venous catheter insertion [107, 108], difficult peripheral arterial and venous catheter insertion [109, 110], arthrocentesis [111], airway management [112], thoracentesis, paracentesis, lumbar puncture, and regional nerve blocks [113]. Using POCUS for procedure guidance helps improve the success rate and decrease the complication rate [110, 113] and is considered the standard of care for central venous catheter insertion [114].

3. Conclusion

The use of POCUS in the ED has grown over the past two decades and has evolved from basic uses (that are discussed in this chapter) to include more advanced applications. Despite the limitation of POCUS, it has numerous advantages that justify its use. The advantages include, but are not limited to, improving the diagnostic accuracy for certain complaints, decreasing ED length-of-stay, improving patient satisfaction, improving procedure success rate, and decreasing procedure complication rates. Any EP practicing in this day and age in a center with POCUS availability has little excuse to justify not utilizing this powerful resource for the best of their patients.

Conflict of interest

All authors declare to have no conflict of interest.

Author details

Irma Faruqi, Maryam Siddiqi and Rasha Buhumaid*

*Address all correspondence to: rbuhumaid@seha.ae

Emergency Department, Sheikh Khalifa Medical City, Abu Dhabi, United Arab Emirates

References

[1] Mateer J, Plummer D, Heller M, Olson D, Jehle D, Overton D, et al. Model curriculum for physician training in emergency ultrasonography. Annals of Emergency Medicine. 1994;**23**(1):95-102

[2] Sanders J, Noble V, Raja A, Sullivan A, Camargo C. Access to and use of point-of-care ultrasound in the emergency department. Western Journal of Emergency Medicine. 2015; **16**(5):747-752

[3] Kendall J, Hoffenberg S, Smith R. History of emergency and critical care ultrasound: The evolution of a new imaging paradigm. Critical Care Medicine. 2007;**35**(5):S126-S130

[4] ACEP Policy Statement. Ultrasound Guidelines: Emergency, Point-of-care, and Clinical Ultrasound Guidelines in Medicine [Internet]. 2016. Available from: https://www.acep.org/Clinical---Practice-Management/Ultrasound-Guidelines--Emergency,-Point-of-care,-and-Clinical-Ultrasound-Guidelines-in-Medicine/?__taxonomyid=471332 [Accessed: 2017-11-2]

[5] CDC National Center for Health Statistics. Emergency Department Visits. 2017. Available from: https://www.cdc.gov/nchs/data/nhamcs/web_tables/2014_ed_web_tables.pdf [Accessed: 2017-12-12]

[6] Melniker L, Leibner E, McKenney M, Lopez P, Briggs W, Mancuso C. Randomized controlled clinical trial of point-of-care, limited ultrasonography for trauma in the emergency department: The first sonography outcomes assessment program trial. Annals of Emergency Medicine. 2006;**48**(3):227-235

[7] Arrillaga A, Graham R, York J, Miller R. Increased efficiency and cost-effectiveness in the evaluation of the blunt abdominal trauma patient with the use of ultrasound. The American Surgeon. 1999;**65**:31-35

[8] McCarter F, Luchette FA, Molloy M, Hurst J, Davis K, Johannigman J, Frame S, Fischer J. Institutional and individual learning curves for focused abdominal ultrasound for trauma: Cumulative sum analysis. Annals of Surgery. 2000;**231**(5):689-700

[9] Boulanger B, McLellan B, Brenneman F, Ochoa J, Kirkpatrick A. Prospective evidence of the superiority of a sonography-based algorithm in the assessment of blunt abdominal injury. The Journal of Trauma. 1999;**47**(4):632-637

[10] Amer M, Ashraf M. Role of FAST and DPL in assessment of blunt abdominal trauma. The Professional Medical Journal. 2008;**15**:200-204

[11] Adeyinka A. Accuracy of the fast exam: A retrospective analysis of blunt abdominal trauma patients. Emergency Medicine: Open Access. 2015;**6**(1)

[12] Nandipati K, Allamaneni S, Kakarla R, Wong A, Richards N, Satterfield J, Turner J, Sung K. Extended focused assessment with sonography for trauma (EFAST) in the diagnosis of pneumothorax: Experience at a community based level I trauma center. Injury. 2011;**42**(5):511-514

[13] Sauter T, Hoess S, Lehmann B, Exadaktylos A, Haider D. Detection of pneumothoraces in patients with multiple blunt trauma: Use and limitations of eFAST. Journal of Emergency Medicine. 2017;**34**:568-572

[14] Medscape. Focused Assessment with Sonography in Trauma (FAST) [Internet]. 2017. Available from: https://emedicine.medscape.com/article/104363-overview?pa=x%2BhBzeRQuBsVbIfG%2F%2BPqyWuwzkM1A35BtfSIktWdH1J3FerFHEPLSCUAf8s%2FdVOA9rwpxt0deiB2TrZfl8JfrUeb0T8SAO%2FpBjZvSxPL9fk%3D [Accessed: 2017-12-12]

[15] Helling T, Wilson J, Augustosky K. The utility of focused abdominal ultrasound in blunt abdominal trauma: A reappraisal. The American Journal of Surgery. 2007;**194**(6):728-732 732-3

[16] Brooks A, Davies B, Smethhurst M, Connolly J. Prospective evaluation of non-radiologist performed emergency abdominal ultrasound for haemoperitoneum. Emergency Medicine Journal. 2004;**21** e5

[17] Brenchley J, Walker A, Sloan J, Hassan T, Venables H. Evaluation of focussed assessment with sonography in trauma (FAST) by UK emergency physicians. Emergency Medicine Journal. 2006;**23**:415-415

[18] Ding W, Shen Y, Yang J, He X, Diagnosis ZM. Of pneumothorax by radiography and ultrasonography: A meta-analysis. Chest. 2011;**140**(4):859-866

[19] Rothlin M, Naf R, Amgwerd M, Candinas D, Frick T, Trentz O. Ultrasound in blunt abdominal and thoracic trauma. The Journal of Trauma. 1993;**34**(4):488-495

[20] Dulchavsky S, Schwarz K, Kirkpatrick A, Billica R, Williams D, Diebel L, Campbell R, Sargysan A, Hamilton D. Prospective evaluation of thoracic ultrasound in the detection of pneumothorax. The Journal of Trauma. 2001;**50**(2):201-205

[21] Kirkpatrick A, Sirois M, Laupland K, Liu D, Rowan K, Ball C, Hameed S, Brown R, Simons R, Dulchavsky S, Hamiilton D, Nicolaou S. Hand-held thoracic sonography for detecting post-traumatic pneumothoraces: The extended focused assessment with Sonography for trauma (EFAST). The Journal of Trauma. 2004;**57**(2):288-295

[22] Ma O, Mateer J. Trauma ultrasound examination versus chest radiography in the detection of hemothorax. Annals of Emergency Medicine. 1997;**29**(3):312-315

[23] Leone K, Gisondi M. Chest and abdominal trauma. In: Amnieva-Wang N, editor. A Practical Guide to Pediatric Emergency Medicine: Caring for Children in the Emergency Department. Cambridge University Press; 2011. p. 681-686

[24] ACEP. Tips and Tricks: First Trimester Pregnancy Ultrasound – Trans-abdominal Pelvis [Internet]. 2016. Available from: https://www.acep.org/content.aspx?id=98218#sm.000rcvzgk1aidwo10rv2ccbp2rblg [Accessed: 2017-12-10]

[25] Durham B, Lane B, Burbridge L, Subramaniam B. Pelvic ultrasound performed by emergency physicians for the detection of ectopic pregnancy in complicated first-trimester pregnancies. Annals of Emergency Medicine. 1997;**29**(3):338-347

[26] Houry D, Salhi B. Acute Complications of Pregnancy. In: Walls R, Hockberger R, Gausche-Hill M, editors. Rosen's Emergency Medicine – Concepts and Clinical Practice. Philadephia: Elsevier; 2017. p. 2282-2299

[27] Doubilet P, Benson C, Bourne T, Blaivas M, Barnhart K, Benacerraf B, Brown D, Filly R, Fox J, Goldstein S, Kendall J, Lyons E, Porter M, Pretorius D, Timor-Tritsch I. Diagnostic criteria for nonviable pregnancy early in the first trimester. The New England Journal of Medicine. 2013;**369**(15):1443-1451

[28] Wilson S, Connolly K, Lahham S, Subeh M, Fischetti C, Chiem A, Aspen A, Anderson C, Fox J. Point-of-care ultrasound versus radiology department pelvic ultrasound on emergency department length of stay. World Journal of Emergency Medicine. 2016;**7**(3):178-182

[29] Arntfield R, Millington S. Point of care cardiac ultrasound applications in the emergency department and intensive care unit - a review. Current Cardiology Reviews. 2012;**8**(2): 98-108

[30] Doniger S. Focused cardiac ultrasound. In: Doniger S, editor. Pediatric Emergency and Critical Care Ultrasound. Cambridge: Cambridge University Press; 2013. p. 57-70

[31] Gaspari R, Weekes A, Adhikari S, Noble V, Nomura J, Theodoro D, Woo M, Atkinson P, Blehar D, Brown S, Caffery T, Douglass E, Fraser J, Haines C, Lam S, Lanspa M, Lewis M, Liebmann O, Limkakeng A, Lopez F, Platz E, Mendoza M, Minnigan H, Moore C, Novik J, Rang L, Scruggs W, Raio C. Emergency department point-of-care ultrasound in out-of-hospital and in-ED cardiac arrest. Resuscitation. 2016;**109**:33-39

[32] Farsi D, Hajsadeghi S, Hajighanbari J, Mofidi M, Hafezimoghadam P, Rezai M, Mahshidfar B, Abiri S, Abbasi S. Focused cardiac ultrasound (FOCUS) by emergency medicine residents in patients with suspected cardiovascular diseases. Journal of Ultrasound. 2017;**20**(2):133-138

[33] ClinicalGate. Emergency Cardiac Ultrasound: Evaluation for Pericardial Effusion and Cardiac Activity [Internet]. 2015. Available from: https://clinicalgate.com/emergency-cardiac-ultrasound-evaluation-for-pericardial-effusion-and-cardiac-activity/#bib1 [Accessed: 2017-12-13]

[34] Jones A, Tayal V, Sullivan D, Kline J. Randomized, controlled trial of immediate versus delayed goal-directed ultrasound to identify the cause of nontraumatic hypotension in emergency department patients. Critical Care Medicine. 2004;**32**(8):1703-1708

[35] Tayal V, Kline J. Emergency echocardiography to detect pericardial effusion in patients in PEA and near-PEA states. Resuscitation. 2003;**59**(3):315-318

[36] Dresden S, Mitchell P, Rahimi L, Leo M, Rubin-Smith J, Bibi S, White L, Langlois B, Sullivan A, Carmody K. Right ventricular dilatation on bedside echocardiography performed by emergency physicians aids in the diagnosis of pulmonary embolism. Annals of Emergency Medicine. 2014;**63**(1):16-24

[37] Russell F, Rutz F, Pang P. Focused ultrasound in the emergency department for patients with acute heart failure. Cardiac Failure Review. 2015;**1**(2):83-86

[38] Rozycki G, Feliciano D, Ochsner M, Knudson M, Hoyt D, Davis F, Hammerman D, Figueredo V, Harviel J, Han D, Schmidt J. The role of ultrasound in patients with possible penetrating cardiac wounds: A prospective Multicenter study. The Journal of Trauma and Acute Care Surgery. 1999;**46**(4):543-552

[39] Plummer D, Brunette D, Asinger R, Ruiz E. Emergency department echocardiography improves outcome in penetrating cardiac injury. Annals of Emergency Medicine. 1992;**21**(6):709-712

[40] Gaspari R, Weekes A, Adhikari S, Noble V, Nomura J, Theodoro D, Woo M, Atkinson P, Blehar D, Brown S, Caffery T, Douglass E, Fraser J, Haines C, Lam S, Lanspa M, Lewis M, Liebmann O, Limkakeng A, Lopez F, Platz E, Mendoza M, Minnigan H, Moore C, Novik J, Rang L, Scruggs W, Raio C. A retrospective study of pulseless electrical activity, bedside ultrasound identifies interventions during resuscitation associated with improved survival to hospital admission. A REASON study. Resuscitation. 2017;**120**:103-107. DOI: 10.1016/j.resuscitation.2017.09.008

[41] Kochanek K, Xu J, Murphy S, Minino A, Kung H. Deaths: Final data for 2009. National Vital Statistics System (US). 2011;**60**(3):1-116

[42] Ernst C. Abdominal aortic aneurysm. The New England Journal of Medicine. 1993; **328**:1167-1172

[43] Medscape. Abdominal Aortic Aneurysm [Internet]. 2017. Available from: https://emedicine.medscape.com/article/1979501-overview [Accessed: 2017-12-11]

[44] Fink H, Lederle F, Roth C, Bowles C, Nelson D, Haas M. The accuracy of physical examination to detect abdominal aortic aneurysm. Archives of Internal Medicine. 2000; **160**(6):833-836

[45] Singh M, Koyfman A, Martinez J. Abdominal Vascular Catastrophes. In: Graham A, Martinez J, editors. Abdominal and Gastrointestinal Emergencies. Pennsylvania: Elsevier; 2016. p. 327-340

[46] Walker A, Brenchley J, Sloan J, Lalanda M, Venables H. Ultrasound by emergency physicians to detect abdominal aortic aneurysms: A UK case series. Emergency Medicine Journal. 2004;**21**:240-242

[47] Kuhn M, Bonnin R, Davey M, Rowland J, Langlois S. Emergency department ultrasound scanning for abdominal aortic aneurysm: Accessible, accurate, and advantageous. Annals of Emergency Medicine. 2000;**36**(3):219-223

[48] Dent B, Kendall R, Boyle A, Atkinson P. Emergency ultrasound of the abdominal aorta by UK emergency physicians: A prospective cohort study. Emergency Medicine Journal. 2007;**24**(8):547-549

[49] EB Medicine. Ultrasound for Abdominal Aortic Aneurysm [Internet]. 2018. Available from: http://www.ebmedicine.net/topics.php?paction=showTopicSeg&topic_id=252&seg_id=4863 [Accessed: 2018-06-01]

[50] ACEP. Focus On: Bedside Biliary Ultrasound [Internet]. 2010. Available from: https://www.acep.org/Content.aspx?id=64648#sm.000rcvzgk1aidwo10rv2ccbp2rblg [Accessed: 2017-12-11]

[51] Woo M, Taylor M, Loubani O, Bowra J, Atkinson P. My patient has got abdominal pain: Identifying biliary problems. Ultrasound. 2014;**22**(4):223-228

[52] Scruggs W, Fox J, Potts B, Zlidenny A, McDonough J, Anderson C, Larson J, Barajas G, Langdorf M. Accuracy of ED bedside ultrasound for identification of gallstones: Retrospective analysis of 575 studies. Western Journal of Emergency Medicine. 2008;**9**(1):1-5

[53] Degerli V, Korkmaz T, Mollamehmetoglu H, Ertan C. The importance of routine bedside biliary ultrasonography in the management of patients admitted to the emergency department with isolated acute epigastric pain. Turkish Journal of Medical Sciences. 2017;**47**:1137-1143

[54] Blaivas M, Harwood R, Lambert M. Decreasing length of stay with emergency ultrasound examination of the gallbladder. Academic Emergency Medicine. 1999;**6**(10):1020-1023

[55] Adhikari S, Morrison D, Zeger W, Chandwani D, Krueger A. Utility of point-of-care biliary ultrasound in the evaluation of emergency patients with isolated acute non-traumatic epigastric pain. Internal and Emergency Medicine. 2014;**9**(5):583-587

[56] Fwu C, Eggers P, Kimmel P, Kusek J, Kirali Z. Emergency department visits, use of imaging, and drugs for urolithiasis have increased in the United States. Kidney International. 2013;**83**(3):479-486

[57] Pearle M, Calhoun E, Curhan G. Urologic diseases in America project: Urolithiasis. The Journal of Urology. 2005;**173**(3):848-857. DOI: 10.1097/01.ju.0000152082.14384.d7

[58] Innes G, Scheuermeyer F, Law M, McRae A, Weber B, Boyda H, Lonergan K, Andruchow J. Sex-related differences in emergency department renal colic management: Females have fewer computed tomography scans but similar outcomes. Academic Emergency Medicine. 2016;**23**(10):1153-1160

[59] ACEP. Focused Renal Sonography [Internet]. 2012. Available from: http://www.acepnow.com/article/focused-renal-sonography/?singlepage=1 [Accessed: 2017-12-12]

[60] Sheafor D, Hertzberg B, Freed K, Carroll B, Keogan M, Paulson E, DeLong D, Nelson R. Nonenhanced helical CT and US in the emergency evaluation of patients with renal colic: Prospective comparison. Radiology. 2000;**217**(3):792-797

[61] Smith-Bindman R, Aubin C, Bailitz J. Ultrasonography Vs CT for suspected nephrolithiasis. The New England Journal of Medicine. 2014;**371**:1100-1110

[62] Leo M, Langlois B, Mitchell P. Bedside Ultrasound versus Computed Tomography in Diagnosing Renal Colic and Predictors of 30 Day Return Visits. Annals of Emergency Medicine. October 2014;**64**(4):S25

[63] Edmonds M, Yan J, Sedran R. The utility of renal ultrasonography in the diagnosis of renal colic in emergency department patients. Canadian Journal of Emergency Medicine. 2010;**12**(3):201-206

[64] Park Y, Jung R, Lee Y. Does the use of bedside ultrasonography reduce emergency department length of stay for patients with renal colic? A pilot study. Clinical and Experimental Emergency Medicine Journal. 2016;**3**(4):197-203

[65] Riddel J, Case A, Wopat R. Sensitivity of emergency bedside ultrasound to detect hydronephrosis in patients with computed tomography-proven stones. The Western Journal of Emergency Medicine. 2014;**15**(1):96-100

[66] Gaspari R, Horst K. Emergency ultrasound and urinalysis in the evaluation of flank pain. Academic Emergency Medicine. 2005;**12**(12):1180-1184

[67] EB Medicine. Ultrasound For Deep Venous Thrombosis [Internet]. Available from: http://www.ebmedicine.net/topics.php?paction=showTopicSeg&topic_id=252&seg_id=4864 [Accessed: 2017-12-12]

[68] Nunn K, Towards TP. Evidence based emergency medicine: Best BETs from the Manchester Royal Infirmary. Using the ultrasound compression test for deep vein thrombosis will not precipitate a thromboembolic event. Emergency Medicine Journal. 2007 Jul; **24**(7):494-495

[69] Bernardi E, Camporese G, Buller H. Serial 2-point ultrasonography plus D-dimer vs whole-leg color-coded Doppler ultrasonography for diagnosing suspected symptomatic deep vein thrombosis: A randomized controlled trial. Journal of the American Medical Association. 2008;**300**(14):1653-1659

[70] Ageno W, Camporese G, Riva N. Analysis of an algorithm incorporating limited and whole-leg assessment of the deep venous system in symptomatic outpatients with suspected deep-vein thrombosis (PALLADIO): A prospective, multicentre, cohort study. The Lancet Hematology. 2015;**2**(11):e474-e480

[71] Zuker-Herman R, Ayalon D, Berant R. Comparison between two-point and three-point compression ultrasound for the diagnosis of deep vein thrombosis. Journal of Thrombosis and Thrombolysis. 2018;**45**(1):99-105

[72] Poley R, Newbigging J, Sivilotti M. Estimated effect of an integrated approach to suspected deep venous thrombosis using limited-compression ultrasound. Academic Emergency Medicine. 2014;**21**(9):971-980

[73] Hunter F. BET 1: Emergency physician performed 2-point bedside compression ultrasound for deep venous thrombosis. Emergency Medicine Journal. 2014;**31**:944-946

[74] Lubna F, Laura H, Derek W. Sonographic diagnosis of pneumothorax. Journal of Emergencies, Trauma and Shock. 2012;**5**(1):76-81

[75] Lichtenstein D, Goldstein I, Mourgeon E. Comparative diagnostic performances of auscultation, chest radiography, and lung ultrasonography in acute respiratory distress syndrome. Anesthesiology. 2004;**100**(1):9-15

[76] Al Deeb M, Barbic S, Featherstone R. Point-of-care ultrasonography for the diagnosis of acute cardiogenic pulmonary edema in patients presenting with acute dyspnea: A systematic review and meta-analysis. Academic Emergency Medicine. 2014;**21**(8):843-852

[77] Martindale J, Wakai A, Collins S. Diagnosing acute heart failure in the emergency department: A systematic review and meta-analysis. Academic Emergency Medicine. 2016; **23**(3):223-242

[78] Subramaniam S, Bober J, Chao J. Point-of-care ultrasound for diagnosis of abscess in skin and soft tissue infections. Academic Emergency Medicine. 2016;**23**(11):1298-1306

[79] Barbic D, Chenkin J, Cho D. In patients presenting to the emergency department with skin and soft tissue infections what is the diagnostic accuracy of point-of-care ultrasonography for the diagnosis of abscess compared to the current standard of care? A systematic review and meta-analysis. British Medical Journal. 2017;**7**:e 013688

[80] Mercier E, Bedside M-CF. Ultrasound for the diagnosis of necrotising fasciitis. Emergency Medicine Journal. 2014;**31**(8):692-693

[81] Adhikari S, Blaivas M. Utility of bedside sonography to distinguish soft tissue abnormalities from joint effusions in the emergency department. Journal of Ultrasound in Medicine. 2010;**29**:519-526

[82] Vieira R, Levy J. Bedside ultrasound to identify hip effusion in pediatric patients. Annals of Emergency Medicine. 2010;**55**(3):284-289

[83] Barata I, Spencer R, Suppiah A. Emergency ultrasound in the detection of pediatric long-bone fractures. Pediatric Emergency Care. 2012;**28**(11):1154-1157

[84] Chartier L, Bosco L, Lapointe-Shaw L. Use of point-of-care ultrasound in long bone fractures: A systematic review and meta-analysis. Canadian Journal of Emergency Medicine. 2017 Mar;**19**(2):131-142

[85] Wang CC, Linden KL, Hansel J. Otero sonographic evaluation of fractures in children. Journal of Diagnostic Medical Sonography. 2017;**33**(3):200-207

[86] Dubrovsky A, Kempinska A, Bank I. Accuracy of ultrasonography for determining successful realignment of pediatric forearm fractures. Annals of Emergency Medicine. 2015;**65**(3):260-265

[87] Gottlieb M, Cosby K. Ultrasound-guided hematoma block for distal radial and ulnar fractures. Journal of Emergency Medicine. 2015;**48**(3):310-312

[88] Eckert K, Janssen N, Ackermann O. Ultrasound diagnosis of supracondylar fractures in children. European Journal of Trauma and Emergency Surgery. 2014;**40**(2):159-168

[89] Adhikari S, Marx J, Crum T. Point-of-care ultrasound diagnosis of acute Achilles tendon rupture in the ED. American Journal of Emergency Medicine. 2012;**30**:634.e3-634.e4, 634.e4

[90] Nesselroade R, Nickels L. Ultrasound diagnosis of bilateral quadriceps tendon rupture after statin use. Western Journal of Emergency Medicine. 2010;**11**(4):306-309

[91] Berg K, Peck J, Boulger C, Bahner D. Patellar tendon rupture: An ultrasound case report. British Medical Journal Case Report. 2013:bcr2012008189

[92] Jarraya M, Hayashi D, de Villiers R. Multimodality imaging of foreign bodies of the musculoskeletal system. AJR. American Journal of Roentgenology 2014;203(1):W92-102

[93] Friedman D, Forti R, Wall S. The utility of bedside ultrasound and patient perception in detecting soft tissue foreign bodies in children. Pediatic Emergency Care. 2005;**21**(8):487-492

[94] Nienaber A, Harvey M, Cave G. Accuracy of bedside ultrasound for the detection of soft tissue foreign bodies by emergency doctors. Emergency Medicine Australasia. 2010;**22**(1):30-34

[95] Taylor M, Lalani N. Adult small bowel obstruction. Academic Emergency Medicine. 2013;**20**(6):528-544

[96] Pongpornsup S, Tarachat K, Srisajjakul S. Accuracy of 64 sliced multi-detector computed tomography in diagnosis of small bowel obstruction. Journal of the Medical Association of Thailand. 2009;**92**(12):1651-1661

[97] Frager D, Medwid S, Baer J. CT of small-bowel obstruction: Value in establishing the diagnosis and determining the degree and cause. American Journal of Roentgenology. 1994;**162**(1):37-41

[98] Mallo R, Salem L, Lalani T. Computed tomography diagnosis of ischemia and complete obstruction in small bowel obstruction: A systematic review. Journal of Gastrointestinal Surgery. 2005;**9**(5):690-694

[99] Suri S, Gupta S, Sudhakar P. Comparative evaluation of plain films, ultrasound and CT in the diagnosis of intestinal obstruction. Acta Radiologica. 1999;**40**(4):422-428

[100] Jang T, Schindler D, Kaji A. Bedside ultrasonography for the detection of small bowel obstruction in the emergency department. Emergency Medicine Journal. 2011;**28**(8):676-678

[101] Unluer E, Yavasi O, Eroglu O. Ultrasonography by emergency medicine and radiology residents for the diagnosis of small bowel obstruction. European Journal of Emergency Medicine. 2010;**17**(5):260-264

[102] Babineau M, Sanchez L. Ophthalmologic procedures in the emergency department. Emergency Medicine Clinics of North America. 2008;**26**(1):17-34 v-vi

[103] Jacobsen B, Lahham S, Retrospective Review PA. Of ocular point-of-care ultrasound for detection of retinal detachment. The Western Journal of Emergency Medicine. 2016;**17**(2):196-200

[104] Nagaraju R, Ningappa R. Bhimarao. Role of high resolution ultrasonography in the evaluation of posterior segment lesions. In The Eye Journal of Evidence Based Medicine and Healthcare. 2015;**2**(2):97-112

[105] Lee S, Hayward A, BellamKonda V. Traumatic lens dislocation. International Journal of Emergency Medicine. 2015;**8**:16

[106] Major R, Girling S, Boyle A. Ultrasound measurement of optic nerve sheath diameter in patients with a clinical suspicion of raised intracranial pressure. Emergency Medicine Journal. 2011;**28**(8):679-681

[107] Karakitsos D, Labropoulos N, De Groot E. Real-time ultrasound-guided catheterisation of the internal jugular vein: A prospective comparison with the landmark technique in critical care patients. Critical Care. 2006;**10**(6):R162

[108] Hind D, Calvert N, McWilliams R. Ultrasonic locating devices for central venous cannulation: Meta-analysis. British Medical Journal. 2003;**327**(7411):361

[109] Stolz L, Stolz U, Howe C. Ultrasound-guided peripheral venous access: A meta-analysis and systematic review. The Journal of Vascular Access. 2015;**16**(4):321-326

[110] Barr L, Hatch N, Roque P. Basic ultrasound-guided procedures. Critical Care Clinics. 2014;**30**(2):275-304 vi

[111] Finoff J, Hall M, Adams E. American medical Society for Sports Medicine position statement: Interventional musculoskeletal ultrasound in sports medicine. Clinical Journal of Sport Medicine. 2015;**25**(1):6-22

[112] Chou E, Dickman E, Tsou P. Ultrasonography for confirmation of endotracheal tube placement: A systematic review and meta-analysis. Resuscitation. 2015;**90**:97-103

[113] Hatch N, Wu T, Barr L. Advanced ultrasound procedures. Critical Care Clinics. 2014; **30**(2):305-329 vi

[114] Rupp S, Apfelbaum J, Blitt C. Practice guidelines for central venous access: A report by the American Society of Anesthesiologists Task Force on central venous access. Anesthesiology. 2012;**116**(3):539-573

Chapter 7

The Evolving Role of Ultrasound in Emergency Medicine

Laura Ann Galdamez

Additional information is available at the end of the chapter

http://dx.doi.org/10.5772/intechopen.74777

Abstract

Ultrasound has dramatically influenced the practice of emergency medicine in the twenty-first century. From its introduction to the medical landscape in the 1950s, it has been studied and utilized in various diagnostic exams and procedural guidance. Bedside ultrasound allowed emergency physicians easy access to immediate imaging, giving them the means to make management decisions quicker and improve quality of care. Ultrasound has demonstrated utility in examination of the heart, lungs, kidneys, liver, biliary system, uterus, ovaries, testicles, eyes and many other structures in the body. It decreases unsuccessful attempts and post-procedural complications in peripheral and central venous cannulation, pericardiocentesis, thoracentesis and other procedures. It has become a vital component of emergency medicine education and physicians now graduating with increased skills in ultrasound will continue to refine and develop its role in the emergent care of critically ill patients.

Keywords: ultrasound, POCUS, point of care ultrasound, echocardiography, FAST

1. An introduction to ultrasound

Ultrasound was first introduced in the early 1950s; however, individual units were not available for use until the 1960s. Its initial application was primarily experimental, and it did not enter a clinical role until the 1970s. The first ultrasound machines were large, complex and required the subject to be immersed in water. The images were difficult to interpret, requiring extensive training. Technological improvements led to a more compact device and better software that decreased the delay from signal acquisition to image display. This optimized real-time scanning and opened the door for widespread clinical use to develop [1]. In the

1970s, studies were performed to evaluate the utility of bedside ultrasound to detect artificially instilled fluid into a cadaver's peritoneal cavity, and within 1 year of this research, the first case of ultrasound used to detect hemoperitoneum was published. The first publication on ultrasound use by an emergency medicine physician appeared in 1988, and research into its use in bedside trauma evaluation began in multiple centers across the globe [1].

In the 1990s, additional advancements included color Doppler mode, the transvaginal transducer and multifrequency probes. The American College of Emergency Physicians (ACEP) offered its first emergency ultrasound course in 1990 and, along with the Society of Academic Emergency Medicine, published the first supporting position paper regarding emergency ultrasound in 1991 [2, 3]. ACEP then published the *Emergency Ultrasound Guidelines* in 2001, defining the scope of practice for emergency ultrasound and included recommendations for credentialing, quality assurance and standards for the examinations [4].

An emergency medicine ultrasound examination, also termed point-of-care ultrasound (POCUS) should be quick, focused, and performed for a specific condition for which it has proven utility. POCUS should be easily learned and attempt to demonstrate only a few easily recognizable findings at the bedside [1]. POCUS has continued to gain popularity due to the significant value it adds in decision-making, the immediate availability to imaging and the advancing technology with further device miniaturization and greater resolution [1]. In prehospital medicine, it is being investigated for its utility in expediting care prior to arrival and has demonstrated the ability to accurately assess trauma patients, allowing early communication of necessary resources to hospitals [5, 6]. It has also demonstrated significant utility in aeromedical evacuation and field assessment of remote-access trauma [7–10]. However, the remainder of this chapter will focus on the utility of POCUS in the hospital and its developing role in emergency department evaluation.

2. Ultrasound machine basics

Ultrasound uses probes that act as transducers for the ultrasound waves. Each transducer uses a piezoelectric crystal material that converts electricity to ultrasound waves, and then converts the returning waves to an electrical signal that is interpreted by the machine to create the two-dimensional image we recognize as the internal structures [11, 12]. The interchangeable probes vary by the ultrasound wave frequency emitted, which provides an array of image acquisition capabilities that favor resolution in different areas. The curvilinear probe emits a lower frequency of 2–5 MHz, providing greater lateral resolution and better penetration for deeper structures. The linear transducer emits higher frequencies of 7–13 MHz, providing much higher resolution for superficial structures. The phased array probe lies between these two, emitting a frequency of 2.5–5 MHz and providing moderate resolution for superficial structures and good penetration for deep structures [9, 11].

If the ultrasound pulse encounters a structure that reflects most waves, it will appear bright white and is termed hyperechoic. If the pulse encounters a structure that does not reflect much or any of the waves, it appears darker or black and is termed hypoechoic or anechoic, respectively [13].

There are also various ultrasound modes that allow us to address specific questions related to movement or flow. "B" mode (brightness mode) is primarily used for diagnostic imaging with two-dimensional displays in gray-scale based on the tissues echogenicity. "M" (motion) mode depicts the motion through time of structures along a single vertical line within the B-mode image. This mode is frequently used to look for subtle movement in images or better characterize the degree of movement experienced by a structure like as a heart valve [12]. Color flow mode depicts direction and flow velocity of fluids, such as blood within the heart or vessels. Power Doppler mode emits short bursts of waves, allowing more accurate localization of echo sources and is more sensitive in measuring flow velocity in low-flow states [12, 13].

3. Diagnostic ultrasound

3.1. Cardiac ultrasound

The phased array probe is typically used in cardiac evaluation, and four basic views are obtained. Parasternal long view visualizes the mitral valve, left ventricle and right ventricle. Apical four view is demonstrated just infero-lateral to the nipple, and demonstrates both atria and ventricles. A pericardial effusion can be easily demonstrated using ultrasound. An acute pericardial effusion of as little as 50 mL can lead to tamponade and requires immediate intervention [14, 15]. Small effusions usually occur in the posterior and inferior areas, and as they grow they extend to the apex. Moderate effusions are defined as 10–20 mm (anterior plus posterior) separation from the pericardial sac and the myocardium, and a large effusion is >20 mm [12]. The effusion will appear as a dense anechoic or hypoechoic area surrounding the heart, between the muscle and the hyperechoic pericardial sac [12]. It is important to determine if an effusion is causing tamponade, a condition when fluid accumulation in the pericardial sac increases the pressure enough to overcome the diastolic pressure of the right heart and prevent sufficient filling [14, 16]. Using ultrasound, visualization of right ventricle (RV) collapse during diastole is more reliable to determine the presence of tamponade, with a sensitivity of 48–100% and specificity of 72–100%. Right atrial collapse has a sensitivity of 50% in early tamponade and 100% in late tamponade, but a poor specificity of 33–100% [14, 17]. If the effusion has pus, blood or fibrin, it can appear less hypoechoic than expected. It is important to differentiate these more obscure pericardial effusions from the "epicardial fat pads" that some patients will have, and performing the ultrasound in a supine position will help as fluid should collect posteriorly and a hypoechoic layer only apparent anteriorly most likely represents fat [12].

The FOCUS (focused cardiac ultrasound) exam was created to protocolize a comprehensive exam looking for pericardial effusion, relative chamber size, global cardiac function and volume status (via left ventricle size, ventricle function or inferior vena cava size and change with respirations) [15]. In the hands of skilled practitioners, this exam can lead to decreased morbidity and mortality in blunt and penetrating trauma [15].

In determining the left ventricle (LV) function, there are three parameters used to give a rough estimate of "good," "moderate" or "poor" ejection fraction. All parts of the ventricle wall should contract equally and symmetrically toward the its center, the myocardia must be thicken during systole and the mitral valve must approximate the septum, demonstrating normal mobility [12]. These three data points allow a rough approximation of LV function, but there are more specific ways to estimate function. Simpson's method involves estimating the LV end-systolic volume (by tracing the two-dimensional area of the LV during a freeze-frame of systole) and end-diastolic volume, using the ultrasound software to perform the calculation [11]. End point septal separation (EPSS) has also been used to estimate cardiac function. EPSS uses the measured distance from the anterior mitral valve leaflet to the ventricular septum in early diastole in the parasternal long view. A value greater than 7 mm indicates poor LV function and likely low ejection fraction [18].

Cardiac ultrasound has recently been incorporated into cases of cardiac arrest and has shown utility in the difficult determination of continued cardiopulmonary resuscitation when it may be futile. Survival of cardiac arrest in the field is less than 5%, and cardiac activity which demonstrates no kinetic cardiac activity suggests only a 1–2% probability of return of spontaneous circulation [19]. Using the ultrasound criteria of no flickering of the ventricle walls or valves lowers the false negative rates even further [19–21]. It is important to hold artificial respirations and medication infusion during ultrasound as these small movements may be misinterpreted as movement of heart muscle [12]. The presence of cardiac contractility does not demonstrate the same prognostic significance, as in these cases, return of spontaneous circulation occurred in only 50% of cases [19].

Cardiac ultrasound can also be used to assess for right heart strain in cases of known or suspected pulmonary embolism. The right ventricle (RV) is typically less than 2/3 the size of the LV, but in acute right heart strain, the RV will appear the same size or larger than the LV [12]. The enlarged RV will put pressure on the septum, causing it to bow in and give the LV a "D" shape on the parasternal short axis view. Enlargement of the RV can also occur with chronic conditions such as pulmonary hypertension from chronic lung disease, so it is important to have a good background and clinical context when looking for this finding [12].

3.2. Pulmonary ultrasound

Air is a poor ultrasound wave transducer, as air molecules scatter ultrasound waves. Historically, sonographers believed that ultrasound could not be used to derive useful information about the lungs; however, artifacts created by normal lungs are helpful, mainly by their absence in pathologic lungs. A linear probe is typically used in the midclavicular area of anterior chest, oriented in the sagittal plane to capture ribs and the intercostal spaces between them [11]. Ultrasound is used commonly to look for pleural sliding, which is absent in a pneumothorax [22–24]. "B" mode can be used to examine the hyperechoic pleural line and look for bright white dots that appear to move along the surface, known as "ants marching on a log." "M" mode can be used as well, with the normal finding being a uniform gray sheet below the hyperechoic pleura, known as the "seashore sign." In the absence of pleural sliding, there will be numerous straight lines in sequence below the pleural line, giving a barcode appearance [11, 12]. Compared to chest radiography, anterior lung ultrasound has a higher sensitivity (59–80%) and comparable specificity (89–99%) [25, 26]. False negatives occur primarily in smaller, clinically insignificant pneumothoraces [27]. The transition point on lung ultrasound images where features of a normal lung and of a pneumothorax converge is known as the "lung point." This finding is controversial, but some sources report a specificity of 100% for this finding in diagnosis of a pneumothorax [23, 28, 29].

Pleural effusions can be visualized using the phased array or abdominal probe in the coronal plane of the right upper quadrant (RUQ) and left upper quadrant (LUQ). In these views, the diaphragm is visible as a hyperechoic, curvilinear line, with the liver or spleen inferior, and the lungs superior [11]. In normal lungs, the lung tissue superior to the diaphragm has the same echogenicity as the liver or spleen due to a "mirroring" phenomena caused by ultrasound waves refracting off the diaphragm. In pleural effusions, this is replaced with a hypoechoic or anechoic signal, and it is possible to visualize the vertebral bodies at the bottom of the screen due to improved penetration of the ultrasound waves through the fluid [29]. The lung border is typically identified in the fluid and will move during inspiration and expiration [24, 30]. Like pneumothoraces, lung ultrasound is superior to chest radiography in detecting clinically significant pleural effusions, with higher sensitivity (91 vs. 74%) and specificity (100 vs. 31%) [31–33].

The lung parenchyma can also be assessed using ultrasound. Ultrasound has demonstrated similar diagnostic reliability as computed tomography (CT) for detecting atelectasis [23, 30]. Overall, it has a sensitivity of 90–93% and specificity of 89–100% for complete atelectasis [23, 34]. The most common ultrasound finding is the "shred sign," the appearance of irregularities, similar to shredded tissue, at the inferior pleural margin in the RUQ and LUQ views [34, 35]. Other findings noted in atelectatic lung include visualization of cardiac activity in the tissue (normally prevented by sliding pleura), lung tissue with similar echogenicity to the liver ("lung hepatization"), mediastinal shift toward collapsed lung, or hemidiaphragm elevation [23, 24, 30]. Lung contusions and pneumonia can mimic atelectasis; however, air artifacts will be present within the tissue in contusion, and in pneumonia, air can be visualized moving within the bronchioles, known as dynamic air bronchograms (intermittent bright white spots within the small airways). Both of these findings will be absent in complete atelectasis [22, 24, 36]. The lung parenchyma can also be assessed for volume overload termed pulmonary edema. The phased array or abdominal probe is used in the lateral, anterior or posterior approach, and the parenchyma is visualized to a depth of >16 cm, looking for "B" lines. These are spotlight-like artifacts that appear bright white and traverse the lung vertically to a depth of at least 16 cm. The presence of three or more "B" lines in a lung field has an overall sensitivity of 94.1% and specificity of 92.4% for pulmonary edema, outperforming chest radiography [12, 37, 38].

Other less utilized exams related to the thoracic area include airway edema and diaphragm rupture. Smoke inhalation can lead to significant endotracheal injury and resultant respiratory distress. A case study has demonstrated that ultrasound can visualize thickening of the anterior tracheal wall following inhalational injury and allow responders to potentially anticipate the need for airway protection [39]. Acute diaphragm rupture can occur in severe trauma and, because clinical manifestations vary, the diagnosis can be challenging without quick access to a CT scanner. Ultrasound has been investigated for its potential to rule out diaphragmatic rupture. Inability to visualize the spleen or heart due to herniated bowel overlying these organs, poor movement of the diaphragm with respirations, and subphrenic effusions are all associated with diaphragm ruptures. Unfortunately, ultrasound is neither sensitive nor specific for rupture, and if suspected, a CT scan should be performed immediately [30, 40].

3.3. Abdominal ultrasound

In modern trauma evaluation, the FAST (focused assessment with sonography for trauma) exam is a regular part of the secondary survey. It is a rapid evaluation looking for fluid within the abdominal, pericardial and pelvic cavities, using the subxiphoid, RUQ, LUQ and suprapubic views [31, 41, 42]. In RUQ and LUQ views, fluid will appear first within the hepatorenal and subdiaphragmatic recesses. It is critical to visualize the entire hepatorenal area on the right, including the inferior pole of the kidney, and the subdiaphragmatic margin above the spleen on the left, to maximize the sensitivity for finding intraperitoneal fluid [12]. In the transverse suprapubic view, fluid accumulation is visualized as anechoic collections to the left or right of the bladder. The longitudinal view is more sensitive for free fluid in this area, because it better captures the most dependent region adjacent to the posterior bladder wall [12]. This exam provides reliable detection of hemoperitoneum and hemopericardium (96–98% specificity, 99% accuracy), which outperforms physical exam (57% accurate) and hemodynamic monitoring [31, 41, 42]. Portable ultrasound has slightly lower sensitivity (60–85%) in the detection of these abnormalities compared to bedside ultrasound [31, 42]. Given the low sensitivity of the exam, experts recommend using only a positive finding to guide triage or management decisions. However, serial exams can be used to improve sensitivity for an evolving or occult injury [43].

Ultrasound has long been the study of choice for the biliary system, and moving it to a bedside POCUS exam provides quick, actionable information. The curvilinear probe is used in this exam and is typically placed in the right or anterior infracostal margin. The gallbladder will appear as a small sac with a hyperechoic lining and hypoechoic interior. Lying the patient in left lateral decubitus and having them take deep breath will help bring the gallbladder closer to the abdominal wall and into view [11]. Gallstones are hyperechoic masses that tend to fall to the most dependent part of the gallbladder [13]. When one of these stones becomes impacted in the gallbladder neck, it can lead to cholecystitis (inflammation of the gallbladder). Typical ultrasound findings indicative of cholecystitis includes the presence of gallstones, pericholecystic fluid (thin, anechoic layer surrounding gallbladder wall) and thickening of the anterior wall, which is normally less than 3 mm [13]. Gallstones can also become lodged in the common biliary duct and lead to distension of the extra- and intrahepatic biliary system, a condition known as choledocholithiasis [12]. The common biliary duct can be measured using ultrasound, evaluating for this pathology. However, the duct's diameter must be interpreted in clinical context as the normal internal diameter can range from 0.6 mm to 1 cm, increasing with age [12]. Measurements greater than 1 cm can usually be assumed to be pathologic [11].

Though not routinely performed, the pancreas can be visualized using ultrasound to investigate for signs of pancreatitis such as pseudocyst formation, peripancreatic fluid and areas of necrosis which would appear as focal, hypoechoic areas [11]. An ultrasound exam of the appendix could reveal signs of appendicitis although this is typically reserved for children. It can be difficult to visualize the appendix well due to the presence of bowel gas, especially in its normal state. The diameter of the normal appendix should be less than six millimeters and it is compressible. Evidence of appendicitis on images obtained using ultrasound includes a larger diameter of over six millimeters, periappendiceal fluid, inability to compress the lumen and in one-third of cases a fecalith can be visualized [13].

3.4. Renal and genitourinary tract ultrasound

Ultrasound can be used to evaluate the genitourinary system for pathology. The major organs of interest in this system are the kidneys and bladder. The normal kidney appears oblong with a hypoechoic outer ring, the cortex, and a hyperechoic central area that contains the collecting system. Ultrasound is often used to evaluate for hydronephrosis, which generally occurs secondary to some downstream obstruction, such as a ureteral stone [13]. Hydronephrosis will appear as increased hypoechoic dilations within the renal pelvis and is graded as mild, moderate or severe depending on the integrity of the remaining structure, the calyceal separation and involvement of the renal pelvis [11, 13]. Renal stones may be visualized within the collecting system as hyperechoic structures that cause shadowing (hypoechoic artifact beyond the stone due to its highly reflective surface). Ultrasound is not sensitive for demonstrating ureteral stones, but the appearance of bilateral ureteral jets in the bladder can help exclude a diagnosis of obstructive uropathy secondary to a stone [11–13]. The renal parenchyma can also be analyzed for changes such as increased echogenicity which occurs in the early stages of medical renal disease [13]. The bladder volume can likewise be analyzed to determine if a patient is retaining secondary to an obstructive process or neurogenic process such as cauda equina [12].

3.5. Aortic ultrasound

Ruptured aortic aneurysms have a high mortality, and the size of the aneurysm is related to its risk of rupture [13]. Most abdominal aortic aneurysms occur below the level of origin of the renal arteries. Ultrasound is effective in visualizing the abdominal aorta. It is the choice screening study in asymptomatic patients and can provide life-saving information in an unstable patient who cannot be transported safely to a CT scanner. The abdominal aorta is normally less than three centimeters in diameter, but as the diameter passes five centimeters, the risk of rupture increases over 25% [13]. One difficulty with obtaining the necessary views is bowel gas that scatters the ultrasound waves and obscures the deeper structures. To minimize the artifact, apply slow steady pressure or jiggle the probe while pressing to encourage peristalsis and movement of the gas out of the bowel segment. Imaging from an angle or turning the patient on their left side to use the liver as an acoustic window can also help [12]. A false negative can occur with this scan if a mural thrombus is present in the periphery of the aneurysm, causing an internal wall that will decrease the diameter of the measured aorta. For this reason, it is important to measure from outer wall to outer wall of the aorta [13]. Aortic dissection can also be detected using these views, and will appear as a free flap within the lumen of the aorta. However, ultrasound is not nearly as accurate or sensitive as CT and should not be used to rule out a dissection [12].

3.6. Pelvic ultrasound

Ultrasound is the choice study for investigating female pelvic organs, especially in pregnancy. One of the most common questions related to a pregnant female in emergency medicine: Is this an intrauterine pregnancy? The definition of intrauterine pregnancy is the presence of a gestational sac with a yolk sac or fetal pole, within the uterus [12, 13]. A physician can use the ultrasound with either a curvilinear transabdominal or a transvaginal (more sensitive) probe to image the female pelvic organs. In conjunction with human chorionic gonadotropin (hCG) levels, ultrasound can be used to determine the likelihood of an ectopic pregnancy. Discriminatory zones refer to the hCG levels at which an intrauterine pregnancy should be apparent on ultrasound, if present [12]. For transabdominal pregnancies, this would be between 4000 and 6500 IU/mL, but for transvaginal ultrasound, it is 1500 IU/mL, due to the higher frequency and better resolution [12]. If hCG is measured above these levels and no intrauterine pregnancy can be visualized, an ectopic pregnancy should be assumed until proven otherwise. The potential deadly consequence of an ectopic pregnancy is its rupture and subsequent massive hemorrhage into the peritoneal cavity, which can go undetected if not specifically investigated. Using ultrasound, the pelvic, RUQ, and LUQ views of a FAST exam can be performed to look for evidence of a ruptured ectopic pregnancy by evaluating for fluid in the peritoneal cavity [12, 13].

A general fetal ultrasound exam can also be performed bedside. While the formal obstetric ultrasound includes many different measurements and assessing for various fetal abnormalities, these considerations are out of the purview of emergency medicine. The principle measurements that are taken bedside typically include the fetal heart rate, which is depicted in M mode, and the estimated gestational age [11, 13]. The fetal heart rate is obtained by placing the line in M mode through the fetal heart and obtaining the tracing of the movement through time. It is important to note that pulsed Doppler mode should not be used on the fetus at any time, as it is believed to have adverse effects on fetal development [11]. The estimated age can be calculated using specific measurements depending on the trimester. In the first trimester, crown-rump-length has been shown to be very accurate (within 3 days for 42–70 days and within 5 days for 70–90 days) and have great correlation between measurements performed by emergency physicians and those performed by obstetricians [44, 45]. In the later part of the first trimester and the second, additional measurements can be used such as femur length, abdominal circumference and transcranial diameter [13].

Molar pregnancies can also be demonstrated on a pelvic ultrasound. Suspicion for a molar pregnancy should arise, if hCG levels exceed 100,000 mIU/mL, with cases of sever hyperemesis gravidarum, or with vaginal bleeding in pregnancy. Ultrasound findings of a molar pregnancy include an enlarged uterus with echogenic material within the endometrial cavity ("snowstorm pattern"), numerous small cystic spaces within the tissue (hydropic villi) and enlarged, cyst-filled ovaries [13, 46].

Outside of pregnancy, ultrasound is used to visualize the female pelvic organs to demonstrate other infectious or structural abnormalities. Transvaginal ultrasound of the normal uterus will appear as a normoechoic outer layer of myometrium with a hyperechoic interior endometrium [13]. Ultrasound can demonstrate intrauterine abnormalities such as endometrial thickening (potentially indicative of endometrial hyperplasia or endometrial carcinoma) or fibroids, which may provide clues to the etiology of new or increased vaginal bleeding [13]. The endometrial cavity appears as a thin, bright line on the interior of the uterus. When performing a transabdominal study of the uterus, a full bladder provides an acoustic window and increases image resolution. However, a full bladder will impede the views of a transvaginal study, which is performed with a higher frequency probe that is better for superficial structures [13].

One of the most common gynecologic emergencies is ovarian torsion, and the consequence of missing this pathology is potential infertility. The presentation is not straightforward, and ultrasound is the best noninvasive technology to investigate the likelihood of torsion [47]. It is difficult to visualize normal ovaries on a transabdominal ultrasound; however, on a transvaginal study, they appear like large chocolate chip cookies, with the chocolate chips being small cystic follicles inside the larger, circular ovary [13]. The most common finding in ovarian torsion is ovarian enlargement [47]. Doppler ultrasound or color ultrasound modes can be used during a transvaginal exam to differentiate venous and arterial blood flow within the ovaries, and ensure that both are present. As torsion can be intermittent, a scan demonstrating adequate flow does not necessarily rule out torsion, and has a high false-negative rate. However, specificity of inadequate blood flow has been quoted from 91 to 97% and is a reliable determinant of torsion [47].

In a similar manner, power Doppler can be used to examine the testicles for potential torsion, but with the same principles of sensitivity and specificity. Each testicle should be examined separately and within the same image, as the most common finding is testicular enlargement and hypoechoic color change compared to the contralateral testicle. Other findings on a scrotal exam include hydrocele (a large fluid collection around the testicles), varicocele (large collection of tortuous and dilated veins appearing next to the testicle), spermatocele and epididymitis. Epididymitis is the most common cause of scrotal pain in postpubertal males, and will appear as increased blood flow posterior to the testicle compared to the contralateral side [48–50]. Following scrotal trauma, hemorrhage can be visualized within the testicle. As a general principal, any abnormality in the traumatized testicle compared to the other side represents testicular rupture until proven otherwise [48–50].

3.7. Ocular ultrasound

Ocular ultrasound has many applications within emergency medicine. All structures of interest are superficial and therefore the linear probe is the probe of choice. The structure of the eye is easy to delineate using ultrasound. The fluid-filled globe is separated into the anterior and posterior chamber, with the lens visible as an oval echogenic structure just posterior to the ciliary body [51]. Lens dislocation will appear as displacement of the small, oblong structure from this usual resting place into the anterior or posterior chamber, and has been well described in ophthalmology literature [12]. Retinal detachment has also been well described and will appear as a flat, worm-like structure in the posterior chamber that moves with eye movement and is attached at one or two points to the posterior wall. Emergency physicians were found to have a 97–100% sensitivity and 83–99.7% specificity for detection of retinal detachment using ultrasound [51]. Vitreous hemorrhage will also appear in the posterior chamber as a heterogeneous mass of swirling gray material within the black globe, often likened to seaweed swaying in the waves with eye movement [11, 12, 51].

A relatively new application of ocular ultrasound is to indirectly assess for increased intracranial pressure (ICP) due to processes such as traumatic brain injury, intracranial bleeding, hydrocephalus or a hypertensive emergency. Various studies have demonstrated that the optic nerve sheath diameter (ONSD) is an accurate diagnostic sign of increased ICP and outperforms CT scan [11, 52, 53]. The globe provides a good acoustic window for visualization of the optic nerve, which appears as a large hypoechoic stripe posterior to the globe. ONSD is measured 3 mm posterior to the optic disc and is normally less than 5 mm. Using a stricter cutoff of greater than 5.8 mm for increased ICP (>20 mmHg) yields a sensitivity of 90% and specificity of 84% [51]. ONSD has mixed reviews for real-time trending of ICP. For increased ICP that is sudden onset, it has been shown that immediate intervention to decrease ICP also leads to resolution of the ultrasound findings [54]. However, for sustained increases in ICP, ONSD does not appear to normalize in real time with measures to decrease ICP [53].

Ocular injuries are a common presentation to the emergency department, and foreign bodies are involved in many cases. Sonography can detect foreign bodies within the globe, which typically appear as a twinkling object and a comet-tail-shaped reverberation artifact posteriorly. Ocular ultrasound has a sensitivity of 87.5% and a specificity of 85.2% for foreign bodies, and is more reliable in the detection of metallic material. However, care must be taken to avoid pressure on a potential open globe secondary to a foreign body. If open glove is suspected, other imaging modalities such as CT are preferred [51]. Lesser utilized ocular exams include demonstration of the ocular vasculature using color Doppler to evaluate for central retinal artery and central retinal vein occlusion, and evaluation of the posterior orbital space for hemorrhage (hypoechoic area) or distortion/flattening of the posterior globe ("guitar pick sign"), indicative of a retrobulbar hematoma [51].

3.8. DVT ultrasound

Deep venous thrombosis (DVT) is commonly asymptomatic, however suspicion for the pathology increases with unilateral pain and swelling of an extremity. Ultrasound is the exam of choice for the initial evaluation of an extremity for DVT. The highest yield exam is for a symptomatic patient, and it has much lower sensitivity for asymptomatic extremities. As the clinical relevance of isolated calf DVT is controversial, most radiology performed and POCUS DVT exams focus on the larger vessels above the knee [12, 13]. However, those who advocate for whole leg ultrasound point out that finding the isolated calf DVT obviates the need for a repeat scan at a later time, which is recommended with a negative two-point compression scan [12].

Two-point compression studies involve complete compression of the common femoral and greater saphenous vein in the inguinal area, and of the popliteal vein in the popliteal fossa of the posterior knee. The veins should compress to a very thin line, and inability to fully compress may indicate a DVT. False positives can occur if structures such as a lymph node, Baker's cyst or pseudoaneurysm, are mistaken for a noncompressible vessel. These structures can be better characterized by placing color Doppler over the structure and evaluating for flow. In low-flow states, squeezing the calf can help to provide extra venous return and allow easier identification [12].

3.9. Soft tissue and bone ultrasound

Ultrasound exams of soft tissue and bone focus on superficial structures, utilizing the linear probe. The different components of soft tissue are easy to differentiate. Skin will be the hyperechoic layer just below the transducer surface, subcutaneous tissue is the hypoechoic layer below the skin, muscle will appear relatively hypoechoic (more than subcutaneous tissue) and feather-like with linear striations, tendons are hyperechoic and fibrillary, and bone is linear and hyperechoic with shadowing posteriorly [11].

On a soft tissue exam, "cobblestoning" or fluid tracking throughout the subcutaneous layer is indicative of cellulitis or edema of the tissues. This is differentiated from a frank fluid collection indicative of an abscess, which will require incision and drainage, versus cellulitis, which is managed using antibiotics alone [12]. Two views can be helpful as the purulent material within an abscess can have increased echogenicity and a collection may be missed, especially if it is a thin collection in the anterior-posterior plane. Sonography can be used to demonstrate nearby vasculature prior to incision and drainage of an abscess to determine optimal incision location [11, 12].

Evaluation of tendons for potential rupture can be performed bedside, and will appear as a break in the normal linear appearance, potentially with hypoechoic hemorrhage separating the two parts [12]. A similar finding is noted in fractures. Ultrasound evaluation of bones clearly demonstrates the hyperechoic, linear cortex. In a suspected fracture, the ultrasound probe is scanned along the bone looking for defects or discontinuity of the cortex. Patient history and physical examination have poor accuracy in determining the presence of a fracture in trauma. Ultrasound has up to 90–95% sensitivity in fracture detection, making it useful to rule out a fracture, but has lower specificity and usually cannot reliably rule in a fracture [9, 11, 55]. Ultrasound is less accurate if a fracture occurs close to a joint, but additional evidence such as soft tissue swelling or a hypoechoic hematoma adjacent to the bone provide clues that a fracture may be present [9, 11].

4. Procedural ultrasound

When the ultrasound is used for procedural guidance, precautions are taken to keep the probe sterile. A probe cover and sterile gel are used for this purpose, and some procedural kits are found where ultrasound guidance has become more standardized. Since most procedures using ultrasound guidance involve superficial structures, the linear probe is regularly utilized. The orientation of the probe becomes critical, as movements of equipment on the screen, such as needles, need to correlate with movement relative to the patient [11]. There are two general methods for procedure guidance using ultrasound: static and dynamic. Static guidance usually entails either visualization of internal structures before the procedure to mark the ideal entry site, or post-procedure to verify success. Dynamic guidance entails visualization during the actual procedure [12].

4.1. Venous cannulation

Insertion of intravenous catheters using visual guidance is one of the most common procedural uses for the ultrasound [56–58]. Ultrasound-guided peripheral and central line placement is nearly always performed dynamically, watching the needle advance until there is successful cannulation of the vein. Peripheral vein cannulation uses either 1.5-inch cannulated needle, or a longer angiocath for deeper veins. Ultrasound guidance is most useful in patients with difficult IV access, such as obese, young, IV drug abusing or prior chemotherapy patients. In patients with difficult to obtain IV access, ultrasound-guided IV placement was demonstrated to be consistently twice as fast and decrease the total number of punctures needed by an average of two, but still had variable success (80–90%) [9]. Physicians with greater ultrasound experience have more than 60% increased success rates between ultrasound and landmark guidance compared to novice practitioners with no ultrasound background [9, 56, 59].

In general, there are two methods to visualize dynamic IV placement. In the transverse approach, the probe is held perpendicular to the vessel. The probe can be used to apply compression and differentiate artery from vein. The depth of the desired vessel is measured and needle is inserted at the same distance distal to the ultrasound probe at a 45° angle. This allows visualization of the needle tip, which appears as a bright, white dot, just as it enters the vessel below the ultrasound probe [11]. The other technique is to place the probe in line with the needle so that the vessel is visualized running across the screen from left to right, and the entire length of the needle can be visualized as it tracks through the skin and soft tissue to the vessel [11].

Central line placement follows the same principles and ultrasound has become routinely used in internal jugular and common femoral vein cannulation. While advancing the needle during central line placement, just as in landmark-based techniques, applying slight negative pressure to the syringe allows you to feel when you have punctured the vein rather than relying only on ultrasound visualization. Once blood is withdrawn, the ultrasound probe is set aside in the sterile field while the wire is inserted. Ultrasound can then be used to verify the placement of the wire within the lumen of the vein and not the adjacent artery. The use of ultrasound in central line placement has led to reduction in complications by 78%, reduction in attempts needed by 40% and reduction in unsuccessful cannulation by 64% [9, 12].

4.2. Paracentesis and thoracentesis

Paracentesis can be performed for both diagnostic sampling and/or therapeutic drainage. Although the landmark-based approach has generally been safe, ultrasound allows several advantages including the ability to find the deepest fluid pocket and avoid inadvertent puncture of the internal organs, visualization of overlying or underlying vasculature or abnormal anatomy to avoid, and confirmation that the abdominal distension is secondary to ascites and not another disease process [60, 61]. Physical exam itself has poor reliability in the diagnosis of ascites, and ultrasound demonstrated improved sensitivity (94% compared to 50%) and specificity (82 vs. 29%) in detection [62]. In landmark-based paracentesis, success is determined mainly by the overall volume of ascites, success rates are 44% for 300 mL and 78% for 500 mL, but virtually never successful with volume is less than 50 mL [63]. A prospective, randomized study involving inexperienced emergency medicine residents performing ultrasound-guided paracentesis compared to this landmark-based technique demonstrated higher success rates (95 vs. 61%, P = 0.0003) [64]. Another retrospective study demonstrated the association of ultrasound guidance with lower adverse events rates such as post-paracentesis infection, hematoma, and seroma (1.4 vs. 4.7%, p = 0.01) [65].

http://dx.doi.org/10.5772/intechopen.74777

The abdominal or phased array probe is typically used in a static exam, finding the best fluid pocket with the patient supine or in left lateral decubitus, marking that spot on the skin and then placing the ultrasound aside for needle insertion. The practitioner should avoid the upper quadrants, given the proximity of the liver and spleen to the abdominal wall. They should also avoid 11 and 2 o'clock angles of the abdomen to prevent inadvertently puncturing the inferior epigastric arteries, a known cause of hemorrhagic complications [66]. A pocket of 3–4 cm between the abdominal wall and the free-floating loops of bowel is adequate and is usually found in the lateral-most aspect of the abdomen [11].

Thoracentesis follows similar principles and can be used for diagnostic or therapeutic collection. Ultrasound guidance for bedside thoracentesis has resulted in overall shorter hospital stays, less overall cost and fewer complications [67]. Specifically, ultrasound reduces the rates of iatrogenic pneumothorax by 29%, which complicates 20–39% of physical exam-guided thoracenteses [68]. In cases of iatrogenic pneumothorax, ultrasound guidance also reduced the number of those ultimately requiring tube thoracostomy [69]. Ultrasound increases the accuracy of site selection by 26% and decreases the number of unsuccessful attempts [70]. It can also be used to estimate the size of a pleural effusion which helps to predict the utility of drainage. In patients with a pleural effusion greater than 500 mL, successful drainage leads to improvement in their oxygen saturation to inspired oxygen ratio [27]. With the patient supine, a distance from the thoracic wall to the visceral pleura over 5 cm at the posterior axillary line can identify an effusion larger than 500 mL (90% specificity and 100% sensitivity) [24, 71].

Similar to a paracentesis, a phased array transducer is used with the patient either supine or sitting up, and a static exam is performed to demonstrate the deepest fluid pocket within the thoracic cavity. The diaphragm should be visualized and care should be taken to avoid the needle tip coming in close proximity to it. A depth of 15 mm between the visceral and parietal pleura over three sequential intercostal spaces is adequate to perform the procedure. Real-time ultrasound guidance can also be used to actively visualize the needle passing through the pleura and into the fluid [11].

Ultrasound can be used in tube thoracostomy pre-procedure to optimize site selection and decrease complications, or post-procedure to quickly verify correct placement. Pre-procedure ultrasound lowers the rate of iatrogenic pneumothorax (4–30 to 1.3–6.7%), helps avoid intercostal vessels and allows visualization of aberrant anatomy that can lead to complications. Post-procedure ultrasound can be used to detect complications such as a misplaced tube, iatrogenic pneumothorax and re-expansion pulmonary edema [22, 72, 73]. Extra-thoracic placement of chest tubes is estimated to complicate 0.5–2.6% of attempts, and ultrasound has demonstrated a sensitivity of 83–100% and specificity of 83–100% for differentiating intra- and extra-thoracic placement [74]. When viewing the thorax with ultrasound, a correctly placed chest tube will disappear as it enters the thorax, but an extra-thoracic tube can be viewed in its entirety [74].

4.3. Pericardiocentesis

The significant drop in cardiac output in tamponade can be life-threatening, and emergent pericardiocentesis can be life-saving. As previously mentioned, ultrasound can be used to diagnose pericardial effusion and tamponade and can help in its immediate management. Ultrasound guidance allows visualization of the area of maximum fluid accumulation and real-time needle guidance to decrease complications such as inadvertent puncture of the internal mammary artery or the neurovascular bundle at the inferior edge of the ribs [11, 75, 76]. The traditional technique involved a subxiphoid approach and blind needle advancement until blood or fluid was withdrawn. Using ultrasound, the initial approach in over 80% of patients was changed to an apical puncture site due to better fluid accumulation here [75, 77].

The procedure is performed with the curvilinear or phased array transducer and can be placed either subxiphoid or in the parasternal position for viewing the pericardial effusion. The ideal site for needle placement is where the effusion has maximal depth, is closest to the skin and farthest from structures the needle could damage, such as the liver or lung. The ultrasound beam is used to simulate the needle tract, so if the liver or lung lies above the pericardium on the screen, the needle will penetrate these structures [11]. The placement of the pericardiocentesis catheter can be confirmed using ultrasound. After the needle or catheter is deemed likely to be in the pericardial sac, a syringe filled with agitated saline can be connected and injected while viewing with the ultrasound. A "snow-storm" of bubbles, showing as white dots, will be seen within the pericardial sac if the catheter is correctly placed, or may be apparent within the ventricle if the myocardium was penetrated during the procedure [9, 11].

4.4. Lumbar puncture

The complication rate for lumbar punctures is exceedingly low; yet in patients with increased body-mass-index and excess soft tissue, the success rates can vary greatly. Anesthesia literature from Russia first mentioned the concept of ultrasound guidance used during lumbar punctures in 1971 [78]. Following this publication, further anesthesia literature has documented a reduced number of unsuccessful attempts, fewer interspaces punctured, and decreased needle repositioning within the skin when using pre-procedure ultrasound guidance [79–81]. Ultrasound was recently demonstrated to be a preferred rescue method in failed neonatal lumbar punctures [82]. Likewise, a 2005 case series demonstrated its utility in localization in three failed adult lumbar punctures performed by experienced physicians [83]. In patients with difficulty to palpate landmarks, ultrasound has proven value to identify the lumbar vertebral landmarks as well as other relevant structures that help to guide a lumbar puncture [84, 85].

As the best utility in ultrasound guidance is experienced in patients with a high amount of overlying soft tissue, a curvilinear transducer will typically be the choice probe to gain a greater amount of depth. The transducer is placed parallel to the vertebral column at first to view the spinous processes and the desired para-vertebral space. The spinous processes will be hyperechoic and rounded, and there will be a notable gap where the space occurs. Ultrasound allows alignment in both the vertical as well as the horizontal axis, providing an exact point for needle puncture to optimize success. Real-time guidance is generally not performed given the difficulty of needle insertion with one hand while holding the probe, and typically static guidance and skin marking are sufficient [11].

4.5. Endotracheal intubation confirmation and tracheostomy

Intubation is a common procedure performed in emergency medicine and has high rates of first pass success [86]. However, one of the well-known complications is accidental endobronchial intubation which would result in ventilation of only one lung, or intra-esophageal intubation which would result in neither lung being ventilated. As many as 55% of these endobronchial intubations are missed by auscultation of the bilateral lung fields alone, and in cases of poor cardiac output (e.g., cardiac arrest), patients may lack sufficient circulation to the lungs to expel enough carbon dioxide for accurate capnography [87]. Ultrasound has demonstrated utility in verifying the correct placement of the endotracheal tube (ETT) directly and indirectly [9, 88]. Indirect verification involves demonstration of pleural sliding in the anterior, midclavicular line bilaterally once the ETT is placed. This technique would be limited in the setting of a pneumothorax [31, 87]. Direct verification involves real-time visualization during intubation with the probe placed midline over the trachea in the suprasternal notch. Evidence of successful intubation is seen as a single air artifact, and unsuccessful, esophageal intubation would be apparent as a double air artifact (air in the tube and the trachea). The direct method has overall sensitivity of 98.9, with 100% specificity in noncardiac arrest patients, and 75% specificity in cardiac arrest patients [89]. This technique is limited if the trachea lies directly over the esophagus, as it would obscure visualization of the air artifact within the esophagus [88].

If intubation is ultimately unsuccessful, ultrasound can also provide guidance in cricothyroidotomy [9]. Inaccurate landmark identification using digital palpation is one of the leading causes of cricothyroidotomy failure and complication [90]. Excess soft tissue in the neck can result in significant difficulty palpating and identifying the thyroid and cricoid cartilage. Ultrasound has demonstrated increased reliability in identification of the cricothyroid membrane and its use has the potential to decrease moderate-severe injuries to the trachea and larynx by up to one third compared to landmark-based technique [90].

5. Conclusion

Ultrasound has helped to transform the practice of emergency medicine by providing an efficient and powerful tool that allows rapid information acquisition and subsequently informed, quick decision-making. Its utility continues to expand and, with technological advancements, it will continue to become more versatile and widespread in its use, not only in the emergency department, but in the prehospital and more austere settings. It allows the emergency physician to expedite care by decreasing time needed to obtain imaging and speak with consultants or to order additional tests or treatments based on the findings. It decreases procedural complications by allowing real-time guidance of needles along specific tracts, avoiding inadvertent organ or vessel injury.

Ultrasound education is established as an essential part of all emergency medicine residencies, as well as some general surgery residencies, and is offered as an accredited fellowship. As physicians graduate from these training programs, the expectations of their ultrasound skills will grow. Bedside ultrasound is increasingly available, and emergency medicine physicians will continue to refine and optimize its use.

Acknowledgements

I would like to thank Ann Hudgins Chastain of Strategic Discussions for providing proofreading, language and technical editing.

Conflicts of interest

I have no conflicts of interest to declare.

Author details

Laura Ann Galdamez

Address all correspondence to: laura@outdoorem.com

Department of Emergency Medicine, Baylor College of Medicine, Houston, TX, United States of America

References

[1] Kendall J, Hoffenberg S, Smith R. History of emergency and critical care ultrasound: The evolution of a new imaging paradigm. Critical Care Medicine. 2007;**35**(5):126-130

[2] United States, Emergency Medicine Practice Committee, American College of Emergency Physicians. Use of Ultrasound for Emergency Department Patients.1991

[3] Society for Academic Emegency Medicine. Ultrasound Position Statement [Internet]. 1991. Available from: http://www.saem.org

[4] American College of Emergency Physicians. ACEP Emergency Ultrasound Guidelines [Internet]. 2001. Available from: http://www.acep.org

[5] Walcher F, Kirschning T, Müller MP, Byhahn C, Stier M, Rüsseler M, et al. Accuracy of prehospital focused abdominal sonography for trauma after a 1-day hands-on training course. Emergency Medicine Journal. 2010;**27**:345-349

[6] Heegaard W, Hildebrandt D, Spear D, Chason K, Nelson B, Ho J. Prehospital ultrasound by paramedics: Results of field trial. Academic Emergency Medicine. 2010;**17**:624-630

[7] Jakobsen L, Bøtker M, Lawrence L, Sloth E, Knudsen L. Systematic training in focused cardiopulmonary ultrasound affects decision-making in the prehospital setting – Two case reports. Scandinavian Journal of Trauma, Resuscitation and Emergency Medicine. 2014;**22**:29

[8] Ketelaars R, Hoogerwerf N, Scheffer GJ. Prehospital chest ultrasound by a dutch helicopter emergency medical service. The Journal of Emergency Medicine. 2013;**44**(4):811-817

[9] Galdamez LA, Clark JB, Antonsen EL. Point-of-care ultrasound utility and potential for high altitude crew recovery missions. Aerospace Medicine and Human Performance. Feb 2017;**88**(2):128-136

[10] Press GM, Miller SK, Hassan IA, Alade KH, Camp E, Del Junco D, et al. Prospective evaluation of prehospital trauma ultrasound during aeromedical transport. The Journal of Emergency Medicine. 2014;**47**(6):638-645

[11] Killu K, Dulchavsky S, Coba V. The ICU Ultrasound Pocket Book. 1st ed. 2010

[12] Noble VE, Nelson BP. Manual of Emergency and Critical Care Ultrasound. 2nd ed. New York, NY: Cambridge University Press; 2011

[13] Herring W. Learning Radiology: Recognizing the Basics. 2nd ed. Philadelphia, PA: Elsevier; 2012

[14] Perera P, Lobo V, Williams SR, Gharahbaghian L. Cardiac echocardiography. Critical Care Clinics. 2014;**30**(1):47-92

[15] Labovitz AJ, Noble VE, Bierig M, S a G, Jones R, Kort S, et al. Focused cardiac ultrasound in the emergent setting: A consensus statement of the American Society of Echocardiography and American College of Emergency Physicians. Journal of the American Society of Echocardiography. 2010;**23**(12):1225-1230

[16] Yoshino S, Minagoe S, Yu B, Kosedo I, Yamashita M, Ishizawa M, et al. Cardiac tamponade due to rupture of coronary artery fistula to the coronary sinus with giant aneurysm of coronary artery: Usefulness of transthoracic echocardiography. Heart and Vessels. 2013;**28**(4):536-540

[17] Guntheroth WG. Sensitivity and specificity of echocardiographic evidence of tamponade: Implications for ventricular interdependence and pulsus paradoxus. Pediatric Cardiology. 2007;**28**:358-362

[18] Secko MA, Lazar JM, Salciccioli LA, Stone MB. Can junior emergency physicians use E-point septal separation to accurately estimate left ventricular function in acutely dyspneic patients? Academic Emergency Medicine. 2011;**18**(11):1223-1226

[19] Blyth L, Atkinson P, Gadd K, Lang E. Bedside focused echocardiography as predictor of survival in cardiac arrest patients: A systematic review. Academic Emergency Medicine. 2012;**19**(10):1119-1126

[20] Breitkreutz R, Price S, Steiger HV, Seeger FH, Ilper H, Ackermann H, et al. Focused echocardiographic evaluation in life support and peri-resuscitation of emergency patients: A prospective trial. Resuscitation. 2010;**81**(11):1527-1533

[21] Salen P, Melniker L, Chooljian C, Rose JS, Alteveer J, Reed J, et al. Does the presence or absence of sonographically identified cardiac activity predict resuscitation outcomes of cardiac arrest patients? The American Journal of Emergency Medicine. 2005;**23**(4):459-462

[22] Lyn-Kew KE, Koenig SJ. Bedside ultrasound for the interventional pulmonologist. Clinics in Chest Medicine. 2013;**34**(3):473-485

[23] Stefanidis K, Dimopoulos S, Nanas S. Basic principles and current applications of lung ultrasonography in the intensive care unit. Respirology. 2011;**16**(2):249-256

[24] Xirouchaki N, Magkanas E, Vaporidi K, Kondili E, Plataki M, Patrianakos A, et al. Lung ultrasound in critically ill patients: Comparison with bedside chest radiography. Intensive Care Medicine. 2011;**37**(9):1488-1493

[25] Lubna F Husain LH, Carmody KA. Sonographic diagnosis of pneumothorax. Journal of Emergencies, Trauma, and Shock. 2012;**5**(1):76-81

[26] Jalli R, Sefidbakt S, Jafari SH. Value of ultrasound in diagnosis of pneumothorax: A prospective study. Emergency Radiology. 2013;**20**(2):131-134

[27] Ashton-Cleary DT. Is thoracic ultrasound a viable alternative to conventional imaging in the critical care setting? British Journal of Anaesthesia. 2013;**111**(2):152-160

[28] Kline JP, Dionisio D, Sullivan K, Early T, Wolf J, Kline D. Detection of pneumothorax with ultrasound. AANA Journal. 2013;**81**(4):265-274

[29] Piette E, Daoust R, Denault A. Basic concepts in the use of thoracic and lung ultrasound. Current Opinion in Anaesthesiology. 2013;**26**(1):20-30

[30] Brun P-M, Bessereau J, Levy D, Billeres X, Fournier N, Kerbaul F. Prehospital ultrasound thoracic examination to improve decision making, triage, and care in blunt trauma. The American Journal of Emergency Medicine. 2014;**32**(7):817.e1-817.e2

[31] Wagner MS, Garcia K, Martin DS. Point-of-care ultrasound in aerospace medicine: Known and potential applications. Aviation, Space, and Environmental Medicine. 2014;**85**(7): 730-739

[32] Schleder S, Dornia C, Poschenrieder F, Dendl L, Cojocaru L, Bein T, et al. Bedside diagnosis of pleural effusion with a latest generation hand-carried ultrasound device in intensive care patients. Acta Radiologica. 2012;**53**(9):556-560

[33] Lisi M, Cameli M, Mondillo S, Luzzi L, Zacà V, Cameli P, et al. Incremental value of pocket-sized imaging device for bedside diagnosis of unilateral pleural effusions and ultrasound-guided thoracentesis. Interactive Cardiovascular and Thoracic Surgery. 2012;**15**(4):596-602

[34] Acosta CM, Tusman G, Jacovitti D, Maidana G, Belaunzarán A, Cereceda S, et al. Anesthesia-induced atelectasis assessed by lung sonography. Critical Ultrasound Journal. 2014;**6**(Suppl 1):A13

[35] Xirouchaki N, Kondili E, Prinianakis G, Malliotakis P, Georgopoulos D. Impact of lung ultrasound on clinical decision making in critically ill patients. Intensive Care Medicine. 2014;**40**(1):57-65

[36] Lichtenstein D, Mezière G, Seitz J. The dynamic air bronchogram. A lung ultrasound sign of alveolar consolidation ruling out atelectasis. Chest. 2009;**135**(6):1421-1425

[37] Al Deeb M et al. Point-of-care ultrasonography for the diagnosis of acute cardiogenic pulmonary edema in patients presenting with acute dyspnea: A systematic review and meta-analysis. Academic Emergency Medicine. 2014;**21**:843

[38] Lichtenstein D, Meziere G. Relevance of lung ultrasound in the diagnosis of acute respiratory failure: The BLUE protocol. Chest. 2008;**134**:117-125

[39] Kameda T, Fujita M. Point-of-care ultrasound detection of tracheal wall thickening caused by smoke inhalation. Critical Ultrasound Journal. 2014;**6**(1):11

[40] Gangahar R, Doshi D. FAST scan in the diagnosis of acute diaphragmatic rupture. The American Journal of Emergency Medicine. 2010;**28**(3):387.e1-387.e3

[41] Jørgensen H, Jensen CH, Dirks J. Does prehospital ultrasound improve treatment of the trauma patient? A systematic review. European Journal of Emergency Medicine. 2010;**17**(5):249-253

[42] Carrié C, Delaunay F, Morel N, Revel P, Janvier G, Biais M. Ability of a new pocket echoscopic device to detect abdominal and pleural effusion in blunt trauma patients. The American Journal of Emergency Medicine. 2013;**31**(2):437-439

[43] Stengel D, Bauwens K, Rademacher G, Ekkernkamp A, Güthoff C. Emergency ultrasound-based algorithms for diagnosing blunt abdominal trauma. Cochrane Database Systematic Review. 2013;**7**

[44] Bailey C, Carnell J, Vahidnia F, Shah S, Stone M, Adams M, et al. Accuracy of emergency physicians using ultrasound measurement of crown-rump length to estimate gestational age in pregnant females. The American Journal of Emergency Medicine. 2012;**30**(8):1627-1629

[45] Saul T, Lewiss RE, Rivera MDR. Accuracy of emergency physician performed bedside ultrasound in determining gestational age in first trimester pregnancy. Critical Ultrasound Journal. 2012;**4**:22

[46] Abdi A, Stacy S, Mailhot T, Perera P. Ultrasound detection of a molar pregnancy in the emergency department. The Western Journal of Emergency Medicine. 2013;**14**(2):121-122

[47] Morton MJ, Masterson M, Hoffman B. Case report: Ovarian torsion in pregnancy – Diagnosis and management. The Journal of Emergency Medicine. 2013;**45**(3):348-351

[48] Blaivas M, Brannam L. Testicular ultrasound. Emergency Medicine Clinics of North America. 2004;**22**(3):723-748

[49] Blaivas M, Sierzenski P, Lambert M. Emergency evaluation of patients presenting with acute scrotum using bedside ultrasound. Academic Emergency Medicine. 2001;**8**(1):90-93

[50] Blaivas M, Sierzenski P. Emergency ultrasonography in the evaluation of the acute scrotum. Academic Emergency Medicine. 2001;**8**(1):85-89

[51] Kilker BA, Holst JM, Hoffman B. Bedside ocular ultrasound in the emergency department. European Journal of Emergency Medicine. 2014;**21**(2):246-253

[52] Ohle R, McIsaac SM, Woo MY, Perry JJ. Sonography of the optic nerve sheath diameter for detection of raised intracranial pressure compared to computed tomography. Journal of Ultrasound in Medicine. 2015;**34**:1285-1294

[53] Hiles LA, Donoviel DB, Bershad EM. Noninvasive brain physiology monitoring for extreme environments: A critical review. Journal of Neurosurgical Anesthesiology. 2015 Oct;**27**(4):318-328

[54] Maissan IM, Dirven PJ, Haitsma IK, Hoeks SE, Diederik G, Stolker RJ. Ultrasonographic measured optic nerve sheath diameter as an accurate and quick monitor for changes in intracranial pressure. Journal of Neurosurgical Anesthesiology. 2015;**123**:743-747

[55] Joshi N, Lira A, Mehta N, Paladino L, Sinert R. Diagnostic accuracy of history, physical examination, and bedside ultrasound for diagnosis of extremity fractures in the emergency department: A systematic review. Academic Emergency Medicine. 2013;**20**(1):1-15

[56] Costantino TG, Parikh AK, Satz WA, Fojtik JP. Ultrasonography-guided peripheral intravenous access versus traditional approaches in patients with difficult intravenous access. Annals of Emergency Medicine. 2005;**46**(5):456-461

[57] Balls A, LoVecchio F, Kroeger A, Stapczynski JS, Mulrow M, Drachman D. Ultrasound guidance for central venous catheter placement: Results from the central line emergency access registry database. The American Journal of Emergency Medicine. 2010;**28**(5):561-567

[58] Stein J, George B, River G, Hebig A, McDermott D. Ultrasonographically guided peripheral intravenous cannulation in emergency department patients with difficult intravenous access: A randomized trial. Annals of Emergency Medicine. 2009;**54**(1):33-40

[59] Bauman M, Braude D, Crandall C. Ultrasound-guidance vs. standard technique in difficult vascular access patients by ED technicians. The American Journal of Emergency Medicine. 2009;**27**(2):135-140

[60] Williams J, Simel D. The rational clinical examination. Does this patient have ascites? Journal of the American Medical Association. 1992;**267**(19):2645-2648

[61] Goldberg B, Clearfield H, Goodman G. Ultrasonic determination of ascites. Archives of Internal Medicine. 1973;**131**(2):217-220

[62] Cattau Jr E, Benjamin S, Knuff T, Castell D. The accuracy of the physical examiation in the diagnosis of suspected ascites. Journal of the American Medical Association 1982; **247**(8):1164

[63] Giacobene J, Silver V. Evaluation of diagnostic abdominal paracentesis with experimental and clinical studies. ournal of Surgery, Obstetrics, and Gynecology. 1960;**110**:676-686

[64] Nazeer S, Dewbre H, Miller A. Ultrasound-assisted paracentesis performed by emergency physicians vs the traditional technique: A prospective, randomized study. The American Journal of Emergency Medicine. 2005;**23**(3):363-367

[65] Patel P, Ernst F, Gunnarsson C. Evaluation of hospital complications and costs associated with using ultrasound guidance during abdominal paracentesis procedures. Journal of Medical Economics. 2012;**15**(1):1-7

[66] Sharzehi K, Jain V, Naveed A, Schreibman I. Hemorrhagic complications of paracentesis: A systematic review of the literature. Gastroenterology Research and Practice. 2014:1-6

[67] Patel P, Ernst F, Gunnarsson C. Ultrasonography guidance reduces complications and costs assocaited with thoracentesis procedures. Journal of Clinical Ultrasound. 2012;**40**(3):135-141

[68] Grogan D, Irwin R, Channick R. Complications associated with thoracentesis: A prospective randomized study comparing three different methods. Archives of Internal Medicine. 1990;**150**:873-877

[69] Barnes T, Morgenthaler T, Olson E. Sonographically guided thoracentesis and rate of pneumothorax. Journal of Clinical Ultrasound. 2005;**33**:442-446

[70] Diacon A, Brutsche M, Soler M. Accuracy of pleural puncture sites: A prospective comparison of clinic examination with ultrasound. Chest. 2003;**123**:436-441

[71] Roch A, Bojan M, Michelet P. Usefulness of ultrasonography in predicting pleural effusions >500 mL in patients receiving mechanical ventilation. Chest. 2005;**127**(1):224-232

[72] Salamonsen M, Dobeli K, McGrath D, Readdy C, Ware R, Steinke K, et al. Physician-performed ultrasound can accurately screen for a vulnerable intercostal artery prior to chest drainage procedures. Respirology. 2013;**18**(6):942-947

[73] Sachdeva A, Shepherd RW, Lee HJ. Thoracentesis and thoracic ultrasound: State of the art in 2013. Clinics in Chest Medicine. 2013;**34**(1):1-9

[74] Salz TO, Wilson SR, Liebmann O, Price DD. An initial description of a sonographic sign that verifies intrathoracic chest tube placement. The American Journal of Emergency Medicine. 2010;**28**(5):626-630

[75] Tirado A, Wu T, Noble VE, Huang C, Lewiss RE, J a M, et al. Ultrasound-guided procedures in the emergency department-diagnostic and therapeutic asset. Emergency Medicine Clinics of North America. 2013;**31**(1):117-149

[76] Osranek M, Bursi F, O'Leary P, Bruce C, Sinak L, Chandrasekaran K, et al. Hand-carried ultrasound-guided pericardiocentesis and thoracentesis. Journal of the American Society of Echocardiography. 2003;**16**(5):480-484

[77] Perera P, Mailhot T, Riley D, Mandavia D. The RUSH exam: Rapid ultrasound in SHock in the evaluation of the critically lll. Emergency Medicine Clinics of North America. 2010;**28**(1):29-56

[78] Bogin I, Stulin I. Application of the method of 2-dimensional echospondylography for determining landmarks in lumbar punctures. Zhurnal Nevropatologii i Psikhiatrii Imeni S.S. Korsakova. 1971;**71**(12):1810-1811

[79] Cork R, Kryc J, Vaughan R. Ultrasonic localization of the lumbar epidural space. Anesthesiology. 1980;**52**(6):513-516

[80] Grau T, Leipold R, Conradi R, Martin E, Motsch J. Efficacy of ultrasound imaging in obstetric epidural anesthesia. Journal of Clinical Anesthesia. 2002;**14**(3):169-175

[81] Grau T, Leipold R, Conradi R, Martin E, Motsch J. Ultrasound imaging facilitates localization of the epidural space during combined spinal and epidural anesthesia. Regional Anesthesia and Pain Medicine. 2001;**26**(1):64-67

[82] Coley B, Shiels 2nd W, Hogan M. Diagnostic and interventional ultrasonography in neonatal and infant lumber puncture. Pediatric Radiology. 2001;**31**(6):399-402

[83] Peterson M, Abele J. Bedside ultrasound for difficult lumbar punctures. The Journal of Emergency Medicine. 2005;**28**(2):197-200

[84] Stiffler K, Jwayyed S, Wilber S, Robinson A. The use of ultrasound to identify pertinent landmarks for lumbar puncture. The American Journal of Emergency Medicine. 2007; **25**(3):331-334

[85] Ferre R, Sweeney T. Emergency physicians can easily obtain ultrasound images of anatomical landmarks relevant to lumbar puncture. The American Journal of Emergency Medicine. 2007;**25**(3):291-296

[86] Lascarrou JB, Boisrame-Helms J, Bailly A, Le Thuaut A, Kamel T, Mercier E, et al. Video laryngoscopy vs direct laryngoscopy on successful first-pass orotracheal intubation among ICU patients: A randomized clinical trial. Journal of the American Medical Association. Feb 2017;**317**(5):483-493

[87] Sim S-S, Lien W-C, Chou H-C, Chong K-M, Liu S-H, Wang C-H, et al. Ultrasonographic lung sliding sign in confirming proper endotracheal intubation during emergency intubation. Resuscitation. 2012;**83**(3):307-312

[88] Chou H-C, Chong K-M, Sim S-S, Ma MH-M, Liu S-H, Chen N-C, et al. Real-time tracheal ultrasonography for confirmation of endotracheal tube placement during cardiopulmonary resuscitation. Resuscitation. 2013;**84**(12):1708-1712

[89] Chou HC, Tseng WP, Wang CH, Ma MHM, Wang HP, Huang PC, et al. Tracheal rapid ultrasound exam (T.R.U.E.) for confirming endotracheal tube placement during emergency intubation. Resuscitation. 2011;**82**(10):1279-1284

[90] Siddiqui N, Arzola C, Friedman Z, Guerina L, You-Ten KE. Ultrasound improves cricothyrotomy success in cadavers with poorly defined neck anatomy: A randomized control trial. Anesthesiology. Nov 2015;**123**(5):1033-1041

Chapter 8

Musculoskeletal Injuries: Types and Management Protocols for Emergency Care

Ahmad Subhy Alsheikhly and
Mazin Subhy Alsheikhly

Additional information is available at the end of the chapter

http://dx.doi.org/10.5772/intechopen.81939

Abstract

These are a common type of human injuries which can result from the damage of muscular or skeletal systems (i.e., bones, muscles, tendons, ligaments, nerves, blood vessels, etc.); they usually occur due to a strenuous and/or repetitive activity and can result into variety of complaints, complications, and deformities causing a big burden on the financial and health system in all societies. They are among the largest category of work-related injuries and are responsible for almost 30% of all worker's compensation costs worldwide. Injuries to the musculoskeletal system occur in 85% of patients who sustain blunt trauma; they often appear dramatic, but rarely cause an immediate life-threatening situation, although these injuries must be assessed and managed accurately so life or limb are not jeopardized. The doctor must be familiar with the anatomy and the injury site to protect his patients from further disability and prevent complications. Major musculoskeletal trauma such as crushed injuries that can cause release of myoglobin resulting in renal tubular injury (acute kidney injury), or can be associated with internal torso injuries like acute compartment syndrome. soft tissue and skeletal system traumas may not be initially recognized, so continued reassessment and evaluation are necessary to identify all injuries.

Keywords: trauma, musculoskeletal, management

1. Introduction

The musculoskeletal system consists of bones, muscles, tendons, ligaments, and intervertebral discs, as well as their associated nerves and blood vessels [1], and is powered by the complex interrelationship between these separate structures, each of which depends on the other to function properly. Musculoskeletal injuries are common and, hence, are routinely seen in the emergency department. This requires the attending physician to have a thorough understanding of human anatomy and to be familiar with the subtypes of these injuries in order to prevent life- or limb-threatening damage, anticipate possible complications, and avoid further disability, any of which might not be clear from the immediate presentation of the injury. Patients may come to the emergency department with a variety of complaints and be in pain, but on examination are found to have a strain (tendon) or sprain (ligament). Many musculoskeletal injuries are overuse injuries resulting from strenuous and/or repetitive activity.

Barring major complications and the potential for long-term deformities, most musculoskeletal injuries are relatively minor and rarely require an immediate life-threatening intervention. However, in patients who sustain blunt trauma, 85% incur musculoskeletal injuries that can be more serious. These patients need to be assessed and managed quickly and correctly. In cases of major musculoskeletal trauma when there are extraordinary forces that cause crushing injuries, the emergency physician may be confronted with more pressing challenges. When major muscle damage occurs, large amounts of myoglobin (a hemeprotein) are released into the bloodstream. When the myoglobin reaches the kidneys, it breaks down into harmful substances that can damage kidney cells, leading to precipitation in the renal tubules and acute kidney injury (AKI). Major musculoskeletal trauma can also result in internal torso injuries; in some cases, the pooling of fluids can form into an intact musculofascial layer with swelling in the space. This can cause complications such as acute compartment syndrome, which can lead to dire consequences if misdiagnosed. Continuous and careful assessment and correct recognition and management of musculoskeletal injuries in the emergency department are the key to successfully preventing further morbidity and reducing mortality.

2. Anatomy of the musculoskeletal system

The human musculoskeletal system (also known as the locomotor system) is a multiple organ system that gives human the ability to move using their muscles, tendons, and bones; it provides form, support, stability, and flexibility to the body as well as protecting vital organs [2]. Also, the skeletal portion of the system serves as the main storage system for calcium and phosphorus and contains critical components of the hematopoietic system [3].

Within the system, bones are connected to muscle fibers via connective tissue like tendons and ligaments. Muscles keep bones in place and also play a role in the movement of bones allowing overall motion; different bones are connected to by joints and cartilage prevents the bone ends from rubbing directly into each other.

There are, however, specific diseases and disorders, which will not be discussed in this chapter, that may adversely affect the function and overall effectiveness of the system. Some of which can be difficult to diagnose and treat in the emergency setting and may require a specialist to handle like an orthopedic surgeon; other issues may require physical rehabilitation which is handled by a physiotherapist.

http://dx.doi.org/10.5772/intechopen.81939

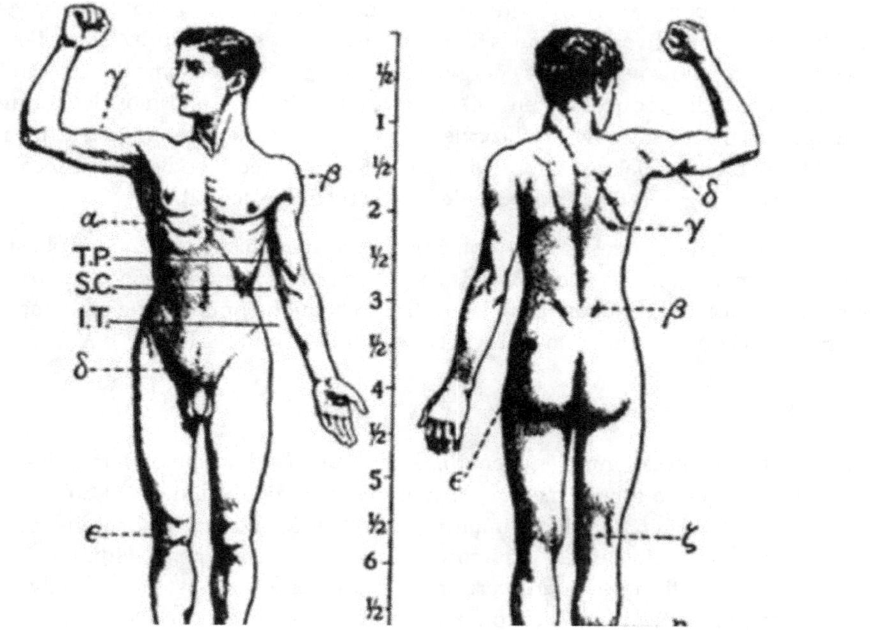

Figure 1. Features of the human activity system from the 1911.

It is of worth to note that previously, the musculoskeletal system used to be called the activity system (**Figure 1**).

2.1. The skeleton

This system serves many important functions; it aids in the shape and morphology of the whole body; it provides support and protection as well as allowing movement. It plays a major role in producing blood for the body and in storage of minerals [4]. The number of bones in the human skeleton is estimated to be around 270 at birth; however, many bones fuse together between birth and maturity. As a result, an average adult skeleton consists of 206 bones. The number of bones varies according to the method used to derive the count. While some consider certain structures to be a single bone with multiple parts, others may see it as a single part with multiple bones [5]. There are five general types of bones: long bones, short bones, flat bones, irregular bones, and sesamoid bones. The human skeleton is composed of both fused and individual bones. It is a complex structure with two distinct divisions; the axial skeleton, which includes the vertebral column, and the appendicular skeleton [2].

The skeletal system serves as a framework for tissues and organs to attach themselves to. This system acts as a protective structure for all vital organs. Major examples of this are the brain being protected by the skull and the heart with the lungs being protected by the rib cage.

Within the long bones are two distinctions of bone marrow (yellow and red). The yellow marrow has fatty connective tissue and is found in the marrow cavity. During starvation, the body uses the fat in yellow marrow for energy [2]. The red marrow of some bones is an important site for blood cell production; here, all erythrocytes, platelets, and most leukocytes form in adults. From the red marrow, erythrocytes, platelets, and leukocytes migrate to the peripheral blood to do their special tasks approximately 2.6 million red blood cells per second in order to replace existing cells that have been destroyed by the spleen [2].

Another function of bones is the storage of certain minerals. Calcium and phosphorus are among the main minerals being stored. The value of this storage "device" helps to regulate mineral balance in the bloodstream. When the fluctuation of minerals is high, these minerals are stored in bone; when it is low, it will be withdrawn from the bone.

2.2. Muscles

There are three types of muscles (smooth, skeletal, and cardiac). Smooth muscles are nonstriated muscles used to control the flow of substances within the lumens of hollow organs like vessels and bowels and are involuntarily controlled [3]. Skeletal and cardiac muscles have striations that are visible under a microscope due to the components within their cells. Only skeletal and smooth muscles are part of the musculoskeletal system and only the skeletal muscles can move the body skeleton. Skeletal muscles are attached to bones and arranged in opposing groups around joints. Cardiac muscles are found in the heart only and used to pump blood; they are like the smooth muscles, involuntarily controlled. Muscles are innervated by nerves which conduct electrical currents from the central nervous system and cause the muscles to contract.

The body contains three types of muscle tissue seen under microscope as shown in (**Figure 2**): (a) skeletal muscle, (b) smooth muscle, and (c) cardiac muscle.

2.3. Joints

Joints, also called articulations, serve two important functions in the human body: holding the skeleton together and allowing it to be mobile. Simply defined as the site where two or more bones meet [2].

There are three types of joints according to its functional classification which measures the amount of movement the joint provides: diarthrosis joints which allow extensive mobility between two or more articular heads; synarthrosis or false joints which are joints that do not provide mobility and amphiarthrosis joints which allow little or very minimal movement.

Structural classification is based on the type of the material binding the bones together. Synovial joints (**Figure 3**) are the joints where the bones are lubricated by a solution called synovial fluid that is produced by the synovial membranes. This fluid lowers the friction between the articular surfaces and is kept within an articular capsule allowing maximum mobility.

http://dx.doi.org/10.5772/intechopen.81939

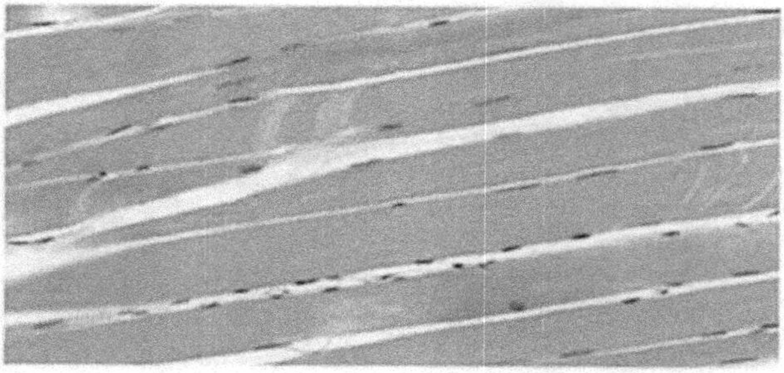

(a)

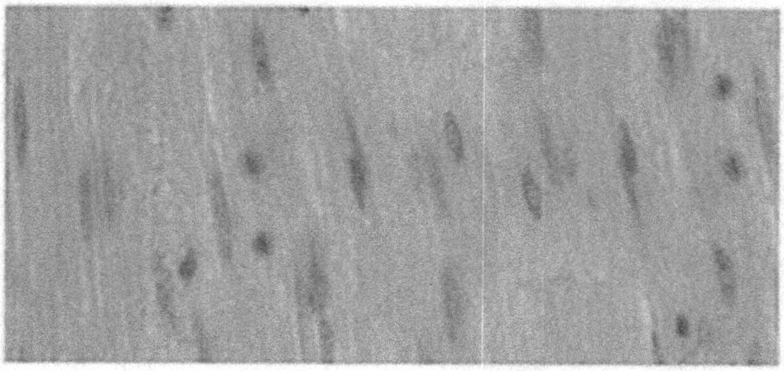

(b)

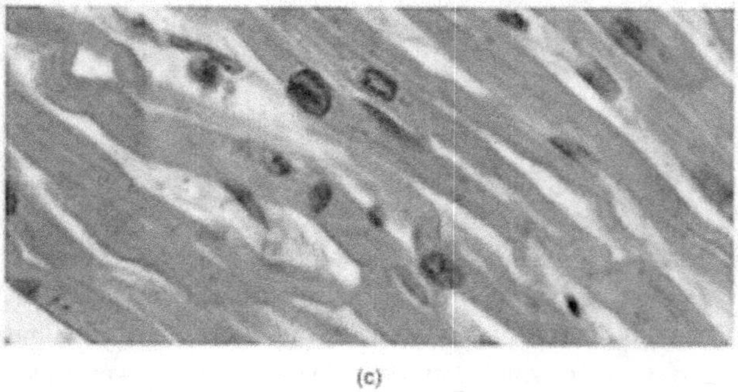

(c)

Figure 2. Muscle tissue under microscope.

Cartilaginous joints are the joints where bone ends are tied by cartilage, and fibrous joints are the joints where the bone ends are united by fibrous tissue; the latter two types vary in mobility according to their subclassifications and position in the body [2].

2.4. Tendons

A tendon is a tough, flexible band of fibrous connective tissue that connects muscles to bones [4]. The extracellular connective tissue between muscle fibers binds to tendons at the distal

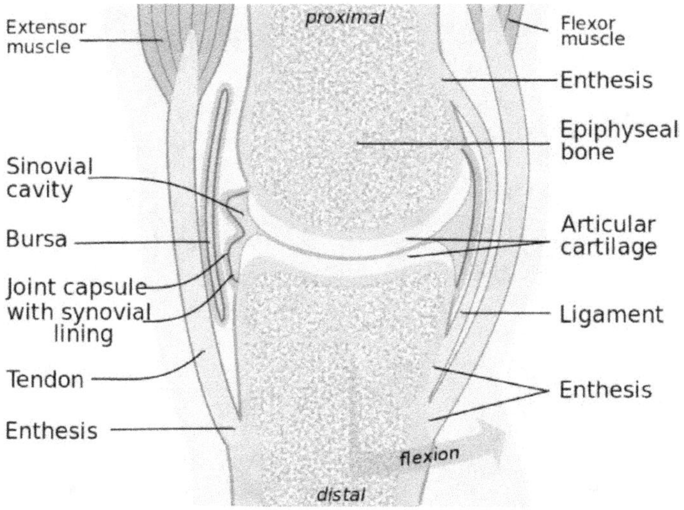

Figure 3. Anatomy of synovial joint.

and proximal ends, and the tendon binds to the periosteum of individual bones at the muscle's origin and insertion. As muscles contract, tendons transmit the forces to the relatively rigid bones, pulling on them and causing movement. Tendons can stretch substantially, allowing them to function as springs during locomotion, thereby saving energy.

2.5. Ligaments

A ligament is a small band of dense, white, fibrous elastic connective tissue [2] that connects both ends of bones together in order to form a joint and they transfer force from one bone to the other allowing movement [6]. Most ligaments limit dislocation or prevent certain movements that can cause injury or tears. Since they are elastic tissue, they increasingly lengthen when under pressure; when the force exceeds the limit of elasticity, the ligament can handle; it becomes susceptible to damage which can result in severe injuries and tears or in an unstable joint movement. Ligaments may also restrict some actions and movements such as hyperextension or hyperflexion that is limited by the ligament ability to prevent this movement to an extent [7].

2.6. Bursa

A bursa is a small synovial fluid-filled sac contained within white fibrous connective tissue which is lined internally with synovial membrane. It provides a cushion between bones and tendons and/or muscles around a joint. The fluid-filled sac can be found in multiple regions in the body mostly around joints [2].

3. Addressing musculoskeletal injuries

It is valuable to have as much insight as possible about the incident, even the site of the incident, as any information may aid in weighing the level of trauma, things like the patient position, causative mechanism of injury (penetrating, blunt, crushing…), bleeding at the scene, exposed bone or fracture ends, open wounds, any deformity or dislocation, motor and/or sensory deficits, delays in transportation, limb function, perfusion, and neurological changes. Other things to keep in mind are to pay special attention to excessive pressure over prominences as they may result in a peripheral nerve compression, compartment syndromes, or crush syndromes.

A thorough history is the first step; always ask about the mechanism of the trauma, it is very essential in the management of musculoskeletal injuries and then past medical history to assess any morbidities, history of medications, any previous injuries, and the last meal the patient had and the timing of it.

Second in line is physical examination. The physical examination in the emergency department for these injuries is based on simple four steps:

1. Inspection (discoloration, swelling, or deformity).
2. Palpation (looking for tenderness and deformity).
3. Assess range of motion (both active and passive) with consideration to the joint above and below the injured part.
4. Neurovascular examination.

This should cover the basic general approach of these injuries.

4. Classification and management of musculoskeletal injuries

4.1. Soft tissue injuries[1]

The soft tissue is a term that encompasses all body tissue except the bones. It includes skin, muscles, vessels, ligaments, tendons, and nerves. Their injuries can range from the trivial, such as a scraped knee, to the critical that includes internal bleeding; those which involve the skin and underlying musculature are commonly divided either as closed or open wounds.

4.1.1. Closed wounds

An injury where there is no open pathway from the outside to the injured site (**Figure 4**) and can be divided into:

[1] This will include soft tissue and connective tissue injuries for the sake of simplification.

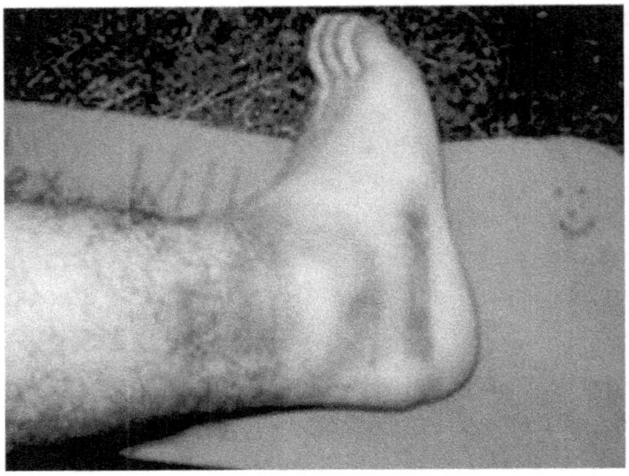

Figure 4. Closed wound.

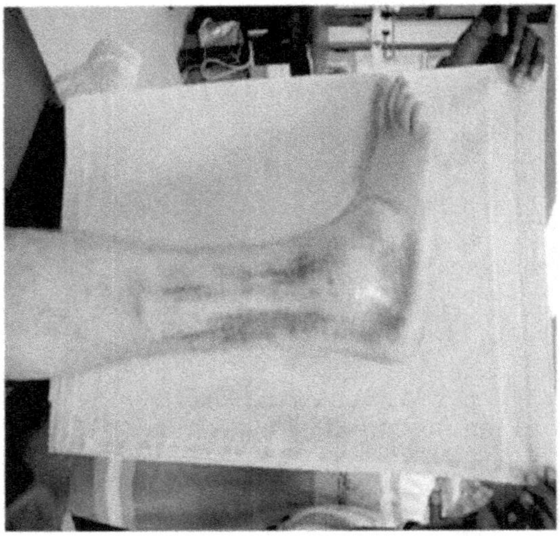

Figure 5. Ankle ligament sprain.

1. Contusion: a traumatic injury to the tissues beneath the skin without a break in the skin.
2. Ecchymosis: discoloration under the skin that is caused when blood leaks out into the surrounding soft tissues causing the skin to turn different colors.
3. Edema: swelling as a result of inflammation or abnormal fluid under the skin.
4. Strain: stretching or tearing of a muscle resulting from overstretching or overexertion. Also known as a pulled muscle or torn muscle [8].
5. Sprain: a joint injury involving damage to supporting ligaments and partial or temporary dislocation of bone ends, partial tearing or stretching of supporting ligaments (**Figure 5**). Also known as a torn ligament [8].

http://dx.doi.org/10.5772/intechopen.81939

4.1.1.1. Managements of closed injuries

Closed injuries can be managed effectively by applying the **R.I.C.E.R.** regime [4]. This involves the application of (**R**) rest, (**I**) ice, (**C**) compression, (**E**) elevation, and obtaining a (**R**) referral for appropriate medical treatment.

4.1.1.1.1. Strains and sprains

A patient with strain and/or sprain usually has pain and edema, a point of tenderness or burning sensation with or without ecchymosis. There may be a mild deformity of the injured joint in addition to complete or near complete loss of movement of joint; treatment consists of pain control, supportive strapping or bandaging, and immobilization by splinting so that affected muscle is in relaxed position. If injury is severe, R.I.C.E.R must be followed [9, 10].

Also, make sure to cover the following:

1. Reassure the patient.
2. Gently support the site.
3. Check circulation, motor, and sensation before and after splinting.
4. Apply ice pack.
5. Splint and immobilize injured limb.
6. Elevate injured limb.
7. Arrange for transport to appropriate care center.

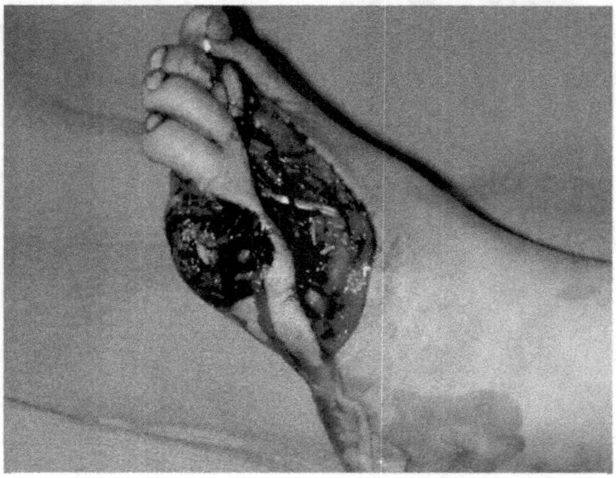

Figure 6. Open wound.

4.1.2. Open wounds

An injury in which the skin is interrupted or broken, exposing the tissues underneath (**Figure 6**) and can be divided into:

1. Abrasions: where the top layer of the skin is removed.
2. Lacerations: these are cuts of the skin with jagged edges.
3. Incisions: which are characterized by smooth edges and resemble a paper cut.
4. Punctures: usually deep, narrow wounds such as a stab wound from a nail or knife.
5. Avulsions: where a flap of skin is forcefully torn from its attachment.
6. Amputations: partial or full detachment of a limb or other appendage of the body which may be iatrogenic or due to trauma.

4.1.2.1. Management of open injuries

4.1.2.1.1. Abrasions

Also called "brush burns," "mat burns," and "road rash" in which some bleeding may result, but usually oozes from injured capillaries. Extremely painful because nerve endings are involved (**Figure 7**).

The management is usually so minimal requiring cleansing of the wound; small bandages may be applied but tactical situations will usually preclude applying field dressings that are needed for more serious injuries. A large amount of dirt may be ground into the wound; therefore, secondary treatment measures should focus on preventing or stopping infections.

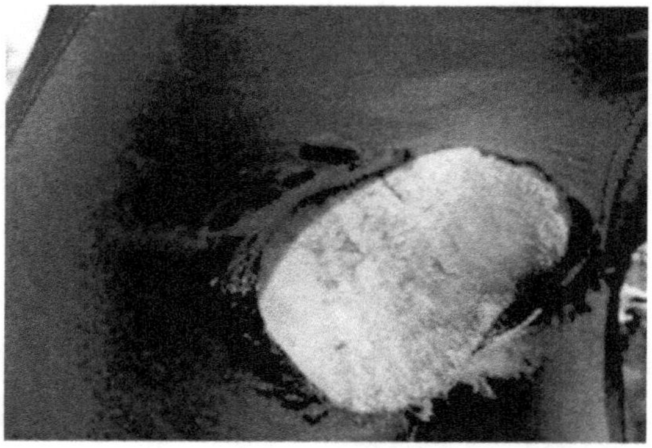

Figure 7. Abrasion post road accident.

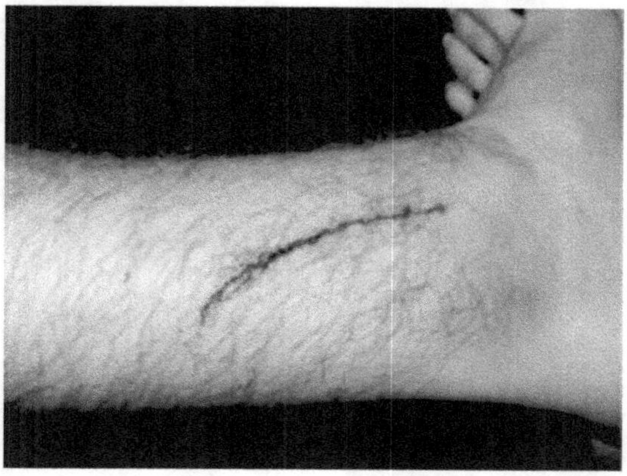

Figure 8. Simple laceration.

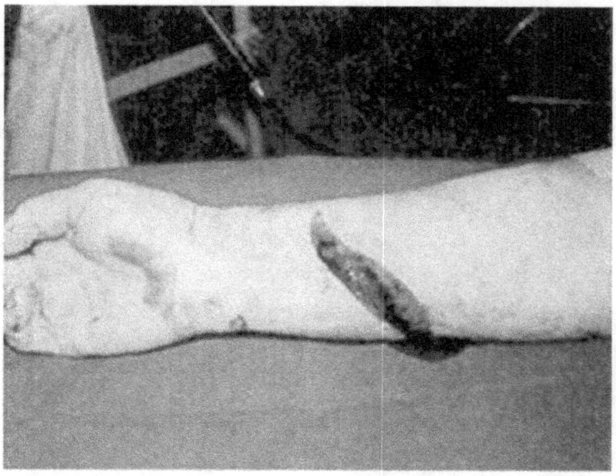

Figure 9. More severe laceration of the forearm.

4.1.2.1.2. Lacerations and incisions

May be smooth or jagged and can be caused by an object with a sharp edge (**Figures 8** and **9**) or may result from a severe blow or impact with a blunt object. Treatment is generally the same as for abrasions. It is very important to remember protecting yourself from disease by using medical gloves, wash or irrigate the injury with warm saline, remove all foreign bodies, control bleeding by applying local compression and dressing, start intravenous fluids when necessary (e.g., in cases of severe bleeding and possible hemodynamic compromise). Insure to keep the patient warm, elevate the injured part of the body. If major tendons and muscles are completely cut, immobilize the limb to prevent further damage.

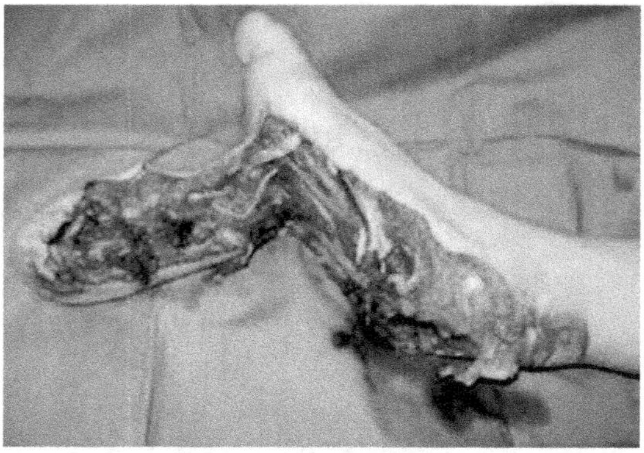

Figure 10. Avulsion.

4.1.2.1.3. Avulsions

These should be assessed carefully to rule out vascular and/or neurological injury (**Figure 10**). Bleeding should be controlled by direct pressure on the bleeding site; the avulsed part should be managed by applying several pressure dressings or an air splint and followed by regular dressing. Contamination should be avoided; ensure avulsed flap is lying flat and that it is aligned in its normal position. If the avulsed part is completely pulled off, make every effort to preserve it. Wrap that part in a saline or water-soaked field dressing, pack wrapped part in ice, and whenever possible be careful to avoid direct contact between the tissue and ice. Transport the avulsed part with the patient but keep it well-protected from further damage and out of view of the patient [4].

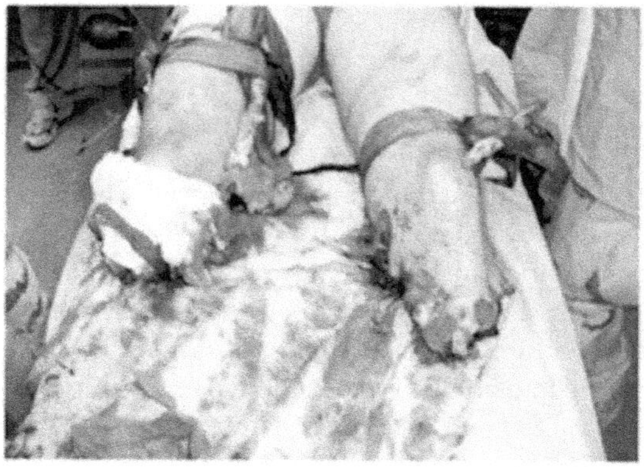

Figure 11. Severe bilateral amputation of the lower limbs.

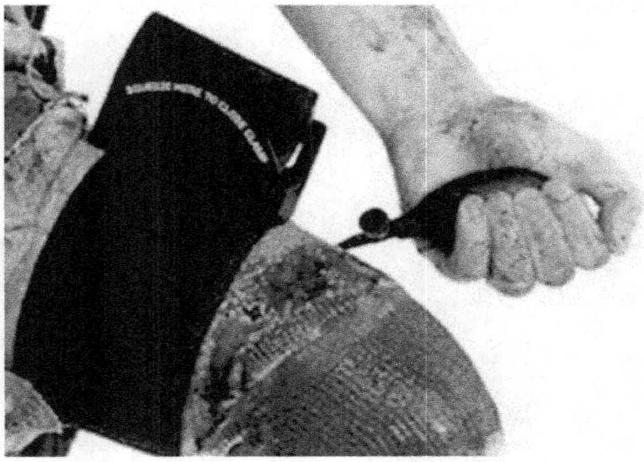

Figure 12. Pneumatic tourniquet in place.

4.1.2.1.4. Amputations

Amputation is a very traumatic event for the patient both physically and psychologically (**Figure 11**). With complete amputations, there is less bleeding than with partial or degloving cases. This is due to elastic nature of blood vessels as they are tended to spaz and retract into the surrounding tissue. It is very important to notice that replantation is performed only with an injury of isolated finger or extremity and should be performed by a skilled surgical team.

Treatment should always be started by ABCDE, which is the management of airway, breathing, circulation, disabilities, and environment in addition to warmth of the patient and control of hemorrhage by direct pressure or application of a tourniquet (**Figure 12**). If a tourniquet is applied, it must occlude arterial inflow, as occluding only venous system can increase bleeding. In severe cases where the patient's life might be at compromise, a tourniquet may remain in place for a prolonged period in order to save the patient's life. The physician must be able to make such decision and be aware that this choice is for life and against limb.

It is helpful to mark the patient's forehead with a "T" (indicating the time it was applied) using a marker to be able to track time of which the tourniquet was applied. Place the patient in shock position (head down, feet elevated). Continue the management by treatment of shock via IV fluids and/or blood transfusion, vasopressors if necessary, pain control, and continuous monitoring of the patient's vitals. Make every effort to preserve the amputated part and transfer the patient to the theater as soon as possible after stabilization of the ABCDE. Wrap the amputated part in a sterile dressing, place in ice and send with patient, and prevent direct contact between tissue and ice as possible [7].

4.2. Fracture and dislocation injuries

4.2.1. Fractures

A break in the continuity of bone which may result in partial or complete disruption of the bone. Fractures are further classified as open or closed.

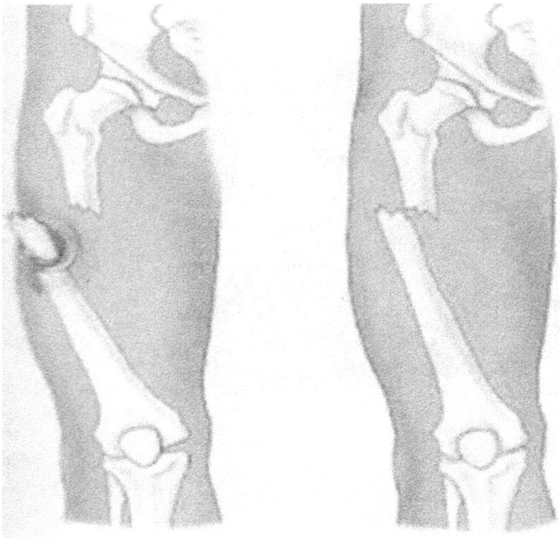

Figure 13. Open versus closed fracture.

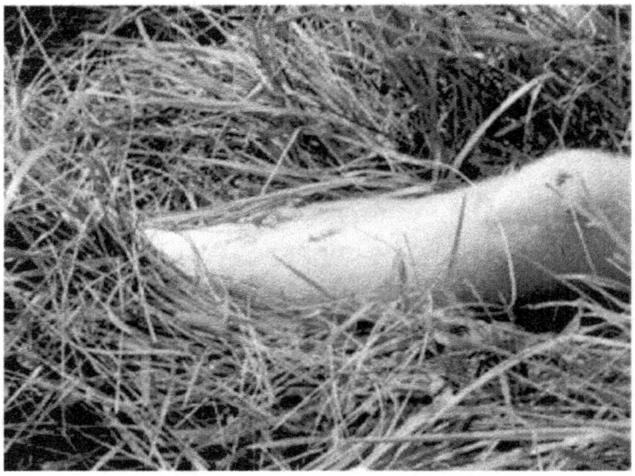

Figure 14. Inside-out open fracture.

Open fractures: in which there is a break through the overlying skin and connective tissue with exposure of the broken bone (**Figure 13**).

It can be **inside-out** (**Figure 14**) where the broken end of the bone breaks through or pierces the skin, or **outside-in** where the external force causes laceration and breaks the layers till the bone. The latter has a higher likelihood of contamination.

Closed fracture: the bone is broken with no skin penetration or connection with the exterior surface (**Figure 13**).

Alternative classification to fractures can be applied in relation to the size of the wound and causative force:

Type I: Small wound (<1 cm), usually clean; low energy.

Type II: Moderate wound (>1 cm), minimal soft tissue damage or loss; low energy.

Type III: Severe skin wound, with extensive soft tissue damage; high velocity impact.

4.2.1.1. Management of fractures

The following guidelines can be applied to any type of fracture, regardless of location:

- Treat as any case of trauma by starting management of airway, breathing, circulation, disabilities, and patients' environment (ABCDE).
- Control hemorrhage.
- Treatment for shock.
- Relieve pain (can include opioids).
- Treat any associated injuries and cover the injured area with sterile dressing.
- Check distal pulses before and after splinting.
- Immobilize the fracture using splints.
- Check pulse, motor, and sensation (PMS).
- Initiate IV antibiotics (usually broad-spectrum type to cover both Gram-positive and Gram-negative bacteria), in addition to tetanus prophylaxis.
- DO NOT re-place protruding bone or explore the wound nor clamp any vessel at the emergency setting and wait for the orthopedic physician.

In general, during clinical examination for suspected fractures, look for the following signs:

- Discoloration.
- Deformity.
- Edema.
- Crepitus.
- Point tenderness.
- Limited range of motion.
- Direct or indirect pain.
- Exposed bone fragments (open fractures).

- Any open wounds over or near a joint should be assumed to extend to the joint till proven otherwise.

Serious complications of open fractures are:

1. Soft tissue infection.
2. Osteomyelitis.
3. Gas gangrene.
4. Tetanus.
5. Crush syndrome.
6. Skin loss.
7. Malunion or Nonunion.

4.2.1.1.1. Splints and splinting

An appliance made of wood, metal, or plaster used for the fixation and protection of an injured part of the body aiming to:

- immobilize the injured body part.
- prevent further damage to muscles, nerves, or blood vessels caused by broken ends of bones.
- prevent a closed fracture from converting into an open fracture.
- decrease and control pain.

4.2.1.1.1.1. General rules for splinting

- Control hemorrhage. Direct pressure and/or pressure dressings will control virtually all external hemorrhage.
- Expose fracture site. Remove jewelry and watches.
- Before splinting, check for distal pulses.
- Splint in the position found unless limb is pulse-less.
- An attempt should be made to straighten a severely deformed limb with gentle traction only if there are no distal pulses, if resistance is felt, stop and splint as it lies.
- Move the fractured part as little as possible while applying the splint.

- DO NOT retract the exposed bone of an open fracture back into the body.
- Pad splint at bony prominence points (elbow, wrist, and ankle).
- Splint the joints above and below the fracture site.
- Reassess circulation and neurological status after splinting.

Common complications that can be seen with splinting include abrasions, sores, neurovascular compromise due to tight fitting splints, contact dermatitis, pressure ulcers, and thermal burns. Splints should be applied by skilled and trained professional, applied splint correctly followed by neurovascular status checkup.

4.2.1.1.1.2. Common types of splints

1. Volar short splint which is used for wrist fractures, fractures of the second to fifth metacarpal bones, carpal tunnel syndrome, and soft tissue injuries (**Figure 15**).
2. Finger splints which are used for phalangeal fractures (**Figure 16**).

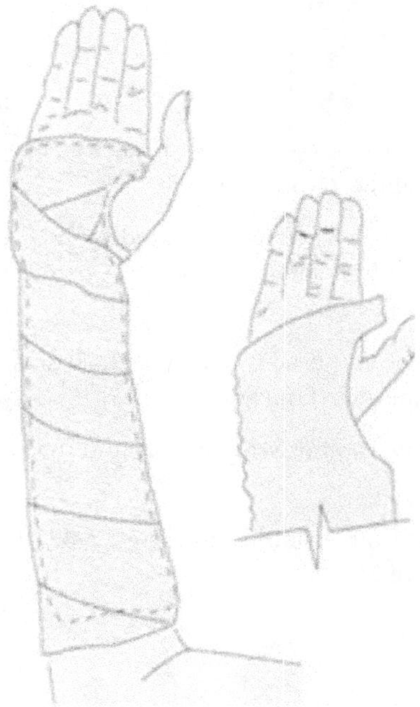

Figure 15.

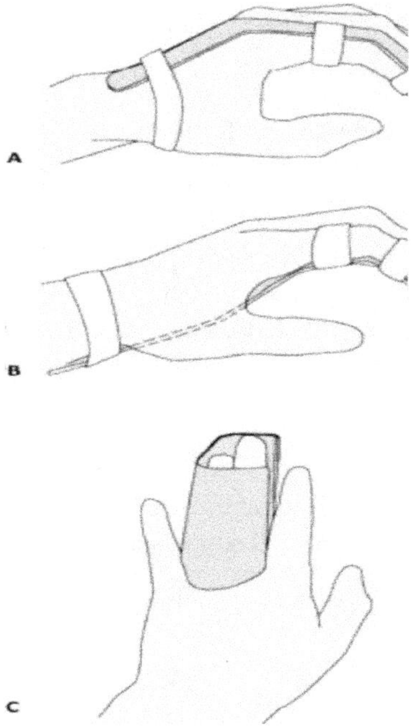

Figure 16.

3. Gutter splint which can be used for phalangeal fractures and metacarpal fractures; these are two types: radial and ulnar (**Figure 17**).
4. Buddy taping of toes used to secure the fractured toe to the adjacent one with adhesive strips; it is necessary to apply a small pad or sheet between toes to prevent maceration (**Figure 18**).
5. Thumb spica splint used for scaphoid fractures, extraarticular fractures of the thumb and ulnar collateral ligament injuries (**Figure 19**).
6. Stirrup splint is a below knee splint wrapping around the ankle to immobilize ankle fractures (**Figure 20**).
7. Posterior leg splint is used for distal leg fractures, ankle fractures, tarsal fractures, and metatarsal fractures (**Figure 21**).

4.2.2. Dislocations

A displacement of bone ends at the joints (**Figures 22–24**) resulting in an abnormal stretching of the ligaments around the joints. Also called luxation, occurs when there is an abnormal separation in the joint where two or more bones meet [9, 10]. Sometimes causes tearing or complete ligament separation; a partial dislocation is referred to as subluxation. They are easily recognized and diagnosed; the impact area may be swollen or look bruised with associated redness

http://dx.doi.org/10.5772/intechopen.81939

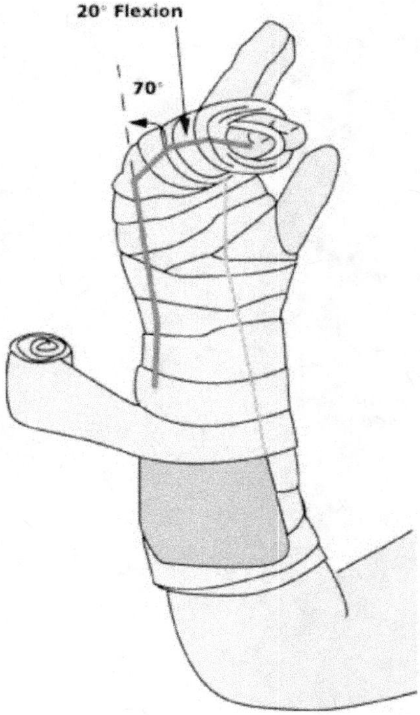

Figure 17.

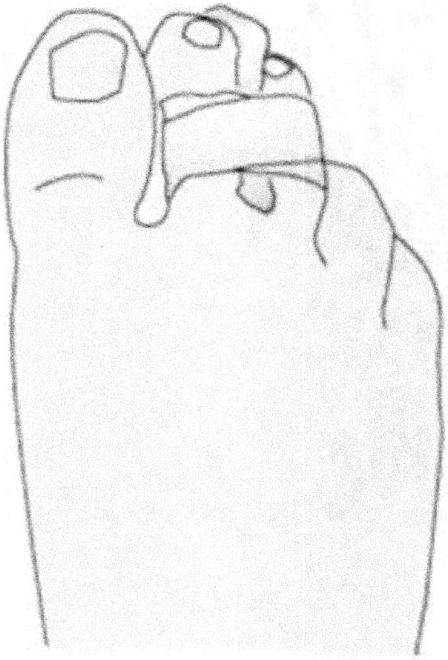

Figure 18.

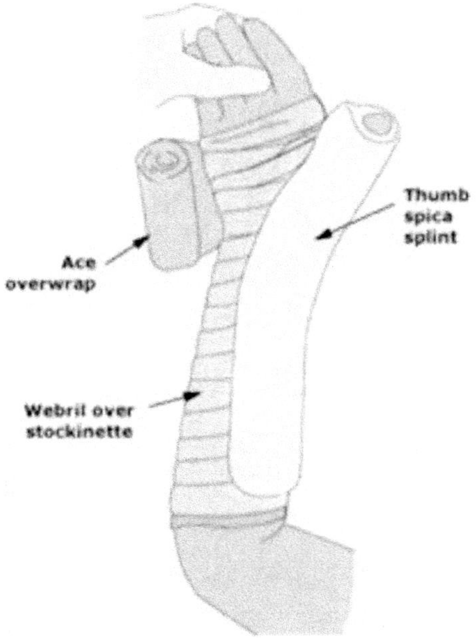

Figure 19.

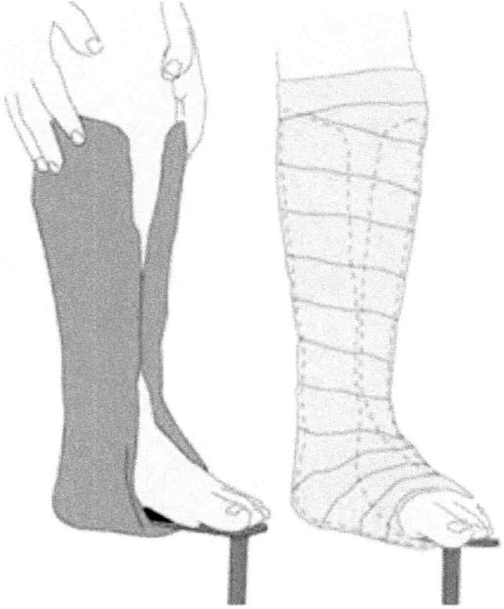

Figure 20.

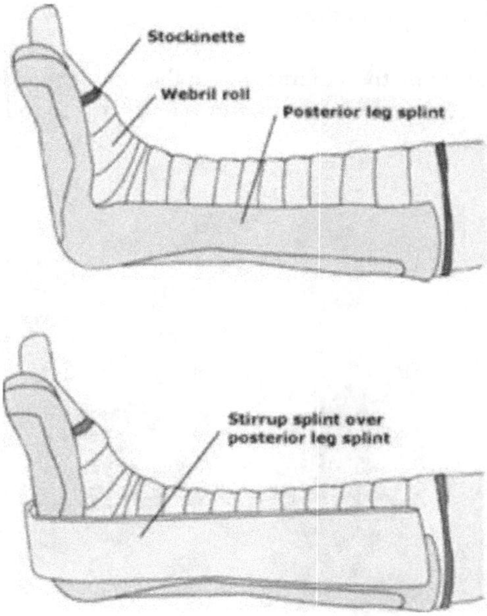

Figure 21.

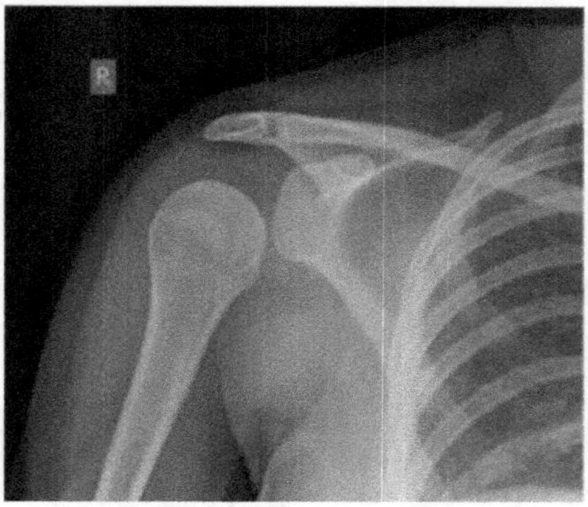

Figure 22. Posterior shoulder dislocation on X-ray.

or discoloration. It may also have a strange shape or be deformed as a result of the unexpected or unbalanced trauma. Some of the other symptoms associated with dislocated joints include:

1. Limited or lost motion.

2. Pain during movement.

3. Numbness around the area.

4. Paresthesia and tingling feeling in the limb.

X-ray is usually the preferred method of imaging in the emergency department, on occasion, special imaging such as an MRI may be required for diagnosis to roll out associated fractures or tear in muscles and ligaments.

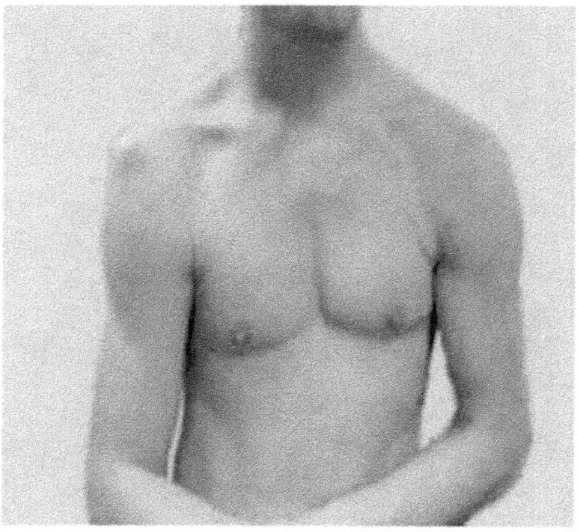

Figure 23. Shoulder dislocation.

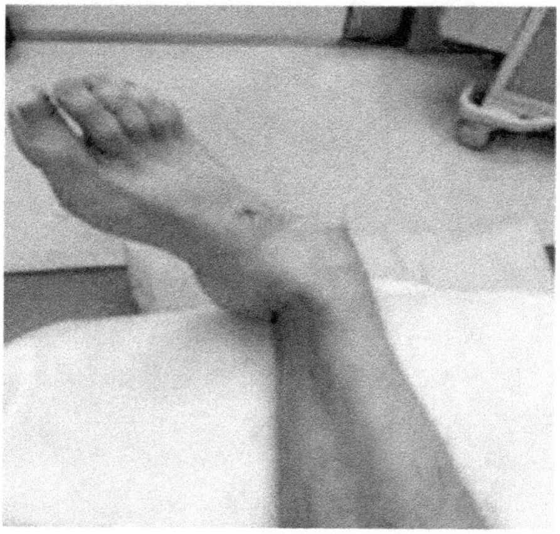

Figure 24. Ankle dislocation.

4.2.2.1. Management of dislocation

Treatment of dislocations and/or subluxations will depend on the site of joint; it may also depend on the severity of injury. According to Johns Hopkins University, initial treatment for any dislocation involves R.I.C.E: rest, ice, compression, and elevation. In some cases, the dislocated/subluxated joint might go back into place naturally after this treatment [11–13].

http://dx.doi.org/10.5772/intechopen.81939

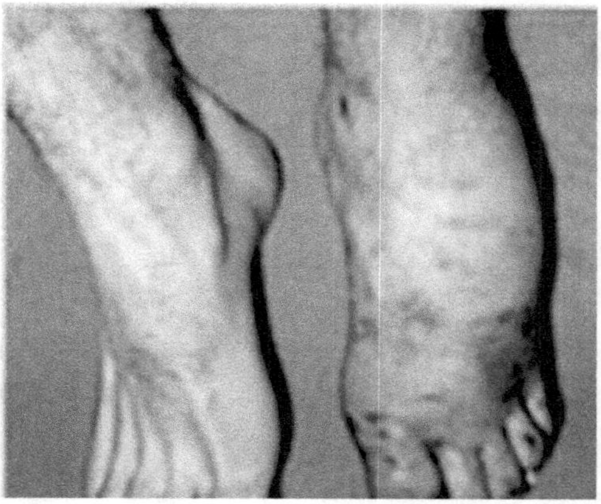

Figure 25. Acute compartment syndrome of the left foot.

If the joint does not return to normal naturally, treatment options should be one or more of the following:

1. Manipulation or repositioning (sedatives or anesthetics are necessary to keep the patient comfortable and also to allow muscles near to the injured joint to relax, which eases the procedure).
2. Immobilization (a sling, splint, or cast for several weeks to prevent recurrence).
3. Medication (a pain reliever or a muscle relaxant).
4. Rehabilitation (to increase the joint's strength and restore its range of motion).
5. Surgery is usually indicated only if there are damaged nerves or blood vessels, or if the doctor is unable to return bones to their anatomical position. Surgery may also be necessary for those who often dislocate the same joints, such as recurrent shoulder dislocations.

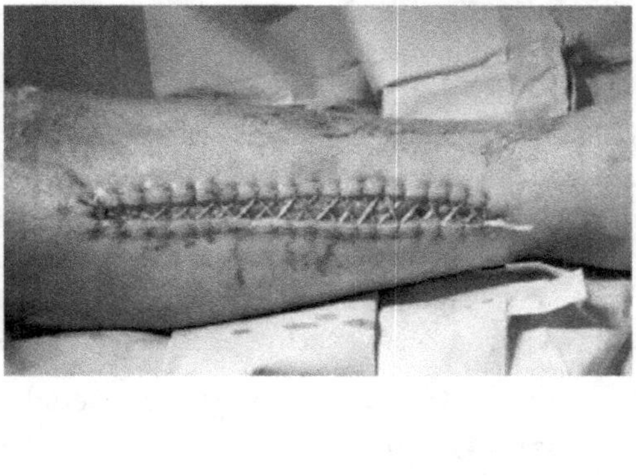

Figure 26. Fasciotomy.

5. Complications of musculoskeletal injury

5.1. Acute compartment syndrome (ACS)

A prolonged elevation of interstitial tissue pressure within an enclosed fascial compartment leading to impaired tissue perfusion and damage. Associated with increased vessel permeability and plasma leak into the intercellular space causing further pressure on muscles and nerves (**Figure 25**); it might result in death if not treated before 8–12 h [14–18].

This serious and critical musculoskeletal complication can be caused by direct blow or contusion, crush injury, burns, snake bites, fractures, hematoma, and prolonged pressure from splinting.

It is characterized by severe pain especially with stretching, tense compartment, tight and shiny skin. Late findings can be paresthesia, loss of pulses, and pain out of proportion.

5.1.1. Management of ACS

Treatment of ACS is urgent surgical exploration with fasciotomy (**Figure 26**).

It should be noted that any case with prolonged ACS of more than 8–12 h can have permanent deformity and limb viability may possibly be lost.

During management, every effort should be used to release all compartments; the main focus is on reducing the dangerous pressure in the body compartment. Dressings, casts, or splints that are constricting the affected body part must be removed. Early recognition and diagnosis, pain control, keeping the body part with ACS below the level of the heart (to improve blood flow into the compartment), treatment of shock, prevention of metabolic acidosis and acute kidney injury (AKI) are all mandatory and crucial to save the patient limb [18–20].

6. Conclusion

The incidence and socioeconomic impact of musculoskeletal diseases globally is increasing due to multiple factors. Prevention of these injuries can be achieved by providing an environment in which the worker has a safe surrounding, improved awareness about what possible danger injuries might occur, a clear path to elevation of such danger in the time of need. Occupational safety measures should always be optimal with nearby kits to aid in on-site management. With the increased demand for building and aiming to touch the clouds with sky-high skyscrapers comes great responsibility to care more about providing a healthy working environment. The frequency of musculoskeletal injury and its concomitant burden on the healthcare system is expected to increase greatly in the coming decades. Physicians are required to keep up with this leap. A well-established basic knowledge of such injuries is very crucial and can be lifesaving and cost-effective especially in the emergency department.

The previous injuries we discussed are not by any chance everything in the musculoskeletal system; we chose the most common and the most essential ones, discussed briefly. We strongly encourage every physician to take this chapter and consider it as a base and build upon it with further reading and practice.

Author details

Ahmad Subhy Alsheikhly[1]* and Mazin Subhy Alsheikhly[2]

*Address all correspondence to: ahmadmomz@yahoo.com

1 Weill Cornell Medical College, Qatar

2 Hamad Medical Corporation, Doha, Qatar

References

[1] Rogers F. Musculoskeletal System [Internet]. National Library of Medicine. PubMed Health. 2017 [cited May 13, 2017]. Available from: https://www.ncbi.nlm.nih.gov/pubmedhealth/PMHT0027058/

[2] Marieb E. Human Anatomy & Physiology. 3rd ed. Redwood City: Benjamin Cummings; 1995

[3] Villa-Forte A. Muscles—Bone, Joint, and Muscle Disorders [Internet]. MSD Manual Consumer Version. 2018 [cited June 14, 2018]. Available from: https://www.merckmanuals.com/home/bone-joint-and-muscle-disorders/biology-of-the-musculoskeletal-system/muscles

[4] Beekley A, Starnes B, Sebesta J. Lessons learned from modern military surgery. Surgical Clinics of North America. 2007;**87**(1):157-184

[5] Mammal Anatomy. New York: Marshall Cavendish Corporation; 2010

[6] Buschmann J, Bürgisser G. Biomechanics of Tendons and Ligaments. Duxford: Matthew Deans; 6 February 2017. pp. 1-22

[7] King RB et al. Evaluation of possible tourniquet systems for use in the Canadian forces. The Journal of Trauma. 2006;**60**(5):1061-1071

[8] Brumitt J, Cuddeford T. Current concepts of muscle and tendon adaptation to strength and conditioning. International Journal of Sports Physical Therapy. 2015;**10**(6):748-759

[9] Warby SA et al. The effect of exercise-based management for multidirectional instability of the glenohumeral joint: A systematic review. Journal of Shoulder and Elbow Surgery. 2014;**23**(1):128-142

[10] Doherty C, Bleakley C, Delahunt E, Holden S. Treatment and prevention of acute and recurrent ankle sprain: An overview of systematic reviews with meta-analysis. British Journal of Sports Medicine. 2017;**51**:113

[11] Simon R, Sherman S, Koenigsknecht S. Emergency Orthopedics: The Extremities. 5th ed. New York: McGraw-Hill; 2006

[12] Schaider J, Simon RR. Clinical Practice of Emergency Medicine. Philadelphia: Lippincott Williams & Wilkins; 2005. p. 1033

[13] Agel J, Rockwood T, Barber R, Marsh J. Potential predictive ability of the orthopedic trauma association open fracture classification. Journal of Orthopaedic Trauma. 2014;**28**(5):300-306

[14] Bagley C, Hunter A, Bacarese-Hamilton I. Patients' misunderstanding of common orthopedic terminology: The need for clarity. Annals of the Royal College of Surgeons of England. 2011;**93**(5):401-404

[15] Chudnofsky C, Byers S. Splinting techniques. In: Roberts J, Hedges J, Chanmugam A, editors. Clinical Procedures in Emergency Medicine. 4th ed. Philadelphia, Pa: Saunders; 2004. p. 989

[16] Boyd AS et al. Principles of Casting and Splinting [Internet]. PubMed-NCBI. Ncbi.nlm.nih.gov. 2018 [cited May 14, 2017]. Available from: https://www.ncbi.nlm.nih.gov/pubmed/19145960

[17] Crespo A, Manoli A, Konda S, Egol K. Development of Compartment Syndrome Negatively Impacts Length of Stay and Cost After Tibia Fracture [Internet]. pubmed. 2018 [cited July 28, 2017]. Available from: https://www.ncbi.nlm.nih.gov/pubmed/25463427

[18] Alessio Giai Via N. Acute Compartment Syndrome [Internet]. PubMed Central (PMC). 2015. Available at: https://www.ncbi.nlm.nih.gov/pmc/articles/PMC4396671/ [Accessed: July 25, 2017]

[19] Dries D. Trauma manual: Trauma and acute care surgery, 3rd edition. Journal of the American College of Surgeons. 2008;**206**(5):200-208

[20] Frink M, Hildebrand F, Krettek C, Brand J, Hankemeier S. Compartment syndrome of the lower leg and foot. Clinical Orthopaedics and Related Research. 2009;**468**(4):940-950

Chapter 9

Systematic Approach to Acute Cardiovascular Emergencies

Shahzad Anjum

Additional information is available at the end of the chapter

http://dx.doi.org/10.5772/intechopen.74682

Abstract

Cardiovascular emergencies and symptoms are one of the most common reasons for patients' attendance in any emergency department (ED). Symptoms are either related to true cardiovascular problems or mimic cardiovascular problems. It becomes very difficult at times to differentiate between them. Many symptoms which mimic the cardiovascular problem may be present due to other systems' involvement. So, there may be an atypical presentation of cardiovascular emergencies or atypical presentation of other system problems presenting as cardiovascular diseases. Missing true cardiovascular emergencies can be a reason for mortality and morbidity cases which puts burden on healthcare services and affects physicians' morale. Here, in this chapter, we will discuss common cardiovascular emergencies and their presentations and approach to deal with them. We will also discuss differential diagnosis, when dealing with such conditions. We will also discuss the best diagnostic modalities and disposition plans which will ensure patient safety.

Keywords: cardiovascular emergencies, approach to common CVS symptoms in ED, approach to CVS emergencies

1. Introduction

Cardiovascular emergencies are one of the most common and serious emergencies presenting to the emergency department. They are notorious in a sense that the signs and symptoms are seen in a huge spectrum of diseases, where some differentials are so benign that they do not require any further investigation. On the other hand, they may present with such vague symptoms that physicians may miss the diagnosis if they do not have a high index of suspicion. Here, in this chapter, we will discuss all the signs and symptoms which any patient with a cardiovascular problem may present. I will also discuss the approach to deal with these symptoms and how to manage them and finally dispose them.

2. Common signs and symptoms in cardiovascular emergencies

The cardiovascular emergencies can present with typical or atypical signs and symptoms. Some patients have so minor complaints that they can be missed if physicians do not have a high index of suspicion. While examining a patient, it is important to have a wide range of differentials in mind. Emergency physicians should examine a patient to pick up signs or symptoms related to cardiovascular emergencies—complications directly or indirectly related to cardiovascular emergencies or signs and symptoms related to underlying diseases which manifest as acute cardiovascular problems at the time of presentation in the emergency department. Physicians with depth of medical knowledge, good skills of history taking and examination will less likely miss serious cardiovascular emergencies.

Following are the signs and symptoms which may indicate cardiovascular problems and need to be evaluated with a high index of suspicion in the emergency department.

A. Typical cardiovascular symptomatology

1. Chest symptoms (chest pain, chest tightness or pressure-like symptoms, discomfort)
2. Breathlessness (orthopnea, paroxysmal nocturnal dyspnea, exertional breathlessness)
3. Palpitation
4. Sweating
5. Pedal edema or generalized edema

B. Atypical symptomatology:

Diagnosis becomes challenging when patients present with atypical symptoms [1]:

1. Pain in the neck, jaw, throat or arm (ischemic pain)
2. Pain in abdomen (related to heart failure/liver congestion or ischemia)
3. Pain or numbness in the leg or cold extremities (related to poor circulation associated with vascular problems or poor cardiac output)
4. Dyspepsia
5. Light headedness or dizziness
6. Pain at the back (ischemia)
7. Fainting (Syncope) or near fainting
8. Fatigability and tiredness
9. Cardiac asthma (cough)

http://dx.doi.org/10.5772/intechopen.74682

C. Important signs of cardiovascular emergencies or problems

1. Hypotension
2. Postural drop
3. Raised jugular venous pressure (JVP)
4. Cyanosis
5. Basal crepitation
6. Muffled/added heart sounds and murmurs
7. Pericardial rub
8. Decreased breath sound
9. Abdominal distension
10. Pedal edema
11. Splinter hemorrhages
12. Osler nodes

D. Signs related to valvular heart diseases

a. Aortic regurgitation signs:

1. Corrigan's pulse
2. De Musset's sign
3. Quincke's sign
4. Traube's sign
5. Duroziez's sign
6. Landolfi's sign
7. Becker's sign
8. Müller's sign

b. Mitral stenosis:

1. Heart failure symptoms, such as dyspnea on exertion, orthopnea and paroxysmal nocturnal dyspnea (PND)
2. Thromboembolism in later stages when the left atrial volume is increased
3. Palpitations
4. Hemoptysis
5. Chest pain

c. Mitral regurgitation:

1. Dyspnea
2. Fatigue
3. Orthopnea
4. Pulmonary edema

d. Infective endocarditis: signs and symptoms of infective endocarditis

E. Signs related to complications of cardiovascular diseases (infective endocarditis)

1. Seizures
2. Stroke
3. Pulmonary embolism
4. Cor pulmonale
5. Kidney damage
6. Enlarged spleen
7. Dissociated abscesses
8. Tender spleen
9. Janeway lesions
10. Petechiae
11. Osler nodes
12. Hematuria

3. Systematic approach to cardiovascular symptoms

3.1. Approach to chest pain in the emergency department

Chest pain is one of the most common symptoms which patients present with in the emergency department. The wide range of differentials and the severity of the consequences of missing serious causes of chest pain and fear of litigation put pressure on physicians to request a wide range of investigations to discharge the patient safely. The lack of confidence in decision-making and unnecessary referrals to other subspecialties are the reasons for delayed disposition, thus adding to the length of stay in the emergency department. In this section we will discuss in detail the common differentials of chest pain in the emergency department and how to investigate and dispose each patient timely and appropriately.

http://dx.doi.org/10.5772/intechopen.74682

3.1.1. Differential diagnosis of atraumatic chest pain

Chest pain is a symptom which could be due to a very serious underlying condition that may be life threatening, or it may be due to very benign condition [2, 3]. Here is the list of conditions which needs to be considered in patients presenting with chest pain [2] **Table 1**.

3.1.2. History taking

The most important key to diagnose serious medical conditions in the emergency department is the accurate history and examination. While taking history, all the important question

Critical diagnosis	Emergent diagnosis
CVS: **1.** Acute MI **2.** Acute Coronary Ischemia **3.** Aortic Dissection **4.** Cardiac Tamponade Pulmonary: **1.** Tension Pneumothorax **2.** Pulmonary Embolism Gastrointestinal: **1.** Boerhaave (Esophageal Rupture)	CVS: **1.** Unstable Angina **2.** Coronary Spasm **3.** Prinzemetal Angina **4.** Cocaine induced Pericarditis/Myocarditis Respiratory: **1.** Mediastinitis **2.** Pneumothorax Gastrointestinal: **1.** Mallory Weiss **2.** Cholecystitis **3.** Pancreatitis
Non-emergent diagnosis Cardiac: **1.** Mitral Valve Prolapse **2.** Valvular Heart Diseases **3.** Aortic stenosis **4.** Hypertrophic cardiomyopathy Pulmonary: **1.** Pneumonia **2.** Pleurisy **3.** Tumor **4.** Pneumomediastinum Gastrointestinal: **1.** Esophageal spasm **2.** Esophageal Reflux **3.** Peptic ulcer disease **4.** Biliary Colic /Musculoskeletal: **1.** Muscle strain **2.** Rib Fracture **3.** Arthritis **4.** Costochondritis **5.** Tumor **6.** Non-Specific pain Neurologic: **1.** Spinal Root Compression **2.** Thoracic outlet **3.** Herpes Zoster **4.** Post herpetic neuralgia	

Table 1. Differential diagnosis of atraumatic chest pain.

should be asked which may help in ruling in or out the important differentials. The important questions to be asked while taking history are:

1. Onset of pain: Sudden onset of severe chest pain may indicate conditions like pneumothorax or aortic dissection. Pain associated with meals may indicate gastrointestinal cause. Cardiac chest pain may occur with exertion or even at rest without any physical activity.

2. Character of pain: The character of pain may give some clue about the underlying condition although a large number of patients with ischemic cause may have non-specific chest pain which may mimic other conditions like dyspepsia. Patients with burning type of chest pain or indigestion may give the impression of gastrointestinal cause but it may be due to cardiac ischemia explaining visceral etiology of pain. Patients with ischemic cardiac disease may have crushing or squeezing chest pain or pressure-like symptoms. Aortic dissection may induce tearing chest pain which migrate from front to back or back to front. Sharp stabbing pain which may increase with breathing may be due to either musculoskeletal cause or pulmonary cause.

3. Severity of pain: The severity of pain may not be linked to severity of underlying diagnosis. Sometimes, peptic ulcer disease may present with a severe type of chest pain mimicking cardiac pain. Patients with ischemic heart disease may present with very vague or mild symptoms. Patients with dissection of aorta may present with severe tearing chest pain.

4. Duration of pain: Pain which is for few days with no change in character is unlikely to be due to cardiac ischemia. Anginal pain is usually less than 30 min in duration whereas pain of myocardial infarction (MI) stays more than 30 min. Pain which stays from few seconds to minutes is unlikely to be cardiac in origin.

5. Associated symptoms: Cardiac chest pain may have associated symptoms like breathlessness, cough, palpitation, sweating and loss of energy and asthenia. Pulmonary embolism or pneumothorax may also present with chest pain, breathlessness and sweating, thus mimicking ischemic cardiac pain. Patients may have a fainting episode or syncope and near syncope before the onset of symptoms. Patients may present with some secondary conditions like road traffic accident or altered sensorium due to the underlying cardiac insult. Nausea and vomiting may be seen with cardiovascular and gastrointestinal causes of chest pain.

6. Radiation of pain: Pain in the chest which radiates to the back may indicate aortic dissection or gastrointestinal causes like perforation, pancreatitis and posterior peptic ulcer. Cardiac chest pain may radiate to the neck, jaw and arm.

7. Location of pain: Pain which is localized and involves a small area is unlikely related to any visceral cause and is due to somatic nerves. Pain involving periphery of the chest is usually due to a pulmonary cause whereas cardiac chest pain is usually in the lower chest or upper abdomen. Gastrointestinal conditions may have the similar area of distribution as cardiac. Cardiac chest pain though is usually in the left precordial area but may also be in right-sided chest.

8. Aggravating or relieving factors: Pain at exertion indicates ischemic coronary syndrome whereas pain at rest indicates conditions like dyspepsia and neuropathic pain.

Musculoskeletal and pulmonary causes of chest pain aggravate with breathing and chest movements.

9. Risk factors: Patients with risk factors like diabetes mellitus, hypertension, smoking, hyperlipidemia, a strong family history of ischemic heart disease, ethnicity and age above 40 years, but patients with no risk factors are not immune to ischemic cardiac disease. The presence of risk factors is the indicator to be more vigilant and careful in discharging patients.

10. Young patients with ischemic character of chest pain: Young patients when having ischemic type of chest pain present a clue to look at the conditions like vasculitis and connective tissue disorders and substance and drug abuse like cocaine.

3.1.3. Examination

Detailed physical examination can give some clue to diagnose the underlying cause. Examination includes general physical examination, abnormalities in vital signs and presence of other signs which may be related to cardiac pathology or complication of ischemic heart disease or an underlying medical condition which is the reason to present as ischemic heart disease. These signs help in the diagnosis of underlying cardiac or other problems. Following are some important findings which must be looked at to diagnose the cause of chest pain.

1. Tachycardia: Presence of tachycardia indicates serious underlying medical conditions. Following are the conditions which cause tachycardia:

MI or coronary ischemia	Cholecystitis
Myocarditis/pericarditis	Diabetic ketoacidosis
Aortic dissection	Pulmonary embolism
Tension pneumothorax	Esophageal rupture
	Mallory Weiss

2. Bradycardia: Bradycardia is a complication of ischemic cardiac problems and is related to heart blocks. It may be seen in

Acute MI	Coronary ischemia	Unstable angina

3. Hypertension: Hypertension may be seen as a stress response to acute cardiac ischemia or it may be the reason to present as acute heart failure or chest pain. Hypertension is seen in conditions like

Acute MI	Coronary ischemia	Aortic dissection

4. Hypotension: Hypotension may be seen as a complication of cardiovascular emergencies. Patient may also present with low BP in conditionwhich mimic cardiovascular emergencies

Severe massive MI	Coronary ischemia
Heart failure	Tension pneumothorax
Aortic dissection	PE
Myocarditis/pericarditis	Esophageal rupture

5. Hypoxemia: Hypoxemia may be seen in acute cardiovascular emergencies or conditions mimicking cardiac emergencies

Heart failure/pulmonary edema	PE
Pneumothorax	Massive effusion

6. Fever: Presence of fever with other serious symptoms like chest pain or breathlessness usually indicates medical emergencies related to other systems. Following are the conditions where fever may be present with other complaints

Myocarditis/pericarditis	Cholecystitis
Mediastinitis	Esophageal rupture
PE	

7. Sweating or diaphoresis: Sweating is an autonomic response to many medical emergencies. It is non-specific symptom or sign but may indicate seriousness of the underlying problem so it must be given importance when present. Following are the differentials which must be considered in a patient presenting with diaphoresis with chest pain or breathlessness.

    - Acute MI
    - Aortic dissection
    - Coronary ischemia
    - Unstable angina
    - PE
    - Cholecystitis
    - Peptic ulcer
    - Esophageal rupture

8. Respiratory distress: Respiratory distress is one of the indications of serious underlying medical problems. Patients who are tachypneic or distressed at presentation in the emergency department should be prioritized and treated. Following are the serious underlying conditions which present with respiratory distress.

    a. Acute MI

    b. PE

http://dx.doi.org/10.5772/intechopen.74682

c. Heart failure/pulmonary edema

d. Tension pneumothorax/simple pneumothorax

9. Cardiovascular system (CVS) examination: When examining CVS, all the differential diagnosis must be kept in mind to elaborate the findings related to these conditions. Each condition may have specific findings which help in reaching diagnosis. The following cardiovascular conditions or conditions which mimic cardiovascular problems must be kept in mind when examining CVS.

   BP difference in upper and lower extremity: Aortic dissection.

   Narrow pulse pressure: Pericarditis with effusion.

   New murmur: Seen in

   a. Acute MI

   b. Coronary ischemia

   c. Aortic dissection

   Gallop (S3/S4)

   a. Acute MI

   b. Coronary ischemia

   Pericardial rub: Pericarditis.

   Raised JVP:

   a. Acute MI

   b. Coronary ischemia

   c. Pericarditis

   d. Tension pneumothorax

   e. PE

10. Respiratory examination: Respiratory system examination is one of the most important examinations in the cardiovascular emergencies as many pulmonary pathologies mimic serious cardiovascular problems, and sometimes differentiating them from cardiac problems is not that easy and needs sophisticated investigations like CT scan in contrast with V/Q scans. Following are the important pulmonary signs which indicate respiratory pathologies mimicking cardiovascular emergencies.

    Unilateral decreased or absent breath sounds:

    - Tension pneumothorax/pneumothorax

    Pleural rub: Pulmonary embolism.

Crepitation:

a. Acute myocardial infarction

b. Coronary ischemia

c. Unstable angina

d. Pneumonia

Subcutaneous emphysema:

a. Tension pneumothorax

b. Simple pneumothorax

c. Esophageal rupture

d. Mediastinitis

Wheezes

- Asthma
- Cardiac asthma

11. Abdominal examination: Many abdominal conditions may mimic cardiovascular emergencies. Sometimes it is difficult to exclude them on the basis of history and examination alone. When examining the abdomen, following signs need to be looked at which indicate abdominal conditions mimicking cardiovascular emergencies.

Epigastric tenderness:

- Esophageal rupture
- Mallory Weiss syndrome
- Cholecystitis
- Pancreatitis

Left upper-quadrant tenderness: Pancreatitis.

Right upper-quadrant tenderness: Cholecystitis.

12. Neurologic examination: Cardiovascular emergencies may have a very atypical presentation when it's a true diagnostic dilemma in the emergency department. Following are the atypical neurological presentations of underlying serious cardiovascular emergencies

Focal neurological findings: Aortic dissection.

Stroke:

- Acute MI
- Coronary ischemia

http://dx.doi.org/10.5772/intechopen.74682

- Aortic dissection
- Coronary spasm

13. Findings of DVT in extremity: PE

3.1.4. Investigations

Patients presenting with chest pain should be investigated for serious underlying medical causes as delay in diagnosis may be catastrophic in many conditions. Following are the important tests needed to diagnose important medical emergencies.

Positive cardiac markers: They give information about myocardial infarction.

ECG

ECG: ECG is the most important bed-side investigations which should be ordered for any patient who comes to the emergency department with chest pain and pain involving lower chest, upper abdomen, neck, arm and jaw in a risky age group. It should be done in the earliest possible (within 10 min of arrival to the emergency department). Delaying in getting ECG done will delay the diagnosis which may result in serious consequences in conditions like acute MI.

Following are the conditions which may have findings on ECG

- Acute MI
- Coronary ischemia
- Coronary spasm
- Aortic dissection
- PE
- Pericarditis/myocarditis
- Arrhythmia

CXR: Chest X-Ray is one of the simplest diagnostic modalities which may give important clues to patients with chest pain and or breathlessness. It may give information about heart, lungs and mediastinum and abdominal and diaphragmatic problems. It is easily available in hospitals and one should have a low threshold in requesting for them if the cause of chest pain and breathlessness is not clear or justified. Following are the conditions which can be seen on CXR.

- Pneumothorax
- Tension pneumothorax
- Pleural effusion (lung and heart pathologies, esophageal rupture)
- Cardiomegaly (CCF, pericardial effusion)
- Pneumomediastinum (esophageal rupture, mediastinitis)

- Widening of mediastinum (aortic dissection)
- Lung masses (malignancies)
- Diaphragmatic problems (paralysis, hernia)

ABG: Arterial blood gases help in diagnosing the cardiac and lung pathologies indirectly by indicating the CO, oxygen, HCO3 levels, PH and A-a gradient. Hypoxemia and A-a gradient may indicate PE. ABG gives information about type 1 and type 2 respiratory failure as well.

Echocardiography: Echocardiography is one of the quickest and easily available modalities in many tertiary care centers where even the ER physicians are experts in using this modality and can get information about patient's conditions [4]. Echocardiography is now one of the most important diagnostic tools in modern emergency medicine practice. Following important information can be taken by using bed-side echo.

- Pericardial effusion
- Wall-motion abnormality
- RV strain
- Dilated right ventricle
- Ejection fraction
- Septal abnormality
- Hypertrophied ventricles and septum
- Valvular problems
- Aortic problems
- IVC
- Left ventricular outflow tract obstruction
- Cardiac masses and thrombi

V/Q scan: V/Q scans are helpful in places where CT scans are not widely available or where due to some reasons CT scans cannot be done or are harmful. V/Q scans help in diagnosing PE.

Spiral CT: Spiral CT helps in diagnosing pulmonary embolism but also gives information about other pulmonary conditions and pathologies which may be the reason for these symptoms.

CT angiography: Computed tomography angiography (CTA) uses an injection of iodine-rich contrast material and CT scan to help diagnose and evaluate blood vessel diseases or related conditions, such as aneurysms or blockage.

Ultrasonography: Ultrasound is a rapidly available important diagnostic tool in many tertiary care centers and is getting more popular in emergency medicine practice. Emergency medicine physicians can use this tool to get important information about many medical conditions and thus can take timely decisions. Following information can be taken by using bed-side ultrasound.

- Pleural effusion and pericardial effusion
- Congestive hepatomegaly
- Inferior vena cava and hydration status
- Pneumothorax
- Pneumonias
- Cholelithiasis, cholecystitis and common bile duct

3.1.5. Management

After taking proper history and doing a detailed examination, the differential diagnosis will be narrowed down. Use of appropriate investigation will help the emergency physician to reach to some conclusion. Serious conditions like tension pneumothorax, pulmonary embolism and acute coronary syndrome need quick attention and referrals to subspecialty for timely management. Each condition has its own management plan which will be discussed later in this chapter.

3.1.6. Disposition

Timely patient disposition is the key to success. Patients presenting with acute coronary syndrome (ACS) and acute myocardial infarction should have timely referral to cardiology for possible early PCI. Patients with moderate to high risk of acute coronary syndrome should be admitted to cardiology care even if the initial labs are normal. Patients with low risk can be discharged with early follow up in the cardiology department. Normal ECG or absence of positive cardiac enzymes is not the criteria to discharge any patient with chest pain who falls in the category of moderate or high risk.

3.2. Approach to breathlessness in the emergency department

Breathlessness is also one of the symptoms which has serious differential diagnosis, which, if not diagnosed and managed timely, can lead to grave consequences. Chest pain and breathlessness are the two serious symptoms which may be due to benign conditions and may be due to serious underlying problems which can lead to death from minutes to hours. Good medical knowledge, anticipation of problems, art of taking good medical history and doing detailed physical examination, choosing the right and appropriate investigation and timely and appropriate disposition help in saving life.

3.2.1. Differential diagnosis of breathlessness

Breathlessness is one of the serious symptoms and should be given due care before we find out the reason for this symptom. Timely patients triaging and intervention is needed to deal with this symptom. Breathlessness may be due to simple problems like anxiety and pregnancy, and it may be related to severe life-threatening conditions like tension pneumothorax. Here we will discuss important differential diagnosis of breathlessness based on the severity of underlying pathology (**Table 2**).

3.2.2. History taking

The most important key to diagnose serious medical conditions in the emergency department is proper history and examination. While taking history, all the important questions should be

Critical diagnosis	**Emergent diagnosis**
CVS:	CVS:
1. Acute MI	**1.** Pericarditis
2. Pulmonary Edema	**2.** Myocarditis
3. Cardiac Tamponade	Respiratory:
Respiratory:	**1.** Pneumothorax
1. Tension Pneumothorax	**2.** Hemothorax
2. Epiglottitis	**3.** Asthma
3. Anaphylaxis	**4.** Pneumonia
4. Ventilatory Failure	**5.** Aspiration
5. Airway Obstruction	**6.** Cor Pulmonale
6. PE	Neuromuscular:
7. Flail Chest	**1.** Multiple Sclerosis
Metabolic/Endocrine:	**2.** Guillian Barre
1. Toxic Ingestion	**3.** Myasthenia Gravis
2. DKA	**4.** Tick Paralysis
Neuromuscular:	Increased Respiratory Effort:
1. CVA	**1.** Mechanical Interference
2. Intracranial Insult	**2.** Hypotension
3. Organophosphate Poisoning	**3.** Bowel Obstruction
Miscellaneous:	**4.** Renal Failure
1. CO Poisoning	**5.** Electrolyte Abnormalities
2. Acute Chest Syndrome	**6.** Metabolic Acidosis
	7. Diaphragmatic Rupture
	8. Anemia
Non-emergent diagnosis:	
Cardiac: Metabolic/Endocrine:	
1. Congenital Heart Disease 1. Thyroid	
2. Cardiomyopathy 2. Fever	
3. Valvular Heart Disease	
Pulmonary: Neuromuscular:	
1. Pleural Effusion 1. ALS	
2. COPD 2. Polymyositis	
3. Pneumonia	
4. Malignancies	
Related to Respiratory Effort:	
1. Pregnancy 5. Rib Fracture	
2. Ascites 6. Panic attack	
3. Obesity 7. Pneumonia	
4. Hyperventilation Syndrome 8. Somatization Disorders	

Table 2. Differential diagnosis of breathlessness.

asked which may help in ruling in or out the important differentials. The onset of breathlessness and duration and severity of breathlessness give a clue about the nature of the underlying disorder and urgency to treat them. The important questions to be asked while taking the history of breathlessness are:

1. Onset of breathlessness: Breathlessness of sudden onset is usually serious and must be addressed immediately. Among the differentials of acute sudden onset breathlessness are pneumothorax and pulmonary embolism. Chocking with foreign bodies should be considered in the extreme of ages as well. Dyspnea which is slowly progressive and becomes serious in few hours to days may be due to conditions like asthma, COPD exacerbation, pneumonia, congestive heart failure, malignancies, recurrent small emboli, pleural effusion and neuromuscular disorders.

2. Duration of breathlessness: Breathlessness of short duration includes acute conditions like asthma exacerbation, infections, allergies, foreign bodies, cardiac dysfunctions and arrhythmias, pulmonary embolism, psychogenic and inhalation of irritants. Chronic and progressive conditions include chronic lung diseases like interstitial lung diseases, chronic heart failure, chronic pleural effusion and chronic cardiac and pulmonary disorders.

3. Related to trauma: Breathlessness related to trauma points to some of the most serious conditions which may be life threatening if not managed early. These include pneumothorax, tension pneumothorax, pulmonary contusion, hemothorax, flail chest, diaphragmatic rupture, cardiac tamponade, pericardial effusion and neurologic injury.

4. Positional changes and aggravating and relieving factors: Patients complaining of orthopnea may be suffering from left-sided heart failure, COPD and asthma exacerbation and neuromuscular disorders affecting the diaphragm which lead to splinting. Paroxysmal nocturnal dyspnea may be due to left-sided heart failure and COPD. Exertional dyspnea may be due to left-sided heart failure, COPD and restrictive and obstructive heart and lung diseases and conditions with abdominal loading. Conditions with abdominal loading include ascites, obesity and pregnancy.

5. Breathlessness with other associated symptoms: Other symptoms like fever, cough, chest pain, palpitation, sweating, weakness and paresthesia, swelling of feet and abdominal distension must be looked for. It helps in differentiating it from underlying cardiac problems or infective pathologies or neuromuscular disorders.

3.2.3. *Examination*

After a detailed history, thorough physical examination helps in finding the underlying cause of breathlessness. The examination includes vital signs, general appearance and detailed physical examination including systemic examinations like CVS, central nervous system (CNS), peripheral nervous system and respiratory system.

1. Tachypnea: Presence of tachypnea may indicate serious underlying medical conditions. Following are the conditions which cause tachypnea:

- Pulmonary edema
- Pneumonia
- Pneumothorax
- Fever
- Psychogenic
- Ascites
- Metabolic causes like diabetic ketoacidosis
- Endocrine disorders
- Infectious causes
- Obstructive and restrictive respiratory and cardiac causes
- Trauma leading to mechanical issues
- Toxins

2. Hypopnea: It can be seen in respiratory depression due to neurologic causes or from toxins.

- Intracranial insult
- Drugs and toxins

3. Tachycardia:

- PE
- Drugs/toxins
- Infections
- Tension pneumothorax
- Tamponade
- Trauma
- Lung contusion
- Hypoxia-causing conditions
- Acidosis and metabolic disorders
- Myocarditis
- Electrolyte and endocrine disorders

4. Hypotension

- Tension pneumothorax
- Cardiac tamponade

http://dx.doi.org/10.5772/intechopen.74682

5. Fever
   - Infective conditions like pneumonia
   - Myocarditis
   - Malignancies
6. General appearance
   - Pregnancy: PE
   - Obesity: Hypoventilation, PE, sleep apnea
   - Cachexia, weight loss: malignancy, chronic diseases like HIV
   - Barrel chest: COPD
   - Sniffing position: epiglottitis
   - Tripod positioning: Severe COPD/asthma
   - Bruises/crepitation/subcutaneous emphysema on chest: Flail chest, rib fracture, hemopneumothorax, lung contusion
7. Skin, nails and hands
   - Wasting of hands: Pancoast tumor
   - Tremors: CO2 retention
   - Tobacco stain: COPD, malignancy, infection
   - Clubbing: Malignancy, shunts (intracardiac), pulmonary vascular anomalies, chronic hypoxia
8. Neck
   - Stridor: Upper airway edema/infection, foreign body, traumatic injury, anaphylaxis
   - JVD: Tension pneumothorax, tamponade, CHF, volume overload, thoracic outlet syndrome, COPD/asthma exacerbation, PE
9. Respiratory
   - Wheeze: CHF, anaphylaxis, bronchospasm
   - Rales: heart failure, pneumonia, PE
   - Hemoptysis: Malignancy, mitral stenosis, infection, CHF, bleeding disorders
   - Rub: Pleurisy
   - Cheyne-stokes breathing: Intracranial insult
   - Subcutaneous emphysema: Pneumothorax, tracheobronchial disruption

10. Cardiac

- Murmur/S3, S4 Gallop, S2 Accentuation: PE
- Muffled heart sound: Tamponade

11. Neurologic

- Focal deficit: Stroke, ICH
- Neuromuscular disease
- Diffuse weakness: Metabolic/electrolyte abnormalities (Ca, Mg, PO4), anemia
- Hyporeflexia: Hypermagnesemia
- Ascending weakness: Guillian Barre syndrome
- Myasthenia Gravis
- ALS

12. Extremities

- DVT
- Edema of legs due to CHF

3.2.4. Investigation

Patients presenting with chest pain should be investigated for serious underlying medical causes as delay in diagnosis may be catastrophic in many conditions. Following are the important tests needed to diagnose important medical emergencies.

CXR: Chest X-Ray is one of the simplest diagnostic modalities which may give important clues in patients with chest pain and or breathlessness. It may give information about heart, lungs and mediastinum and abdominal and diaphragmatic problems. It is easily available in hospitals and one should have a low threshold in requesting them if the cause of chest pain and breathlessness is not clear or justified. Following are the conditions which can be seen on CXR.

ABG: Look for A-a gradient for PE, hypoxia and hypercapnia.

Positive cardiac markers: Myocardial infarction leading to heart failure and presenting with breathlessness can be detected by positive cardiac markers.

VQ Scan: To differentiate PE from other causes.

CT Scan: It helps in identifying pulmonary and mediastinal and intra-abdominal causes and differentiating it from cardiac.

ProBNP: It helps in identifying congestive cardiac failure and complications of MI.

D-Dimer: It gives a clue about PE and negative D-Dimer helps in ruling out PE.

Doppler: It is a modality to look for the source of PE. Sometimes, finding DVT gives indirect information about the cause of breathlessness.

Ultrasound: Look for important Causes of breathlessness and differentiate it from cardiac causes. US may help in detecting or giving a clue about PE, pneumothorax, pleural effusion, pericardial effusion, pneumonia and aortic dissection.

ECHO: It helps in identifying cardiac problems like ejection fraction, fluid overload, aortic dissection, IVC status, wall-motion abnormality, RV strain pattern, pericardial effusion, features of PE and features of CCF.

ECG: ECG is the most important investigation to diagnose the cardiac causes of breathlessness.

- MI/ACS leading to pulmonary edema
- PE: dysrhythmias, right-heart strain
- Pericarditis/myocarditis: heart failure
- Arrhythmias

3.2.5. Management

Serious cardiac emergencies presenting as breathlessness like pulmonary edema, MI, PE and cardiac tamponade should be diagnosed immediately for timely management. The management of individual emergency is discussed further in the chapter.

3.2.6. Disposition

All serious medical emergencies are admitted to the medical ward or in ICU depending on the severity of problem. The individual disposition of each medical diagnosis is discussed further in the chapter.

3.3. Approach to palpitation in the emergency department

Cardiovascular emergencies may present with palpitation in the emergency department. Palpitation is a symptom which could be the manifestation of serious cardiovascular underlying problems. The underlying cause of palpitation may be either ischemic heart disease, metabolic and endocrine disorders, drugs, malignancies, inflammatory and infiltrative disorders, connective disuse disorders and environmental factors like electrocution. Any condition which affects conduction across myocardium may lead to irregular or abnormally fast or slow conduction manifesting as palpitation. On taking an ECG, one may find either very fast or slow rhythm which may be regular or irregular. The other abnormalities which may be seen on the ECG are short PR, prolonged QT, short QT, broad QRS, narrow QRS, abnormalities of P waves and blocks.

3.3.1. Differential diagnosis of palpitation

- Narrow complex tachycardia (regular or irregular)

  AV node independent:

  1. Sinus tachycardia
  2. Atrial tachycardia (unifocal/multifocal)
  3. Atrial fibrillation
  4. Atrial flutter

  AV-node dependent:

  1. AV node re-entry tachycardia
  2. AV re-entry tachycardia
  3. Junctional tachycardia

- Broad complex tachycardia

  1. Ventricular tachycardia
  2. SVT with aberrant conduction

- Bradycardia

  1. Heart tissue damage related to aging
  2. Tissue damage due to ischemic heart disease
  3. Congenital heart diseases
  4. Myocarditis
  5. Heart surgery
  6. Malignancy
  7. Inflammatory and infiltratory diseases
  8. Metabolic and endocrine disorders
  9. Radiations
  10. Toxins, drugs and chemicals

3.3.2. Approach to palpitation

Whenever a patient complains of palpitation, the priority is to look for if the patient is stable or unstable. Immediately, vital signs of patients need to be recorded and the general condition of the patient is looked for. Patients with abnormal vital signs need to be taken to the monitored bed for further management. Patients who are stable hemodynamically can be treated by medication whereas hemodynamically unstable patients require synchronized cardioversion [5]. Patients should be taken to the monitored bed and the IV line is maintained and investigations are sent to look for reversible causes which can be corrected.

3.4. Approach to syncope and fainting episode in the emergency department

Cardiovascular emergencies may present as syncope, pre-syncope and fainting episode in the emergency department [4, 6]. Syncope is defined as a sudden transient loss of consciousness with a loss of postural tone. Any condition which affects cerebral perfusion (cardiac output, systemic vascular resistance, blood volume, regional vascular resistance) can lead to pre-syncope or syncope.

Pre-syncope or syncope may be caused by cardiovascular or CNS conditions. Here are the differential diagnoses of cardiovascular emergencies presenting as syncope:

3.4.1. Differential diagnosis of cardiovascular causes of syncope

- Cardiovascular diseases:
    1. MI
    2. Aortic dissection
    3. Cardiomyopathy
- Outflow obstruction:
    1. Valvular stenosis
    2. HOCM
    3. Atrial Myxoma
    4. PE
    5. Pulmonary hypertension
    6. Cardiac tamponade
    7. Congenital heart disease
- Reduced cardiac output:
    1. Tachycardia
        - I. SVT
        - II. Ventricular tachycardia
        - III. VF
        - IV. WPW
        - V. Torsade de Pointes

2. Bradycardia

    I. Sinus node disease

    II. Heart block (second and third degree)

    III. Prolonged QT

    IV. Pace maker malfunction

    V. ICD malfunction

3. Other cardiovascular diseases

    I. MI

    II. Aortic dissection

    III. Cardiomyopathy

3.4.2. History taking

History taking is the most important in diagnosing the patients presenting with syncope. There are wide differentials of syncope which range from very benign medical conditions like vasovagal attacks to most serious emergencies like aortic dissection or acute MI. History taking helps in narrowing down the differentials to a few in the list and then by detailed examination and suitable investigations physicians may reach to diagnosis or may be comfortable in discharging the patient to appropriate facilities for further management. The important information required in history taking include:

- Presence of chest pain
- Breathlessness
- Cough
- Palpitation
- Onset of symptom
- Pre-syncope symptoms
- Underlying medical conditions and comorbidities
- Use of medication
- Straining factors
- H/O previous such episodes
- Associated symptoms like seizure, loss of consciousness, weakness
- Emotional instability
- Toxins and drugs

3.4.3. *Examination*

Detailed physical examination is required to reach to diagnosis. The examination includes all the important systems which are included in the differential diagnosis of syncope.

- CNS examination:
- Respiratory system examination:

3.4.4. *Investigation*

The emergency physicians must choose important investigations to diagnoses serious underlying medical problems for timely management. Delay in the diagnosis of critical conditions may lead to serious consequences. Following are the important investigations needed in emergency department to diagnose cardiovascular emergencies presenting as syncope.

- ECG: Arrhythmias, ischemic heart diseases, cardiomyopathies
- Cardiac enzymes: Myocardial infarction
- Echocardiogram: Cardiac outflow obstruction, tamponade, aortic dissection, PE, valvular diseases with complications.

3.4.5. *Management*

Underlying cardiovascular problem needs to be treated once diagnosed. Management of individual emergencies is discussed further in the chapter.

4. Quick simple diagnostic and bed-side modalities to rapidly differentiate serious underlying medical emergencies

Patients presenting in the emergency department with chest pain, breathlessness, palpitation or sweating or with pre-syncope or syncope may have a wide range of differentials as a cause. Some of the conditions may be very serious and of grave outcomes if not managed immediately. Emergency physicians can use some important skills, tools and diagnostic tests to pick very serious underlying conditions which are the causes of these presentations. Timely management and disposition of these conditions may impact the overall outcome and prognosis. Here we will mention few tests and investigations which will help in differentiating the cause of cardiovascular symptoms.

a. ECG

1. Ischemic heart disease
2. Cardiomyopathies
3. Blocks

4. Metabolic/electrolyte abnormalities
5. Arrhythmias

b. **Bed-side Ultrasound:**
    1. Pneumothorax
    2. Pneumonia
    3. PE
    4. Pleural effusion

c. **Bed-side Echo**
    1. Wall-motion abnormality
    2. Pericardial effusion/tamponade
    3. PE
    4. Aortic dissection
    5. Valvular heart disease
    6. Ventricular thickening
    7. Ejection fraction
    8. Myxoma/thrombus
    9. Cardiac outflow obstruction

d. **X-Ray**:
    1. Cardiomegaly
    2. CCF/pulmonary edema
    3. Pneumonia
    4. Wide mediastinum
    5. Pleural effusion
    6. Pneumothorax
    7. Lung mass
    8. Diaphragmatic hernia

e. **Cardiac enzymes:** Acute MI

f. **Pro-BNP**: Acute heart failure

g. **ABG**: PE

h. **D-Dimer**: PE

http://dx.doi.org/10.5772/intechopen.74682

5. Management of important cardiac emergencies in the ED

5.1. Acute coronary syndrome

Acute coronary syndrome includes a spectrum of clinical presentations which range from unstable angina to non-ST elevation MI and ST elevation MI. They can be differentiated on the basis of history, ECG changes and blood investigations. The management started should be according to the diagnosis.

5.1.1. Spectrum of ACS

Unstable angina: It is referred to as pre-infarction angina or pre-occlusive syndrome. It is a warning sign of infarction.

Myocardial infarction: It is defined as cell death and necrosis. Below mentioned are the criteria satisfying the diagnosis of acute, evolving or recent MI.

1. Rise and fall of cardiac markers with
   a. Symptoms of ischemia
   b. ECG changes (either Q waves or changes consistent with ischemia like ST or T wave changes)
   c. Coronary artery interventions
2. Pathological findings of acute MI

5.1.2. Diagnosis

Diagnosis is done based on the history and physical examination and finally after diagnostic testing. The diagnostic testing includes ECG, chest X-Ray, serum cardiac markers, echocardiography, scintigraphy and CT angiography depending on the requirement and the availability.

ECG findings of MI:

5.1.3. Management

The management goal is early revascularization and reperfusion using either fibrinolysis or primary angioplasty. In places where PCI is available, quick cardiologist consultation and activation of PCI code are needed so that the cardiologist is involved to decide which pathway to follow. Delay in getting PCI does not justify avoiding thrombolysis. If, for any reason, expected time for PCI is more than 90 min, then thrombolysis is the choice of treatment. Medical management is divided into two categories:

5.1.3.1. Pharmacologic intervention

Oxygen should be administered when blood oxygen saturation is 90% or if the patient is in respiratory distress. In patients whose ischemic symptoms are not relieved by nitrates and beta-blockers, opiate administration is reasonable while waiting for immediate coronary angiography, with the caveat that morphine may slow down the intestinal absorption of oral platelet inhibitors.

- Nitroglycerine: It is a coronary vasodilator and reduces myocardial pre-load and after load.
- Pain management: If the patient is in severe pain and not responding to NTG and beta-blockers.
- Beta-blockers: Early administration of beta-blockers should be avoided in these patients if the ventricular function is unknown and should not be administered in patients with symptoms possibly related to coronary vasospasm or cocaine use, as they might favor spasm by leaving alpha-mediated vasoconstriction unopposed by beta-mediated vasodilation.
- Calcium channel blockers (CCBs): CCBs are recommended for ischemic symptoms when beta-blockers are not successful, are contraindicated or cause unacceptable side effects. Long-acting CCBs and nitrates are recommended for patients with coronary artery spasm. They can be used for rate control in patients with SVT when beta blockers are not tolerable.
- ACE inhibitors: ACE inhibitors should be started and continued indefinitely in all patients with a left ventricular ejection fraction (LVEF) below 40% and in those with hypertension, diabetes mellitus or stable chronic kidney disease (CKD), unless contraindicated.
- **Antiplatelet**: Antiplatelet therapy reduces progression to acute infarction in patients with non-AMI ACS patients. Aspirin or GP11b/111a inhibitors may be used. Antiplatelet treatment reduces mortality.
- **Anticoagulation:** Administer anticoagulation, in addition to antiplatelet therapy, for all patients, irrespective of the initial treatment strategy. Treatment options include the following (all Class I):

  Subcutaneous(SC) enoxaparin for the duration of hospitalization or until PCI is performed (level of evidence: A);

  Bivalirudin until diagnostic angiography or PCI is performed in patients with early invasive strategy only (level of evidence: B);

  SC fondaparinux for the duration of hospitalization or until PCI is performed (level of evidence: B);

  IV unfractionated heparin (UFH) for 48 h or until PCI is performed (level of evidence: B).

5.1.3.2. Reperfusion therapy

Reperfusion therapy, either by using thrombolytics or primary PCI, increases the opportunity to salvage ischemic myocardium. Fibrinolytic therapy improves coronary flow, limits infarct size and improves survival.

5.2. Heart failure

It is defined as the pathophysiologic state in which the heart is not capable of pumping sufficient supply of blood to meet the body requirements or else requires elevated ventricular filling pressures to accomplish this goal.

5.2.1. Pathophysiology of acute pulmonary edema

Cardiogenic pulmonary edema is due to increased capillary hydrostatic pressure secondary to acute ischemia or infarction, cardiomyopathy, valvular heart disease or hypertensive emergencies. Non-cardiogenic pulmonary edema occurs due to alteration in the permeability of pulmonary capillary membrane.

5.2.2. Compensatory mechanisms

The compensatory mechanisms secondary to heart failure include increase in stroke volume in response to increased pre-load, increased systemic vascular resistance and cardiac hypertrophy.

5.2.3. Treatment of heart failure

- stabilization of patient and resuscitation
- identify the underlying and precipitating cause and treat it
- control the symptoms and acute congestive state by reducing the cardiac work load (reducing pre-and after load), controlling excessive salt and water retention and improving cardiac contractility.
- Acute pulmonary edema with adequate perfusion:
    - nitrates
    - morphine
    - loop diuretics
    - nitroprusside
    - noninvasive or invasive ventilation [3, 7]
- Acute pulmonary edema in hypotensive patients
    - vasopressors and inotropes to maintain coronary perfusion
    - manage hypotension due to cardiogenic shock or due to volume depletion (identified by cardiac index and pulmonary artery outflow pressure)
    - judicious fluid challenge if low PAOP (<15 mm Hg)
    - IABP

- Emergency revascularization if ischemic cardiogenic shock

- Treatment of chronic heart failure:
  - Manage hypertension
  - Reverse remodeling by beta-blockers, ACE-I, aldosterone antagonists, ARB
  - Vasodilator therapy (ACE-I, ARB, Nitrates)
  - Diuretics
  - Cautious use of calcium blockers for hypertension, angina and dysrhythmia management
  - Beta-blocker therapy: Carvedilol may be effective agent in chronic HF
  - Digoxin

5.3. Hypertensive emergencies

In the Emergency Department hypertension presents as one of the four varieties:

1. Hypertensive emergency or crisis with acute end organ ischemia
2. Hypertensive urgency: Patients with poorly controlled hypertension
3. Mild hypertension
4. Transient hypertension which is related to anxiety or complaint

Only hypertension crisis requires treatment in the emergency department within 90 min of their presentation. Patients presenting with hypertensive emergencies will have markedly elevated BP and evidence of acute dysfunction in the cardiovascular, neurologic or renal system. Following are the conditions defined as hypertensive crisis:

1. Accelerated or malignant hypertension:
   - Hypertensive encephalopathy
   - Microangiopathic hemolytic anemia
   - Acute renal failure
2. Aortic dissection
3. Eclampsia/pre-eclampsia
4. Severe hypertension in the setting of:
   - Myocardial ischemia
   - LVF
   - Uncontrolled hemorrhage

http://dx.doi.org/10.5772/intechopen.74682

- Systemic reperfusion therapy for stroke or MI
- Postoperative state

Drugs of choice in treatment of hypertensive emergencies: Crack Cast (**Table 3**)

5.4. Dysrhythmias

Dysrhythmias present in the emergency department as chest pain, breathlessness, palpitation, sweating, pre-syncope, syncope and thromboembolic complications [8]. Managing dysrhythmias is very challenging in the emergency department. Timely intervention saves life. The first challenge is to diagnose the type of arrhythmias and categorize them as narrow complex or broad complex tachycardias or brady cardiac. The next step in management is to categorize them as stable or unstable. The type of management depends on the stability of patient as well as emergency physicians' expertise in managing them.

Diagnosis: 12 Lead ECG (see **Images 1**, **2**, **3**, **4** for NCT and WCT)

a. Symptoms and signs of unstable patients in the emergency department includes:

- Hypotension and or features of hypo-perfusion
- Chest pain suggesting myocardial ischemia
- Dyspnea or pulmonary edema
- Altered sensorium (agitation to coma)

Emergencies	Drug of choice	Alternatives
Hypertensive encephalopathy	Nicardipine Labetalol	Esmolol Enalaprilat
Intracranial Hemorrhage	Nicardipine Labetalol	Esmolol
Acute Pulmonary Edema	Nitroglycerine Furosemide Enalaprilat	Nicardipine Sodium Nitroprusside
Aortic Dissection	Esmolol and Sodium Nitroprusside Labetalol	Esmolol and Nicardipine Diltiazem, Verapamil
Ischemic Stroke	Nicardipine Labetalol	Esmolol Enalaprilat
Acute Kidney Injury	Fenoldapam Nicardipine, Clevidipine	Labetalol Sodium Nitroprusside
Preeclampsia/eclampsia	Hydralazine Labetalol	Nicardipine
Sympathetic Crisis	Phentolamine Nitroglycerine	Fenoldapam Clevidipine Nicardipine Sodium nitroprusside

Table 3. Management of hypertensive emergencies (Crack Cast).

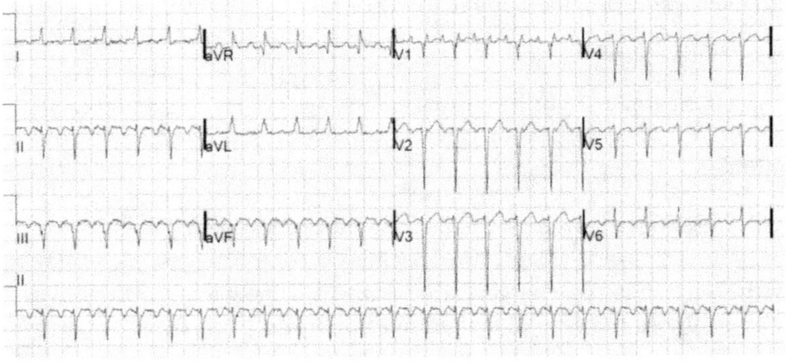

Image 1. Narrow complex tachycardia: Courtesy Dr. smith ECG blog.

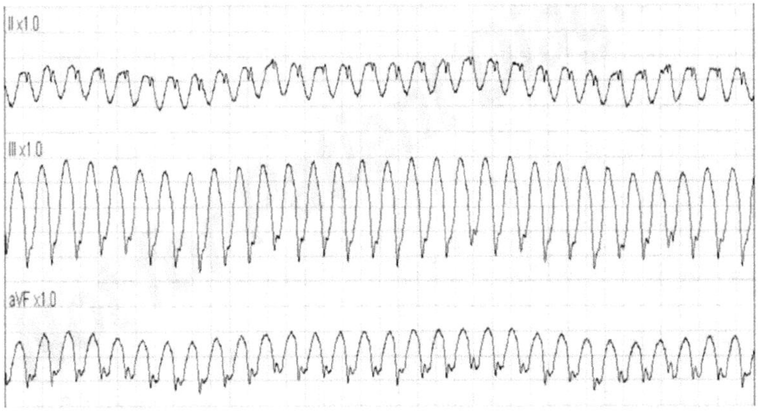

Image 2. Wide complex tachycardia (courtesy Dr smith blog).

b. Management of stable patients: Management of stable patients requires proper assessment and evaluation by detailed history and examination, ECG and then treatment depending on the type of rhythm, whether it's narrow complex or broad complex tachycardias. The treatment options are some maneuvers like vagal or valsalva and medications like adenosine, amiodarone, procainamide, verapamil and diltiazem. Narrow complex tachycardias are treated with drugs which slow AV nodal conduction like class 11 agents (beta-blockers) or class 1 V agents (calcium blockers) and adenosine or Class 1A (procainamide) and 1C (flecainide) drugs which are useful in converting narrow complex tachycardias to a sinus rhythm. See **Table 4** for treatment of NCT and WCT

c. Management of unstable patients: Unstable patients are managed more aggressively. Again, treatment options depend on whether it's narrow complex tachycardias or wide complex tachycardias and an emergency physician's expertise with the drugs and synchronized cardioversion.

http://dx.doi.org/10.5772/intechopen.74682

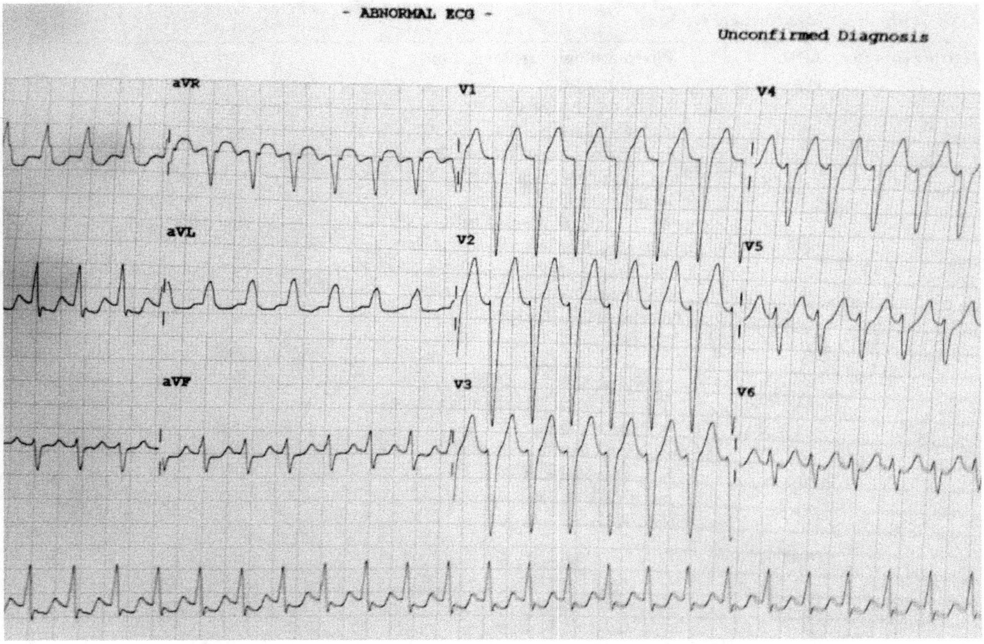

Image 3. SVT with aberrancy: Courtesy the blunt dissection.

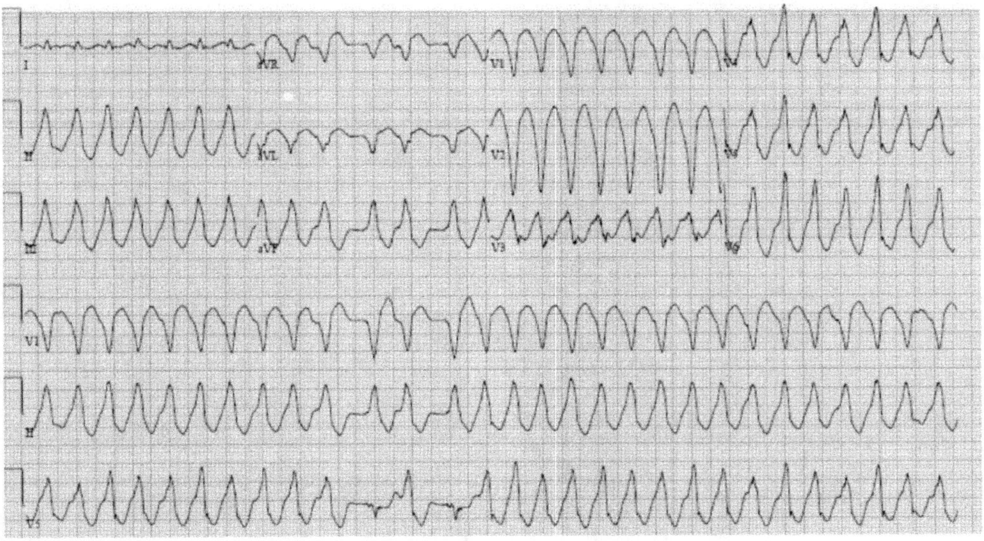

Image 4. Polymorphic V-Tac.

Type of Rhythm	**Management Options**	
Narrow complex	Atrial Fibrillation	**Pharmacologic cardioversion:** **1.** Procainamide (1A) or **2.** Propafenone (1C) or **3.** Flecainide (1C) or **4.** Amiodarone (111) or **5.** Ibutilide (111) **Rate Control:** **1.** A calcium blocker (Verapamil or diltiazem) may be used before type 1A agent **2.** Beta Blockers **Anticoagulation**: anticoagulation in ED is needed depending on whether AF is new or chronic. **Electrical Cardioversion:** (50–100 J)
	SVT (AV nodal)	Vagal Maneuvers Pharmacologic Treatment: **1.** Adenosine **2.** Calcium Blockers **3.** Beta Blockers Electrical Cardioversion: (50-100 J)
	Atrial Flutter	**Pharmacologic:** **a.** **Rate Control:** **b.** Beta Blockers **c.** Calcium Blockers **d.** **Pharmacologic Cardioversion** **e.** Procainamide (1A) **f.** Ibutilide (111) **g.** Amiodarone (111) **h.** **Electrical Cardioversion:** (25-50 J)
Wide Complex	V-Tach (stable)	Monomorphic: **1.** Treat underlying cause **2.** Amiodarone **3.** Procainamide **4.** Lidocaine **5.** Magnesium SO4 Polymorphic with Torsade de Pointes **1.** Treat Underlying Causes **2.** IV MgSO4 **3.** Beta-Adrenergic Infusion **4.** Amiodarone **5.** Overdrive Pacing
	SVT with Aberrancy	Atrial Fibrillation with aberrancy: **a.** Avoid: calcium Blockers Beta Blockers Digoxin **a.** Use: Amiodarone Procainamide **a.** Electrical Cardioversion 50-100 J (increase by 50–100 if no response till 360 J) **b.** If Unstable: Treat as V Tac
	V-Tac (Pulseless)	Treat as Ventricular Fibrillation

Table 4. Treatment of Arrhythmias.

5.5. Aortic dissection

Aortic dissection is one of the most serious cardiovascular emergencies, presenting in ER, mimicking cardiac ischemia [9]. Failure to diagnose is catastrophe for the patient and may lead to death. Thrombolysis is contraindicated. Wrongly diagnosing them as cardiac ischemia and treating as MI may kill the patient.

a. Types: Type A involves ascending aorta; Type B does not involve ascending aorta (Stanford classification)

b. Presentation:

- Chest pain/back pain (interscapular)
- Syncope
- Neurologic symptoms like weakness or change in mental status

c. Physical examination:

- Severe hypertension
- Aortic regurgitation findings on auscultation
- Discrepancy in BP and pulse deficits between limbs
- Findings of stroke
- Ischemic paraparesis or ischemic peripheral neuropathy (dissection of anterior spinal artery)
- Acute inferior or posterior MI (RCA dissection)

d. Diagnostic tests:

- ECG: LVH, MI, ischemia, non-specific ST-T changes
- CXR: Normal or widened mediastinum, calcium sign, double density aorta, obliteration of aortic knob, displaced NG-Tube
- Echocardiography: Transthoracic echo is an insensitive tool but TEE is 98% sensitive and 95% specific. It is operator dependent.
- Helical CT: It's a reliable test for diagnosis. It is almost 100% sensitive and 98% specific.

e. Management: Medical management is needed in Type B, whereas type A requires surgical intervention.

- Pain management
- Blood pressure management: The goal is to reduce blood pressure and to decrease the rate of rise of arterial pulse. The target BP is 100/60 and heart rate of less than 60/m.

- Use beta-blockers with vasodilators to avoid tachycardia. Esmolol is used to control heart rate. Labetalol can be used. Sodium nitroprusside is used as a vasodilator. Nitroglycerin can be used as a vasodilator but needs beta-blocker in conjunction.
- Consultation with thoracic surgery for possible intervention in type A dissection.

5.6. Pulmonary embolism

Pulmonary embolism is the result of clot dislodgement which formed hours, days or weeks earlier in the deep veins and traveled through the venous system to traverse the right-sided heart, finally lodging in the pulmonary vasculatures.

5.6.1. Risk factors

The risk factors for pulmonary embolism are:

- Hypercoagulability like inherited thrombophilia, acquired thrombophilia, carcinomas, estrogen, pregnancy/postpartum
- Inflammation (connective tissue disorders, trauma, surgery, smoking)
- Vascular stasis (limb or generalized immobility)

5.6.2. Signs and symptoms:

Chest Pain	Pulse >100.
Breathlessness	Pulse oximeter reading <95%.
Syncope	Unilateral leg or arm swelling.
Hemoptysis	Signs of right heart failure

5.6.3. Diagnosis:

ECG: ECG may show S1, Q3, T3, non-specific ST-T changes, RV strain pattern, sinus tachycardia, pulmonary Hypertension changes (T inversion in V1-V4), incomplete or complete RBBB.

CXR: It may help in ruling out other causes of chest pain or breathlessness. Features of pulmonary infarction may indicate underlying PE (Hamptons Hump). Rarely an oligemic lung is seen.

Echocardiography: It helps in identifying features of right ventricular strain and right ventricular dilatation (indirect evidence of PE).

D-Dimer: It is used as a screening test. Negative D-Dimer is more helpful than positive D-Dimer which occurs in many other medical conditions as well.

CTPA: It's a gold standard to diagnose or rule out PE.

Doppler Ultrasound can be used to look for the primary source of thrombus when CTPA or V/Q scan is absolutely contraindicated or is considered a high-risk procedure.

V/Q Scan: It is used when CTPA is either contraindicated or not possible to perform.

5.6.4. Management:

- Anticoagulation: Anticoagulation with IV Heparin (bolus then infusion), fractionated heparin (Enoxaparin) or the Factor Xa inhibitor (Fondaparinux) is the current standard treatment for patients presenting with PE.
- Thrombolytic therapy: This is used in patients who present with severe symptoms, with features of massive PE who are not responding to standard treatment and are unstable and or go into cardiac arrest (PEA/asystole). Patients who show evidence of massive PE can be given thrombolytics provided they do not have contraindications of thrombolysis.
- IVC filters: These can be used in patients who have recurrent PE even on treatment.

6. Conclusion

Cardiovascular emergencies present as most challenging emergencies in the emergency department. Presence of atypical signs and symptoms and presentations resembling many other benign medical conditions make it very challenging to timely diagnose them few times. Choosing inappropriate or unnecessary investigations will delay the disposition of the patient which may lead to a busy emergency department. It may lead to prolonged length of stay, delay in diagnosing serious emergencies and discharging patients inappropriately resulting in mortality or morbidity cases. This will compromise the credibility of the department. Taking proper history with systematic and symptomatic approach and doing a detailed examination and choosing the right investigations will reduce the length of stay of patient and on the other hand will help the physician in avoiding inappropriate discharges or referrals to subspecialty. Sound medical knowledge and awareness of differential diagnosis help in avoiding delayed patient disposition.

Author details

Shahzad Anjum

Address all correspondence to: shahzad177@yahoo.com

Hamad Medical Corporation, Doha, Qatar

References

[1] Kim I, Kim MC, Park KH, Sim DS, Hong YJ, Kim JH, Jeong MH, Cho JG, Park JC, Cho MC, Kim JJ, Kim YJ, Ahn Y. Korea acute myocardial infarction registry investigators. Prognostic significance of non-chest pain symptoms in patients with non-ST-segment elevation myocardial infarction. The Korean Journal of Internal Medicine. 2017 Nov 10 PMID: 29117666

[2] Brown A, Dingle HE, Brywczynski J, McKinney JJ, Slovis CM. The 5 deadly causes of chest pain: Recognizing the potentially lethal causes other than myocardial infarction. JEMS: A Journal of Emergency Medical Services. 2017 Jan;**42**(1):55-63 PMID:29206410

[3] Bittencourt HS, Reis HF, Lima MS, Neto GM. Non-invasive ventilation in patients with heart failure: A systematic review and meta-analysis. Arquivos Brasileiros de Cardiologia. 2017 Feb;**108**(2):161-168. DOI: 10.5935/abc.20170001 Epub 2017 Jan 16. Review. English, Portuguese. PMID: 28099587

[4] Wolfe TR, Allen TL. Syncope as an emergency department presentation of pulmonary embolism. The Journal of Emergency Medicine. 1998;**16**:27 [PMID: 9472756]

[5] Goldberger ZD, Rho RW, Page RL. Approach to the diagnosis and initial management of the stable adult patient with a wide complex tachycardia. The American Journal of Cardiology. 2008 May 15;**101**(10):1456-1466. DOI: 10.1016/j.amjcard.2008.01.024 Epub 2008 Mar 21. Review. Erratum in: Am J Cardiol. 2008 Aug 1;**102**(3):374. PMID: 18471458

[6] Mussi C, Ungar A, Salvioli G, et al. Orthostatic hypotension as cause of syncope in patients older than 65 years admitted to emergency departments for transient loss of consciousness. The Journals of Gerontology. Series A, Biological Sciences and Medical Sciences. 2009;**64**: 801 [PMID: 19349588]

[7] Moret Iurilli C, Brunetti ND, Di Corato PR, Salvemini G, Di Biase M, Ciccone MM, Procacci V. Hyperacute hemodynamic effects of BiPAP Noninvasive ventilation in patients with acute heart failure and left ventricular systolic dysfunction in emergency department. Journal of Intensive Care Medicine. 2018 Feb;**33**(2):128–133. DOI: 10.1177/0885066617740849. Epub 2017 Nov 15. PMID: 29141525

[8] Nishizaki M. Life-threatening arrhythmias leading to syncope in patients with vasospastic angina. Journal of Arrhythmias. 2017 Dec;**33**(6):553-561. DOI: 10.1016/j.joa.2017.04.006 Epub 2017 May 10. PMID: 29255500

[9] Alter SM, Eskin B, Allegra JR. Diagnosis of aortic dissection in emergency department patients is rare. The Western Journal of Emergency Medicine. 2015 Sep;**16**(5):629-631. DOI: 10.5811/westjem.2015.6.25752 Epub 2015 Oct 20. PMID:26587083

Chapter 10

Emergency Management of Acute Ischaemic Stroke

Ekanem Philip-Ephraim

Additional information is available at the end of the chapter

http://dx.doi.org/10.5772/intechopen.75305

Abstract

Stroke is a medical emergency with ischaemic stroke being the commonest type worldwide. Hypertension has been identified as the leading modifiable risk factor globally. The management of acute ischemic stroke is fast changing due to the advancement in technology and the introduction of intravenous recombinant tissue plasminogen activator. There is a limited time window for early intervention to salvage the ailing neurons. The first 24 hours of presentation is therefore crucial in management. Early recognition of stroke symptoms with rapid intervention can lead to a favourable outcome. Specialized care during the acute phase in the intensive care or stroke unit can improve the overall prognosis.

Keywords: ischaemic stroke, haemorrhagic stroke, emergency, management

1. Introduction

Stroke has been defined by the World Health Organization as "rapidly developing clinical signs of focal (at times global) disturbance of cerebral function, lasting more than 24hours or leading to death with no apparent cause other than of vascular origin" [1].

Stroke is a neurologic emergency with poorer prognosis in blacks [2, 3]. It represents one of the major causes of morbidity and mortality globally and ranks third as the most common cause of mortality in developed countries resulting in long term disability and accounting for 4.4 million deaths in the world [4, 5]. The severity of stroke varies widely, ranging from full recovery on one hand to both fatal and non-fatal events with neurological deficits and functional disabilities on the other hand [5–7].

Risk factors for stroke have been classified as modifiable and non-modifiable. The non-modifiable factors include sex, age, race, family history, genetic and low birth weight while the modifiable risk factors include hypertension, diabetes mellitus, hyperlipidaemia, atrial fibrillation, smoking, obesity, carotid artery disease, hyperhomocysteinemia, hypercoagulable states and select biomarkers [8].

Stroke increases sharply with age and the incidence of a first time stroke is about 200 per 100,000 annually with a prevalence of 5–12 per 1000 population. Stroke mortality rate is different among countries ranging from 20 to 250 per 100,000 populations annually [9]. In the UK about 90,000 females and 60,000 males die from stroke yearly with the approximate cost of stroke to NHS and social services being £2.3bn annually [10]. The risk of a recurrent stroke is very high among survivors. About 14% of patients who survive a stroke or TIA will have a recurrence in the first year; 22% of males and 25% of females will have mortality in the first year of an initial stroke and more than half of all stroke patients experience mortality within 8 years [5].

2. Classification

Stroke is classified into two major types: Ischaemic and haemorrhagic. Ischaemic stroke is by far the commonest, accounting for 85% of all strokes while haemorrhagic stroke accounts for 15% of strokes - intracerebral 10%, subarachnoid 5% [5].

Ischaemic stroke is the leading worldwide cause of morbidity and mortality in the developed world. About 8–12% of patients die within 30 days of their first stroke and those that survive the first attack are at increased risk of a recurrence [11]. Ischaemic stroke is caused by atherosclerotic vascular disease leading to occlusion and stenosis of major intracranial or extracranial arteries and constriction of small penetrating arteries of the brain. Cardioembolic stroke due to myocardial infarction is usually due to atherosclerosis of the coronary arteries. The resulting ischaemia leads to direct brain insult because of inadequacy of flow, hypoxia and metabolic substrate and institutes a cascade of neurochemical processes causing continuous damage within hours. Treatment of ischaemic stroke has been with the use of drugs such as fibrinolytic agents, anticoagulants and antiplatelets to improve blood supply to the brain. Prevention of stroke both at the primary and secondary levels is now possible because of availability of various safe and successful interventions directed at high risk individuals [5, 12].

3. Clinical presentation

Patients present with abrupt onset of focal neurological deficit such as facial paresis, arm drift, leg weakness and abnormal speech [13]. Although patients with acute ischaemic stroke do present with headache, vomiting, seizures, depressed level of consciousness; these symptoms are commoner in patients with haemorrhagic stroke. It is difficult, on the basis of clinical presentation, to distinguish intracerebral haemorrhage from ischaemic stroke as they may look alike [14]. The duration of stroke onset should be noted as this is crucial in defining treatment options. Past medical and drug history (e.g heroin, amphetamines, and cocaine) should be obtained. History of vascular risk factors such as obesity, hypertension, hyperlipidaemia, diabetes mellitus, and smoking should also be obtained. The initial neurological assessment of the patient should be brief but detailed. Different stroke scales such as National Institutes of Health Stroke Scale (NIHSS) can be employed as this helps in determining the severity of the stroke [15]. Assessment of airway, breathing and circulation may precede a thorough evaluation of the stroke patient. A comprehensive physical examination is carried out by the attending physician or the stroke team. This may reveal an irregular pulse, bradycardia, cardiomegaly or heart murmurs. The blood pressure should also be checked [16].

4. Investigations

Besides doing basic investigations such as carotid Doppler, pregnancy test, full blood count, fasting lipid profile, blood sugar, serum homocysteine, serum electrolyte, urea and creatinine, coagulation studies (PT/INR/PTT), liver function tests, Haemoglobin AIc, electrocardiography (ECG), electroencephalopathy (EEG), toxicology screen, cardiac enzymes (CK,CK-MB, TROPONIN I and T) a brain Computed Tomography/Magnetic Resonance Imaging (CT/MRI) Scan is also required as this is the single most important investigation to help exclude a cerebral haemorrhage and stroke mimics. It confirms the diagnosis of ischaemic stroke allowing for prompt treatment of the condition. Increase in both cardiac Troponin T and Troponin I have been found to be associated with stroke severity and poor clinical outcomes [17, 18].

5. General supportive care

Issues to be focused on include: Airway management, hydration, increased intracranial pressure (ICP), Blood pressure control, Blood sugar control, Temperature.

5.1. Airway management

Coma is uncommon with ischaemic stroke patients. Patients who have neurological decline with reduced level of consciousness have challenges in maintaining their airway due to loss of protective reflexes [19]. This can result in aspiration, hypoxaemia or hypercapnia that may increase intracranial pressure by causing cerebral vasodilatation. The role of oxygen therapy in ischaemic stroke has been controversial due to failure of three clinical trials of hyperbaric oxygen to demonstrate efficacy. Supplemental oxygen can be administered at a dose of 10-15 L/min if there is evidence of hypoxia by pulse oximetry. This was shown to slow down the process of ischaemia and extend the therapeutic time window for thrombolysis [20, 21]. Patients with depressed level of consciousness should be intubated to avoid the risk of aspiration [22].

5.2. Hydration

Patients with ischaemic stroke should be routinely hydrated with isotonic saline. This helps ensure adequate perfusion to the ischaemic penumbra and may prevent infarct extension. Hypotonic solutions should be avoided as this may lead to increased cerebral oedema.

5.3. Increased intracranial pressure (ICP)

The head of the bed should be elevated at 30 degrees. Other measures to reducing ICP include administration of 0.5-1 g/kg of 20% mannitol as a bolus. Infusion of hypertonic saline solution (23.4%) can also be administered at a dose of 0.5–2.0 ml/kg as an alternative to mannitol especially in the setting of hypotension. Hyperventilation to a pCO2 of 28-35 mmHg has also been employed as a measure in reducing ICP.

5.4. Blood pressure management

High blood pressure is a frequent occurrence in acute ischaemic stroke. Although blood pressure declines spontaneously within 90 mins after stroke onset [23], about one third of the patients continue to have hypertension with an increased risk of poor outcome [24, 25]. The mechanisms implicated for the increase in blood pressure are multifactorial and include a previous history of hypertension, release of endogenous catecholamines, raised intracranial pressure (Cushing's reflex), infection, "White coat hypertension effect", prior alcohol intake, pain from urinary retention, impaired baroreceptor sensitivity and stress relating to hospitalization [25–29].

Hypotension, though uncommon in acute stroke, correlates with a poor clinical outcome. Causes implicated include infection, cardiac failure, arrhythmias, hypovolaemia and aortic dissection [30].

Rapid blood pressure reduction in acute ischaemic stroke reduces the cerebral blood flow thereby increasing the area of cerebral infarction and worsening neurological outcome [31]. For over three decades, there has been a controversy regarding the treatment of high blood pressure in the setting of acute ischaemic stroke [32, 33]. Some studies have observed a U-shaped relationship between the admission blood pressure and good clinical outcomes, with an optimal systolic blood pressure ranging from 121 to 200 mm Hg and diastolic blood pressure ranging from 81 to 110 mm Hg [34]. High blood pressure should not be treated in the first 24 hours after ischaemic stroke unless the systolic blood pressure is greater than 220, the diastolic blood pressure is greater than 120, the mean arterial blood pressure is greater than 130 mmHg or there are associated complications such as presence of myocardial infarction, aortic dissection or heart failure. At such times, the goal would be to reduce the blood pressure by 15%.

Recommendations for blood pressure control have been established regarding patients undergoing fibrinolytic therapy. The recommendations include a gradual approach to reducing the pressure below 185/110 mm Hg to qualify for fibrinolytic therapy with intravenous recombinant tissue plasminogen activator (rt-PA). Once intravenous (rt-PA) is given, the blood pressure must be maintained below 180/105 mm Hg to reduce the risk of intracerebral haemorrhage [16].

Antihypertensives given when considering re-perfusion therapy include IV Labetalol 10–20 mg over 1–2 minutes, may be repeated once, IV Nicardipine 5 mg/h, titrating up by 2.5 mg/h every 5–15 minutes, maximum 15 mg/h; when desired BP is reached, adjust to maintain proper BP levels. Other drugs such as hydralazine, enalaprilat, etc. may be considered where necessary. Do not administer rt-PA if the blood pressure is not maintained at or below 185/110 mm Hg. Blood pressure should be monitored every 15 minutes for 2 hours from the start of rt-PA therapy, then every 30 minutes for 6 hours, and then every hour for 16 hours. If the blood pressure still remains uncontrolled or diastolic BP >140 mm Hg, consider IV sodium nitroprusside [16].

5.5. Management of blood sugar

Hyperglycaemia occurs in about 20–40% of acute stroke patients with no previous diagnosis of diabetes mellitus [35]. There is overwhelming clinical evidence that correlates hyperglycaemia at the onset of acute ischaemic stroke with a negative outcome [36]. Hyperglycaemia influences neuronal damage by encouraging anaerobic metabolism and lactic acidosis within the ischaemic tissue, thus worsening outcome and heightening the risk of haemorrhagic transformation after thrombolysis [37]. Hyperglycaemia should be treated with insulin to achieve a blood sugar control between 7.7 and 10.0 mmol/l with close monitoring to avoid hypoglycaemia [16]. Insulin is indicated in the treatment of hyperglycaemia in acute ischaemic stroke because of its ability to reduce neuronal necrosis regardless of its effect on glucose levels [38].

5.6. Temperature control

About one third of patients presenting with stroke develop fever in the first few hours after stroke onset [39]. Increased body temperature of 37.5°C is associated with poor neurological outcome secondary to increased free radical production, increased metabolic demands and increased release of neurotransmitters [39, 40].

The source of the fever should be determined. Some of the possible causes of the fever include aspiration pneumonia and other respiratory infections, urinary tract infections or line infections, infective endocarditis, deep vein thrombosis/pulmonary embolism and cocaine intoxication. The guideline for the early management of acute ischaemic stroke recommends the lowering of temperature during the acute stroke period. Fever is managed strictly with antipyretics and appropriate antibiotics given if infection is suspected. The most frequently used antipyretic is acetaminophen. Aspirin, ibuprofen and indomethacin have also been considered in patients with reduced risk of bleeding [41].

5.7. Antiplatelet therapy

The commonly used antiplatelets include aspirin, clopidogrel and dipyridamole. The use of aspirin in acute ischaemic stroke was examined in CAST (the Chinese Acute Stroke Trial) and IST (the International Stroke Trial). In IST study, aspirin at a dose of 300 mg/day was found to reduce stroke recurrence within the first 14 days with no effect on early mortality. In the CAST study, aspirin 160 mg/day reduced the risk of recurrence and mortality in the first

28 days. Clopidogrel at a dose of 75 mg was found to have a risk reduction of 8.7% in the prevention of cerebrovascular and cardiovascular events [42]. Various studies have shown that the combination of dipyridamole and aspirin is superior to aspirin alone as an antithrombotic therapy after cerebral ischemia of arterial origin [43, 44].

5.8. Anticoagulant therapy

Heparin is not indicated for routine use in the treatment of acute ischaemic stroke. Some of the indications for its use include cerebral venous thrombosis, acute infarct with high grade carotid stenosis, cardiogenic emboli with high risk of recurrence, hypercoagulable states such as protein C deficiency, protein S deficiency, antithrombin III deficiency and antiphospholipid antibody syndrome. Other anticoagulants include warfarin which is useful in the prevention of stroke recurrence in atrial fibrillation patients [45]. Dabigatran has also been found to reduce the occurrence of stroke among non-valvular atrial fibrillation patients [46].

5.9. Statins

Statins have been observed to be efficacious in both primary and secondary prevention of stroke independent of cholesterol levels. This might be due to other beneficial effects of statins such as stabilization of atherosclerotic plaques, improvement of endothelial function, antioxidant properties, increased nitric oxide bioavailability, inhibition of inflammatory responses and immunomodulatory actions [47, 48]. The use of Statin early in stroke patients has been found to be strongly associated with improved post stroke survival, and discontinuation of statin, even for a brief period, has been associated with worsened survival [49].

6. Thrombolysis

The goal of reperfusion therapy for acute ischaemic stroke is prompt restoration of blood flow to regions of brain that are ischemic but not yet infarcted. This reduces the volume of brain damage, reduces oedema and improves outcome. The use of intravenous recombinant tissue plasminogen activator was approved by the US FDA in 1996 for use in acute ischaemic stroke patients presenting within 3 hours of stroke onset [50]. Its use is associated with favourable outcomes although increased risk of intracranial haemorrhage has been observed [16].

Intravenous recombinant tissue plasminogen activator (IV rt-PA) is administered when an acute stroke patient meets all of the inclusion criteria and none of the absolute exclusion criteria. The dose of the IV rt-PA is 0.9 mg/kg (maximum dose 90 mg). Infuse 0.9 mg/kg over 60 minutes, with 10% of the dose given as a bolus over one minute. Patient should be admitted into the intensive care unit or stroke unit for close monitoring. The infusion should be discontinued if the patient develops severe headache, acute hypertension, nausea, or vomiting or has a worsening neurological examination. An emergent CT scan should be requested for. Blood pressure monitoring and neurological assessment are carried out every 15mins during and after the administration of the IV rt-PA infusion for 2 hours, then every 30 minutes for 6 hours, then hourly until 24 hours after IV rt-PA treatment [16].

http://dx.doi.org/10.5772/intechopen.75305

Inclusion criteria

Diagnosis of ischemic stroke causing measurable neurological deficit

Onset of symptoms <3 hours before beginning treatment

Aged ≥18 years

Exclusion criteria

Significant head trauma or prior stroke in previous 3 months

Symptoms suggest subarachnoid haemorrhage

Arterial puncture at non-compressible site in previous 7 days

History of previous intracranial haemorrhage

Intracranial neoplasm, arteriovenous malformation, or aneurysm

Recent intracranial or intraspinal surgery

Elevated blood pressure (systolic >185 mm Hg or diastolic >110 mm Hg)

Active internal bleeding

Acute bleeding diathesis, including but not limited to

Platelet count <100,000/mm^3

Heparin received within 48 hours, resulting in abnormally elevated aPTT greater than the upper limit of normal

Relative exclusion criteria

Recent experience suggests that under some circumstances—with careful consideration and weighting of risk to benefit—patients may receive fibrinolytic therapy despite 1 or more relative contraindications. Consider risk to benefit of IV rt-PA administration carefully if any of these relative contraindications are present:

Only minor or rapidly improving stroke symptoms (clearing spontaneously)

Pregnancy

Seizure at onset with postictal residual neurological impairments

Major surgery or serious trauma within previous 14 days

Recent gastrointestinal or urinary tract haemorrhage (within previous 21 days)

Recent acute myocardial infarction (within previous 3 months)

Adapted from Guidelines for the early management of patients with acute ischaemic stroke. Stroke 2013.

The checklist includes some FDA-approved indications and contraindications for administration of IV rt-PA for acute ischemic stroke. Recent guideline revisions have modified the original FDA-approved indications. A physician with expertise in acute stroke care may modify this list.

Onset time is defined as either the witnessed onset of symptoms or the time last known normal if symptom onset was not witnessed.

In patients without recent use of oral anticoagulants or heparin, treatment with IV rt-PA can be initiated before availability of coagulation test results but should be discontinued if INR is >1.7 or PT is abnormally elevated by local laboratory standards.

In patients without history of thrombocytopenia, treatment with IV rt-PA can be initiated before availability of platelet count but should be discontinued if platelet count is <100,000/mm^3.

aPTT indicates activated partial thromboplastin time; CT, computed tomography; ECT, ecarin clotting time; FDA, Food and Drug Administration; INR, international normalized ratio; IV, intravenous; PT, partial thromboplastin time; rt-PA, recombinant tissue plasminogen activator; and TT, thrombin time.

Table 1. Inclusion and exclusion characteristics of patients with ischemic stroke who could be treated with IV rtPA within 3 hours from symptom onset.

Inclusion criteria	
	Diagnosis of ischemic stroke causing measurable neurological deficit
	Onset of symptoms within 3 to 4.5 hours before beginning treatment
Relative exclusion criteria	
	Aged >80 years
	Severe stroke (NIHSS>25)
	Taking an oral anticoagulant regardless of INR
	History of both diabetes and prior ischemic stroke

INR indicates international normalized ratio; IV, intravenous; NIHSS, National Institutes of Health Stroke Scale; and rt-PA, recombinant tissue plasminogen activator.

Table 2. Additional inclusion and exclusion characteristics of patients with acute ischemic stroke who could be treated with IV rt-PA within 3 to 4.5 hours from symptom onset.

Placement of nasogastric tubes, indwelling bladder catheters, or intra-arterial pressure catheters should be delayed if the patient can be safely managed without them. A follow-up CT or MRI scan should be obtained at 24 hours after IV rt-PA before commencing anticoagulants or antiplatelets (**Tables 1** and **2**).

7. Endovascular treatments

This modality of treatment for acute ischaemic stroke is fast emerging. Mechanical clot retrieval with MERCI device (Mechanical Embolus Removal in Cerebral Ischaemia) has been employed. Other interventions have included mechanical clot aspiration with the Penumbra system. The Penumbra System (PS) is a new embolectomy device specifically designed to remove the thrombus in acute ischemic stroke secondary to large vessel thromboembolism. The device removes the thrombus through two mechanisms: aspiration and extraction [16]. Earlier trials, Trevo versus Merci Retrievers for Thrombectomy Revascularization of Large Vessel Occlusions in Acute Ischaemic Stroke (TREVO 2) and SWIFT, showed significantly higher recanalization rates associated with stent retriever devices compared to the first generation Merci Retriever [51, 52].

8. Complications

Patients who have sustained a stroke are prone to developing complications. About 30–60% of patients after acute ischaemic stroke develop these complications. The most frequent complications include respiratory and urinary tract infections, deep vein thrombosis (DVT) and pulmonary embolism (PE) [53]. Pulmonary embolism occurs in about 10% of patients post stroke. Deep vein thrombosis and pulmonary embolism tend to occur in the first three months post

http://dx.doi.org/10.5772/intechopen.75305

stroke with an incidence of 2.5% and 1.2% respectively [54]. The risk of DVT/PE is increased in immobile and elderly patients with severe stroke [55]. Pressure sores are also common and have been attributed to poor nursing care. Stroke patients should therefore be turned frequently at 2-hourly interval to prevent this complication. Water bed can also be used.

9. Conclusion

Ischaemic stroke remains the commonest type of stroke worldwide. Its successful treatment is dependent on prompt restoration of blood flow to the penumbral tissue. Other supportive therapies have also been helpful in ensuring a favourable outcome. This was an overview of the management of the condition.

10. Intracerebral haemorrhage (ICH)

10.1. Introduction

This refers to bleeding into the brain parenchyma. Intracerebral haemorrhage is a devastating disease with increased morbidity and mortality constituting 15% of all stroke types [56, 57]. Factors associated with increased mortality include large clots, low Glasgow Coma Scale score, intraventricular haemorrhage and haematoma expansion. The causes of haematoma growth include a past history of stroke, liver disease, hyperglycaemia and hypertension [58]. The common sites for ICH include the basal ganglia, thalamus, brain stem and the cerebellum.

10.2. Causes

Causes of ICH have been classified into primary and secondary. Hypertension remains the most common modifiable risk factor for the development of ICH [59, 60] while cerebral amyloid angiopathy is the second most frequent risk factor in ICH leading to lobar haemorrhages . Other risk factors include increasing age, anticoagulation therapy, AV malformations, and aneurysms [61].

10.3. Clinical features

The symptoms are usually sudden in onset; most times occurring during exercise or emotional stress although it can also occur during routine activity [61, 62]. It is difficult, on the basis of clinical presentation, to distinguish ICH from ischaemic stroke as they may look similar.

Presentation of ICH differs depending on the size and location of the ICH. Symptoms that may suggest ICH include severe headache, vomiting, seizures, reduced level of consciousness. Headache is more frequent in patients with large haematomas and has been attributed to raised intracranial pressure and traction on the meningeal pain fibres. Small, deep haematomas rarely present with headache. [61]. About 15–23% of patients tend to have haematoma expansion and neurological deterioration in the first few hours of the event [63, 64].

10.4. Assessment

According to the guideline on the emergency diagnosis and assessment of an ICH patient, the following should be done:

A baseline severity score should be performed as part of the initial evaluation of patients with ICH (Class 1; level of evidence B); rapid neuroimaging with CT or MRI is recommended to distinguish ischaemic stroke from ICH (Class 1, level of evidence A); Computed Tomography Angiography (CTA) and contrast-enhanced CT may be considered to help identify patients at risk for hematoma expansion (Class 11b, level of evidence B) and CTA, CT venography, contrast-enhanced CT, contrast-enhanced MRI, MR angiography and magnetic resonance venography, and catheter angiography can be useful to evaluate for underlying structural lesions including vascular malformations and tumours when there is clinical or radiological suspicion (Class 11a, level of evidence B).

10.4.1. Diagnosis

Rapid diagnosis is essential in the management of the condition. Deterioration in the first few hours after onset has been reported due to haematoma expansion [64].

Initial assessment will include stabilization of patient by maintaining the airway. General physical examination and quick neurological examination should be performed on all patients. Vital signs should be measured. Baseline severity scale score like ICH score, Glasgow coma scale (GCS), NIHSS should be employed. The ICH score is a simple clinical grading scale, reliable and validated for rapid evaluation of ICH severity [63].

10.5. Investigations

Brain non- contrast CT Scan (NCCT) - this is the goal standard in diagnosing ICH. It is convenient and highly sensitive in the detection of ICH [65]. Other useful information that can be extracted from NCCT includes the location of ICH, intraventricular bleed, hydrocephalus, early signs of herniation, lesional oedema, and midline shift. ICH volume, a strong predictor of outcome can also be estimated. Brain MRI can help in identifying the exact neuroanatomic site as well as the aetiology [66]. Other investigations are same as for ischaemic stroke.

10.6. Management

Airway management is similar to that of acute ischaemic stroke.

10.6.1. Peri-haematomal oedema

This occurs in the first few days after intracerebral haemorrhage. It is significantly associated with hematoma expansion, increased intracranial pressure, mass effect, midline shift and brain herniation leading to poor functional outcome of ICH [67–69]. Agents that can reduce peri-haematomal oedema process provide protective effects for ICH. These include the use of osmotic diuretics such as Mannitol. Hypertonic saline can also be used. An earlier retrospective study had reported rapid reversal of transtentorial herniation and decreased intracranial pressure with the use of 23.4% of hypertonic saline [70]. Another study had observed the superiority of hypertonic saline over mannitol in the treatment of increased intracranial pressure [71]. The routine use of mannitol in small ICH and asymptomatic peri-haematoma oedema should be discouraged.

10.6.2. Seizures

These are common in ICH occurring in up to 16% of the cases in the first week with most occurring at onset [72]. Lobar haematomas carry an increased risk of seizures than deep ICH [73]. A recent AHA/ASA guideline for management of spontaneous ICH recommend the use of antiepileptic drugs only in patients with clinical seizures and those with depressed mental status found to have electrographic seizures on EEG [74]. Drugs that have been used include intravenous Lorazepam (0.05–0.1 mg/kg), fosphenytoin (or Phenytoin 15-20 mg/kg), and valproic acid (15-45 mg/kg).

10.6.3. Hyperglycaemia

Hyperglycaemia at presentation portends a worse outcome. This is independent of diabetes mellitus [75]. Treatment involves the use of Insulin. Hypoglycaemia should be avoided.

10.6.4. Deep vein thrombosis

Symptomatic deep vein thrombosis occurs in 1–5% of patients with ICH with pulmonary embolism occurring in about 0.5–2% of such cases. It is therefore crucial to prevent both DVT and PE [76]. Prophylaxis for DVT includes the use of intermittent pneumatic compression devices (IPC) or compression stockings if IPC devices are not available. Subcutaneous low-dose unfractionated heparin can be used when the intracranial bleeding has been controlled within 48 hours of the admission [74].

10.6.5. Blood pressure

Lowering of blood pressure in the setting of ICH has been frequently practiced to reduce haematoma growth. However, the association between elevated BP and hematoma expansion remains controversial. An increasing blood pressure has been associated with haematoma expansion. The AHA/ASA guidelines recommend mean arterial Pressure of 130 mmHg. Titratable antihypertensive drugs such as Intravenous Labetalol (10–20 mg IV bolus, can be repeated up to max of 60 mg) and Nicardipine (5 mg/h up to 15 mg/h) are often used in acute ICH. Nitroprusside should be avoided because of its tendency to increase ICP.

10.6.6. Fever

This is a frequent occurrence in patients with ICH especially in those with intraventricular extension. Patients with persistent fever after ICH tend to have a worse prognosis [77].

10.6.7. Haemostatic therapy

The outcome of ICH is made worse by coagulopathy as this causes expansion of haematoma. Coagulopathy should therefore be reversed. Intravenous Vitamin K 10 mg and fresh frozen plasma 20 ml/kg can be given to patients with Warfarin related ICH. Alternatives to fresh frozen plasma include prothrombin complex concentrate and activated factor VII (Novoseven) [78]. Although recombinant factor VIIa was shown to be efficacious in reducing haematoma growth in phase II trial, it failed to demonstrate consistency in efficacy in subsequent trials. It is often used in patients with ICH associated haemophilia.

10.6.8. Intraventricular haemorrhage and hydrocephalus

About 45% of patients with intracerebral haemorrhage (ICH) develop intraventricular haemorrhage (IVH). ICH often predicts a poor outcome. There are two types of IVH; the primary –confined to the ventricles and secondary due to extension of an ICH. Secondary IVH is the commonest and is related to haemorrhages from hypertension involving the basal ganglia and the thalamus [79]. Treatment involves the use of intraventricular administration of rt-PA or urokinase. This was found to reduce mortality and morbidity by increasing blood clearance and clot lysis [80]. Unfortunately, the procedure was not without the risk of intracranial bleeding [81]. Other treatment options included an endoscopic surgical evacuation and ventriculostomy, ventriculoperitoneal shunting or lumbar drainage for hydrocephalus [82–84].

10.6.9. Surgical intervention

Controversies exist over the role of surgical haematoma evacuation. The International Surgical Trial in Intracerebral haemorrhage (ISTICH) and subsequent STICH 11 demonstrated no improvement for early haematoma evacuation in patients with supratentorial ICH [85, 86]. However in subgroup analysis, patients with superficial haematomas were more prone to a favourable outcome when managed surgically compared to deep ICH. In contrast to supratentorial haematomas, cerebellar ICH is a neurosurgical emergency requiring urgent evacuation as rapid deterioration can occur in the first 24 hours of onset. Indications for surgical intervention include haemorrhages greater than 3 cm and those with brainstem compression or hydrocephalus [87].

10.7. Stroke recovery and rehabilitation

Advancement in the treatment of acute stroke and the establishment of dedicated stroke units has led to an increase in the survival of stroke patients. Many of the survivors experience persistent difficulty in their activities of daily living. Moderate functional impairment has been observed in 40% of stroke patients with about 15–30% having severe disability [88]. Early initiation of effective rehabilitation post stroke has been found to enhance recovery process and minimize functional disability. Stroke rehabilitation is therefore crucial for recovery post stroke.

The services of rehabilitation involve a multidisciplinary approach comprising healthcare providers with training in neurology, rehabilitation nursing, physical therapy, occupational therapy and speech and language therapy. Other health professionals who play key roles in rehabilitation include social workers, psychologists, psychiatrists and counselors [89].

Stroke rehabilitation usually commences during the acute hospitalization when the patient has been stabilized medically and neurologically. The major concern in the acute phase are prevention of a recurrent stroke, prevention of complications, mobilizing the patient, promoting resumption of activities of daily living as well as providing emotional support to the patient and family. Thereafter the focus shifts to evaluation and recovery of any residual physical and cognitive deficits [90].

A patient with stroke is at risk of developing joint and muscle contractures. The reasons for this are multifactorial and include hemiparesis, impaired sensation, reduced level of consciousness, older age, incontinence and pressures sores. Early rehabilitation can reduce the contractures.

10.8. Conclusion

Recent advances in neuroimaging, organized stroke care, dedicated Neuro-ICUs, medical and surgical management have changed the management of ICH. Early airway protection, blood pressure control, rapid reversal of coagulopathy and surgical intervention may increase the chance of survival for patients with severe ICH.

Author details

Ekanem Philip-Ephraim

Address all correspondence to: nneninge@yahoo.com

University of Calabar Teaching Hospital, Calabar, Nigeria

References

[1] Hill MD, Liebeskind DS, Roberts S. Case fatality rates after hospital admission for stroke. BMJ. 2003;**326**:1085-1086

[2] Jones MR, Horner RD, Edwards LJ, Hoff J, Armstrong SB, Smith-Hammond CA, et al. Racial variation in initial stroke severity. Stroke. 2000;**31**:563-567

[3] Gillum RF. Stroke mortality in blacks: Disturbing trends. Stroke. 1999;**30**:1711-1715

[4] Feigin VL, Lawes CM, Bennett DA, Anderson CS. Stroke epidemiology: A review of population-based studies of incidence, prevalence, and case fatality in the late 20th century. Lancet Neurology. 2003;**2**:43-53

[5] Welch KMA. Statins for the prevention cerebrovascular disease: The rationale for robust intervention. European Heart Journal Supplements. 2004;**s6**:c34-c42

[6] Bath PM, Lees KR. ABC of arterial and venous disease: Acute stroke. BMJ. 2000;**320**:920-923

[7] Warlow CP. Epidemiology of stroke. Lancet. 1998;**352**:1-4

[8] Romero JR, Morris J, Pikula A. Stroke prevention: Modifying risk factors. Therapeutic Advances in Cardiovascular Disease. 2008;**2**(4):287-303

[9] Hankey GJ. Preventable stroke and stroke prevention. Journal of Thrombosis and Haemostasis. 2005;**3**:1638-1645

[10] Sani M, Lacey J, Rudd A, et al. The management of stroke. Hospital Pharmacist. 2002;**9**: 37-41

[11] Diener H, Wong P. Developments in secondary stroke prevention. European Neurological Review. 2008;**3**(2):50-57

[12] Adams HP. Secondary prevention of Atherothrombotic events after ischaemic stroke. Mayo Clinic Proceedings. 2009;**84**(1):43-51

[13] Goldstein LB, Simel DL. Is this patient having a stroke? Journal of the American Medical Association. 2005;**293**(19):2391-2402

[14] Goldstein LB. Modern medical management of acute ischaemic stroke. Methodist DeBakey Cardiovascular Journal. 2014;**10**(2):99-104

[15] Lyden P, Raman R, Liu L, Emr M, Warren M, Marier J. National Institute of health stroke scale certification is reliable across multiple venues. Stroke. 2009;**40**:2507-2511

[16] Jauch EC, Saver JC, Adams HP, Bruno A, Connors JJ, et al. Guidelines for the early management of patients with acute ischaemic stroke. Stroke. 2013;**44**:870-947

[17] Ay H, Koroshetz WJ, Benner T, Vangel MG, Melinosky C, Arsava EM, Ayata C, et al. Neuroanatomy correlates of stroke-related myocardial injury. Neurology. 2006;**66**: 1325-1329

[18] Cui Y, Ren H, Lee C, Li S, et al. Characteristics of elevated cardiac Troponin I in patients with acute ischaemic stroke. Journal of Geriatric Cardiology. 2017;**14**(6):401-406

[19] Milhaud D, Popp J, Thouvenot E, Heroum C, Bonafe A. Mechanical ventilation in ischaemic stroke. Journal of Stroke and Cerebrovascular Diseases. 2004;**13**:183-188

[20] Singhai AB. Oxygen therapy in stroke: Past, present and future. International Journal of Stroke. 2006;**1**(4):191-200

[21] Chan YY, Katz M, Moskowitz A, et al. Supplemental oxygen delivery to suspected stroke patients in pre hospital and emergency department setting. Medical Gas Research. 2014;**4**:16

[22] Grotta J, Pasteur W, Khwaja G, Hamel T, Fisher M, Ramirez A. Elective intubation for neurologic deterioration after stroke. Neurology. 1995;**45**(4):640-644

[23] Britton M, Carlsson A, de Faire U. Blood pressure course in patients with acute stroke and matched controls. Stroke 1986;**17**:861-864.

[24] Willmot M, Leonardi-Bee J, Bath PMW. High blood pressure in acute stroke and subsequent outcome: A systematic review. Hypertension. 2004;**43**:18-24

[25] Appleton JP, Sprigg N, Bath PM. Blood pressure management in acute stroke. Stroke and vascular. Neurology. 2016;**1**:e000020

[26] Chamorro A, Amaro S, Vargas M, et al. Catecholamines, infection and death in acute ischaemic stroke. Journal of the Neurological Sciences. 2007;**252**:29-35

[27] Alqadri SL, Sreenivasan V, Qureshi AI. Acute hypertensive response management in patients with acute stroke. Current Cardiology Reports. 2013;**15**:426

[28] Fodstad H, Kelly PJ, Buchfelder M. History of Cushing reflex. Neurosurgery. 2006;**59**: 1132-1137

[29] Robinson TG, James M, Youde J, et al. Cardiac baroreceptor sensitivity is impaired after acute stroke. Stroke. 1997;**28**:1671-1676

[30] Sprigg N, Bath PMW. Management of blood pressure in acute stroke. Practical Neurology. 2005;**5**:218-223

[31] Owens WB. Blood pressure control in acute cerebrovascular disease. Journal of Clinical Hypertension. 2011;**13**:205-211

[32] Spence JD, Del Maestro RF. Hypertension in acute ischaemic strokes. Archives of Neurology. 1985;**42**:1000-1002

[33] Yatsu FM, Ziyin J. Hypertension in acute ischaemic strokes. Archives of Neurology. 1985;**42**:999-1000

[34] Vemmos KN, Tsivgoulis G, Spengos K, Zakopoulos N, et al. U-shaped relationship between mortality and admission blood pressure in patients with acute stroke. Journal of Internal Medicine. 2004;**255**:257-265

[35] Kiers L, Davis SM, Larkins R, Hopper J, Tress B, Rossiter SC, Carlin J, Ratnaike S. Stroke topography and outcome in relation to hyperglycemia and diabetes. Journal of Neurology, Neurosurgery, and Psychiatry. 1992;**55**:263-270

[36] Baker L, Juneja R, Bruno A. Management of hyperglycaemia in acute ischemic stroke. Current Treatment Options in Neurology. 2011;**13**(6):616-628

[37] Yip PK, He YY, Hsu CY, Garg N, Marangos P, Hogen EL. Effect of plasma glucose on infarct size in focal cerebral ischemia-reperfusion. Neurology. 1991;**41**:899-905

[38] Voll CL, Auer RN. Insulin attenuates ischemic brain damage independent of its hypoglycemic effect. Journal of Cerebral Blood Flow and Metabolism. 1991;**11**:1006-1014

[39] Azzimondi G, Bassein L, Nonino F, Fiorani L, et al. Fever in acute stroke worsens prognosis: A prospective study. Stroke. 1995;**26**:2040-2043

[40] Prasad K, Krishnan PR. Fever is associated with doubling of odds of short-term mortality in ischemic stroke: An updated meta-analysis. Acta Neurologica Scandinavica. 2010; **122**:404-408

[41] Wrotek SE, Kozak WE, Hess DC, Fagan SC. Treatment of fever after stroke: Conflicting evidence. Pharmacotherapy. 2011;**31**(11):1085-1091

[42] CAPRIE Steering Committee. A randomised, blinded, trial of clopidogrel versus aspirin in patients at risk of ischaemic events (CAPRIE). Lancet. 1996;**348**(9038):1329-1339

[43] Halkes PH, van Gijn J, Kappelle LJ, Koudstaal PJ, Algra A. Aspirin plus dipyridamole versus aspirin alone after cerebral ischaemia of arterial origin (ESPRIT): Randomised controlled trial. ESPRIT Study Group, Lancet. 2006;**367**(9523):1665-1673

[44] Diener HC, Cunha L, Forbes C, Sivenius J, Smets P, Lowenthal A. European Stroke Prevention Study. 2. Dipyridamole and acetylsalicylic acid in the secondary prevention of stroke. Journal of the Neurological Sciences. 1996;**143**(1-2):1-13

[45] Adjusted-dose warfarin versus low-intensity. Fixed-dose warfarin plus aspirin for high-risk patients with atrial fibrillation. Stroke Prevention in Atrial Fibrillation III randomised clinical trial. Lancet. 1996;**348**(9028):633-638

[46] Connolly SJ, Ezekowitz MD, Yusuf S, Eikelboom J, Oldgren J, Parekh A, Pogue J, Reilly PA, Themeles E, Varrone J, Wang S, Alings M, Xavier D, Zhu J, Diaz R, Lewis BS, Darius H, Diener HC, Joyner CD, Wallentin L. Dabigatran versus warfarin in patients with atrial fibrillation.RE-LY steering committee and investigators. The New England Journal of Medicine. 2009 17;**361**(12):1139-1151

[47] Hong K, Lee JS. Statins in acute ischaemic stroke: A systematic review. Journal of Stroke. 2015;**17**(3):282-301

[48] Montecucco F, Quercioli A, Mrabelli-Badenier M, et al. Statins in the treatment of acute ischaemic stroke. Current Pharmaceutical Biotechnology. 2012;**13**(1):68-76

[49] Flint AC, Kamel H, Navi BB, Rao VA, et al. Statin use during ischaemic stroke hospitalization is strongly associated with improved Poststroke survival. Stroke. 2012;**43**(1):147-154

[50] The National Institute of Neurological Disorders and Stroke rt-PA Stroke Study Group. Tissue plasminogen activator for acute ischemic stroke. The New England Journal of Medicine. 1995;**333**:1581-1587

[51] Saver J, Jahan R, Levy E, et al. Solitaire flow restoration device versus the Merci retriever in patients with acute ischaemic stroke (SWIFT): A randomized parallel-group, non-inferiority trial. Lancet. 2012;**380**:1241-1249

[52] Nogueira R, Lutsep H, Gupta R, et al. Trevo versus Merci retrievers for thrombectomy revascularisation of large vessel occlusions in acute ischaemic stroke (TREVO 2): A randomised trial. Lancet. 2012;**380**:1231-1240

[53] Kumar S, Selim MH, Caplan LR. Medical complications after stroke. Lancet Neurology. 2010;**9**(1):105-118

[54] Indredavik B, Rohweder G, Naalsund E, Lydersen S. Medical complications in a comprehensive stroke unit and an early supported discharge service. Stroke. 2008;**39**:414-420

[55] Desmukh M, Bisignani M, Landau P, Orchard TJ. Deep vein thrombosis in rehabilitating stroke patients: Incidence, risk factors and prophylaxis. American Journal of Physical Medicine & Rehabilitation. 1991;**70**:313-316

[56] Gebel JM, Broderick JP. Intracerebral haemorrhage. Neurologic Clinics. 2000;**18**(2):419-438

[57] Taylor CL, Selman WR, Ratcheson RA. Brain attack: The emergent management of hypertensive haemorrhage. Neurosurgery Clinics of North America. 1997;**8**:237-244

[58] Kazui S, Minematsu K, Yamamoto H, Sawada T, Yamaguchi T. Predisposing factors to enlargement of spontaneous intracerebral hematoma. Stroke. 1997;**28**:2370-2375

[59] Feldstein CA. Early treatment of hypertension in acute ischaemic and intracerebral haemorrhagic stroke: Progress achieved, challenges and perspectives. Journal of the American Society of Hypertension. 2014;**8**(3):192-202

[60] Carpenter AM, Singh IP, Gandhi CD, Prestigiacomo CJ. Genetic risk factors for spontaneous intracerebral haemorrhage. Nature Reviews. Neurology. 2016;**12**(1):40-49

[61] An SJ, Kim TJ, Yoon B. Epidemiology risk factors and clinical features of Intracerebral haemorrhage: An update. Journal of Stroke. 2017;**19**(1):3-10

[62] Kim KS, Brophy GM. Symptomatic venous thromboembolism: Incidence and risk factors in patients with spontaneous or traumatic intracranial hemorrhage. Neurocritical Care. 2009;**11**:28-33

[63] Hemphill JC, Bonovich DC, Besmertis L, Manley GT, Johnson SC. The ICH score: A simple, reliable grading scale for intracerebral hemorrhage. Stroke. 2001;**32**(4):891-897

[64] Rodriguez-Luna D, Pineiro S, Rubiera M, et al. Impact of blood pressure changes and course on haematoma growth in acute intracerebral haemorrhage. European Journal of Neurology. 2013;**20**:1277-1283

[65] Macellari F, Paciaroni M, Agnellia G, Caso V. Neuroimaging in intracerebral haemorrhage. Stroke. 2014;**45**(3):903-908

[66] Rabinstein AA, Resnick SJ. Practical Neuroimaging in Stroke: A Case-Based Approach. Philadelphia: Saunders/Elsevier; 2009

[67] Arima H, Wang JG, Huang Y, et al. Significance of perihematomal edema in acute intracerebral hemorrhage: The INTERACT trial. Neurology. 2009;**73**:i963-i968

[68] Murthy SB, Moradiya Y, Dawson J, et al. Perihematomal edema and functional outcomes in intracerebral hemorrhage: Influence of hematoma volume and location. Stroke. 2015;**46**:3088-3092

[69] Yang J, Arima H, Wu G, et al. Prognostic significance of perihematomal edema in acute intracerebral hemorrhage: Pooled analysis from the intensive blood pressure reduction in acute cerebral hemorrhage trial studies. Stroke. 2015;**46**:1009-1013

[70] Koenig MA, Bryan M, 111 LJL, et al. Reversal of transtentorial herniation with hypertonic saline. Neurology. 2008;**70**:1023-1029

[71] Kamel H, Navi BB, Nakagawa K, et al. Hypertonic saline versus mannitol for the treatment of elevated intracranial pressure: A meta-analysis of randomized clinical trials. Critical Care Medicine. 2011;**39**:554-559

[72] De Herdt V, Dumont F, Henon H, et al. Early seizures in intracerebral hemorrhage: Incidence, associated factors and outcome. Neurology. 2011;**77**:1794-1800

[73] Passero S, Rocchi R, Rossi S, Ulivelli M, Vatti G. Seizures after spontaneous supratentorial intracerebral hemorrhage. Epilepsia. 2002;**43**(10):1175-1180

[74] Morgenstem L, Hemphill C, Anderson C, Berker K, Broderick JP, Connoly ES, et al. Guidelines for the management of spontaneous intracerebral hemorrhage. A guideline for healthcare professionals from the American Heart Association/American stroke association. Stroke. 2010;**41**:2108-2129

[75] Passero S, Ciacci G, Ulivelli M. The influence of diabetes and hyperglycemia on clinical course after intracerebral hemorrhage. Neurology. 2003;**61**:1351-1356

[76] Goldstein JN, Fazen LE, Wendell L, et al. Risk of thromboembolism following acute intracerebral hemorrhage. Neurocritical Care. 2009;**10**:28-34

[77] Schwarz S, Hafner K, Aschoff A, et al. Incidence and prognostic significance of fever following intracerebral hemorrhage. Neurology. 2000;**54**:354-361

[78] Aguilar M, Brott TG. Update in Intracerebral Hemorrhage. The Neurohospitalist. 2011; **1**(3):148-159

[79] Hallevi H, Albright KC, Aronowski J, Barreto AD, Martin-Schild S, Khaja AM, Gonzales NR, Illoh K, Noser EA, Grotta JC. Intraventricular hemorrhage: Anatomic relationships and clinical implications. Neurology. 2008;**70**:848-852

[80] Fountas KN, Kapsalaki EZ, Parish DC, Smith B, Smisson HF, Johnston KW, Robinson JS. Intraventricular administration of rt-PA in patients with intraventricular hemorrhage. Southern Medical Journal. 2005;**98**:767-773

[81] Morgan T, Awad I, Keyl P, Lane K, Hanley D. Preliminary report of the clot lysis evaluating accelerated resolution of intraventricular hemorrhage (CLEAR-IVH) clinical trial. Acta Neurochirurgica. 2008;**105**:217-220

[82] Horváth Z, Veto F, Balás I, Kumlautovér F, Dóczi T. Biportal endoscopic removal of a primary intraventricular hematoma: Case report. Minimally Invasive Neurosurgery. 2000;**43**:4-8

[83] Yilmazlar S, Abas F, Korfali E. Comparison of ventricular drainage in poor grade patients after intracranial hemorrhage. Neurological Research. 2005;**27**:653-656

[84] Huttner HB, Schwab S, Bardutzky J. Lumbar drainage for communicating hydrocephalus after ICH with ventricular hemorrhage. Neurocritical Care. 2006;**5**:193-196

[85] Mendelow AD, Gregson BA, Femandes HM, et al. Early surgery versus initial conservative treatment in patients with spontaneous supratentorial intracerebral haematomas in the international surgical trial in Intracerebral haemorrhage (STICH): A randomised trial. Lancet. 2005;**365**:387-397

[86] Mendelow AD, Gregson BA, Rowan EN, et al. Early surgery versus initial conservative treatment in patients with spontaneous supratentorial lobar intracerebral haematomas (STICH II): A randomised trial. Lancet. 2013;**382**:397-408

[87] Broderick J, Connolly S, Feldmann E, et al. Guidelines for the management of spontaneous intracerebral haemorrhages in adults: 2007 update: A guideline from the American Heart Association/American Stroke Association stroke council, high blood pressure research council, and the quality of care and outcomes in research interdisciplinary working group. Stroke. 2007;**38**(6):2001-2023

[88] American Heart Association. Heart and Stroke Statistical Update—2005. Dallas, Tex: American Heart Association; 2004

[89] Winstein CJ, Stein J, Arena R, Bates B, Cherney LR, et al. Guidelines for adult stroke rehabilitation and recovery. In: A Guidelinefor Healthcare Professionals from the American Heart Association/American Stroke Association. 2016

[90] Duncan PW, Zorowitz R, Bates B, et al. Management of adult stroke rehabilitation care: A clinical practice guideline. Stroke. 2005;**36**:e100-e143

Chapter 11

Toxicology in Emergency Medicine

Ehab Said Aki, Waleed Awad Salem and Jalal Alessai

Additional information is available at the end of the chapter

http://dx.doi.org/10.5772/intechopen.77011

Abstract

Poisoning is a serious worldwide public health problem. Based on WHO data in 2012, almost 190,000 people died worldwide and the number of deaths due to poisoning in 2008 exceeded the number of deaths due to motor vehicular crashes; also, poisoning death rate nearly tripled worldwide. Number of patients presenting to the emergency departments with overdose, had been increased both intentionally and accidentally. All the previous facts make Toxicology an important field in emergency medicine. Management of intoxicated patients has a unique approach because of the challenge in diagnosis and treatment of overdose cases. This chapter is focusing on general approaches for intoxicated patients and initial management and on how the history and physical examinations could help physicians to have what drug have been abused as well as review the mechanism of action, physical finding and treatment of the most common drugs-causing toxicity in addition to the drugs with high mortality morbidity rates.

Keywords: approach, decontamination, toxidrome, acetaminophen, aspirin, cardiac drug toxicity, pesticides, toxic alcohol

1. Introduction

Poisoning is a serious worldwide public health problem. Based on World Health Organization (WHO) data in 2012, almost 190,000 people died worldwide and number of deaths due to poisoning in 2008 exceeded the number of deaths due to motor vehicular crashes; also, poisoning death rate nearly tripled worldwide. Number of patients presenting to the emergency departments with overdose, had been increased both intentionally and accidentally. All the previous facts make Toxicology an important field in emergency medicine [1, 2].

Management of intoxicated patients has a unique approach because of the challenge in diagnosis and treatment of overdose cases. This chapter is focusing on general approaches for intoxicated patients and initial management and on how the history and physical examinations could help physicians to have what drug have been abused as well as review the mechanism of action, physical finding and treatment of the most common drugs-causing toxicity in addition to the drugs with high mortality morbidity rates.

2. General approach to toxicological cases in emergency medicine

Approach for the poisoned patients in emergency includes: resuscitation, history, physical examination and management.

3. Resuscitation

The initial priorities for a poisoned patient presented emergency department are: securing the air-way and breathing and stabilizing the circulation. Inadequate ventilation may need intubation and mechanical ventilation. First-line treatment of hypotension is IV fluid bolus (10–20 mL/kg), if hypotension is not responding to fluid, it may be necessary to add specific antidote. If the patient presented with signs of opioid over dose (low Glasgow coma scale-GCS respiratory depression, meiosis), give him naloxone (0.1–2.0 mg I.V), check blood sugar and treat hypoglycaemia with 50% 50 mL dextrose [3].

4. History

History is very important and can be obtained from the patient, and in case the patient is comatose or cannot give his history, we may take collateral information from family, friends or medical records looking for past psychiatry illness, previous history of suicide or drugs abuse, chronic medication… History must include time, route of entry, quantity, intentional or accidental exposure, availability of drugs at home and if any member of the family has chronic diseases (hypertension, diabetic etc…), missing tablets or any empty pill bottles or other material was found around him [4].

5. Physical examination

Physical examination of poisoned patients may give clues regarding the substance which has been abused and toxidromes. Physical examination includes: general appearance, mental status (agitated or confused), Skin (cyanosis, flashing, physical signs of intravenous drugs abuse (track marks), eyes: (pupil size reactivity lacrimation and nystagmus), odour (garlic, bitter almonds, glue, alcohol etc.…), Oropharynx hyper salivation or dryness, chest: breath sound, bronchorrhea, wheezing, heart rate, rhythm regularity), abdomen(bowel sound, tenderness, and rigidity), limbs(tremors and fasciculation), patient's clothing (looking for any medications, illegal drugs) [3].

http://dx.doi.org/10.5772/intechopen.77011

6. Toxidromes

The term toxidrome was coined in 1970 by Mofenson and Greensher. Toxidromes are group of abnormal physical examination and abnormal vital signs known to present with specific group of medications or substances. Most common toxidromes are Cholinergic, Anticholinergic, Sympathomimetic, opioids, and serotonin syndrome [4, 5].

6.1. Cholinergics

Patients with cholinergic toxidrome present with wet manifestation. SLUDGE+3 killer B's"or DUMBELLS are simple mnemonics for the common clinical symptoms.

"SLUDGE": Salivation, Lacrimation, Urination, Defecation, GI cramping, Emesis + "Killer B's": Bronchorrhea, Bradycardia, and Bronchospasm.

"DUMBELLS": Diarrhoea, Urination, Miosis (small pupils), Bradycardia, Emesis, Lacrimation, Lethargy, and Salivation.

Most common Causes: Organophosphate pesticides, Carbamates, Same type Mushrooms and Sarin (warfare agent) [4].

6.2. Anticholinergics

Patients with Anticholinergic toxidrome with dry manifestation, delirium, tachycardia, dry flushed skin, dilated pupils, clonus, elevated temperature, decreased bowl sounds, urinary retention. Simple mnemonics: "Hot as a Hare, Mad as a Hatter, Red as a Beet, Dry as a Bone, Blind as a Bat".

Most common Causes: Antihistamines, antiparkinsonians, atropine, scopolamine, amantadine, antipsychotics, antidepressants, muscle relaxants and plants (Jimson weed) [4].

6.3. Sympathomimetics

Patient present with CNS stimulation and psychomotor agitation, elevated blood pressure, tachycardia, dilated pupils, hyperthermia, diaphoresis and seizure in severe cases.

Most common causes: cocaine, amphetamine.

6.4. Opioids

Most common clinical presentation of opioids toxidrome are: coma, respiratory depression and meiosis, hypotension, hypothermia, bradycardia and seizure may occur in propoxyphene overdose, but small pupils not always present may present with normal size pupils such in meperidine and, propoxyphene toxicities [4].

6.5. Serotonin syndrome

Patient present with altered mental status, hypertensive, and tachycardia, Myoclonus hyperreflexia, hyperthermia and increase muscles rigidity. Most common causes: SSRI interaction or overdose [4].

7. Decontaminations

Decontamination of poisoned patient means remove the patient from the toxin and remove the toxin from patient, either outside patient's body by gross washing or inside the body by gastrointestinal decontamination or enhance elimination.

7.1. Gross decontamination

Patient must be fully undressed and washed thoroughly with copious amount of water; all the clothing must be removed, and decontamination must be in isolated specific area. Gross decontamination used in chemical, biological and radiation exposure.

7.2. Gastrointestinal decontamination

There are multiple methods used for gastrointestinal decontamination including:

Emesis and gastric Lavage.

Induced vomiting by ipecac syrup and gastric lavage: those methods were used in the past and now rarely indicated because there is no evidence supporting them. They can decrease absorption and they may also increase the risk of complications. Syrup ipecac and gastric Lavage may be considered in conscious, alert patients with ingestion of potentially number of toxic drugs and present in a very short time after ingestion (<1 h). Contradictions includes: unprotected airway, Corrosive/hydrocarbon ingestion and unstable patient status (hypotensive-seizure) [6].

7.3. Activated charcoal

Activated charcoal is super-heating carbonaceous material. Activated charcoal works by reducing the absorption of substance in the gastrointestinal lumen but it is not effective in metal, alcohols, corrosive, and lithium. Most effective action can be achieved when activated charcoal is given within the first hour of ingestion. Contraindications: absent gut motility or perforation, caustic ingestion and unprotected airway (can be given through nasogastric tube if patient intubated).Complications: aspiration of activated charcoal led to pneumonitis, ARDS and other complications such as small bowel obstruction [7].

7.4. Whole-bowel irrigation

Whole-bowel irrigation is a mechanical cleansing of the whole gastrointestinal track reducing toxin absorption. The whole-bowel irrigation can be done by Polyethylene glycol solution. Indication includes: substance with a prolonged absorption phase like sustained released medication, potential toxin not absorbed by activated charcoal such—(metals, lithium) and Body packers or suffers. Adverse effects of whole bowel irrigation could be: vomiting, bloating and rectal irritation. Contradiction: absent bowel sound or perforation [8].

7.5. Enhanced elimination

Enhanced elimination is a method used to increase the rate of toxic removal from the body so reducing the severity and duration of clinical intoxication.

http://dx.doi.org/10.5772/intechopen.77011

Enhanced elimination methods are not routinely used in poisoned patients. The indications for Enhanced elimination include [4]:

- Severe toxicity
- Poor outcome despite supportive care/antidote
- Slow endogenous rate of elimination

There are different techniques to enhance elimination:

Multiple dose activated charcoal (MDAC): it can be used in cases of carbamazepine, Phenobarbital, Dispone sever toxicities,

Urinary alkalinisation:

Can be used in cases of Salicylates Phenobarbitone.

Extracorporeal elimination (e.g. haemodialysis, hemofiltration, and haemoperfusion, plasmapheresis and exchange transfusion:

Can be used in cases of lithium, carbamazepine, salicylates, theophylline, and toxic.

Alcohols: ethylene glycol and methanol metformin.

7.6. Antidotes

Antidote is a substance that can prevent further poisoning from specific substances. The table below showing most common antidote used in emergency department (see **Table 1**) [4].

8. Acetaminophen poisoning

First time acetaminophen had been clinically used was in 1950 and since that time acetaminophen become most common over-the-counter antipyretic and analgesic used in public. Acetaminophen is the most common cause of acute liver failure in the United States [9, 10].

8.1. Mechanism of action

Acetaminophen metabolized in the liver and converted to nontoxic metabolites via glucuronidation (40–67%) and sulfation (20–46%). In therapeutic doses of acetaminophen, the small amount of NAPQI formed which detoxified by conjugation with reduced glutathione (GSH). Glutathione is an important tripeptide which is reduced in a NADPH dependent reaction, and used to reduce oxidants (such as NAPQI).

In large overdoses of APAP, the usual pharmacokinetic pathways are overwhelmed and saturation of the nontoxic pathways occurs. Endogenous glutathione is depleted and NAPQI cannot be detoxified. Leaving excess NAPQI to bind to intracellular proteins, cause cell death [11].

8.2. Clinical features

Symptoms are frequently nonspecific or absent in early Acetaminophen toxicity.

Toxin	Antidote
Acetaminophen	N-acetylcysteine 150 mg/kg dextrose IV over 15–60 min then50 mg/kg NAC IV over 4 h. Then 100 mg/kg NAC IV over 16 h.
Cholinergic (organophosphates, carbamates)	Atropine 1–2 mg every 2–3 mins, until there is drying of secretions
	Pralidoxime (2-PAM) 70 mg/kg IV then infusion at 500 mg/h
Anticholinesterases	Physostigmine 0.5–1 mg IV as a slow push over 5 min and repeat every 10 min
Benzodiazepines	Flumazenil 0.2 Mg repeated max dose 2 mg
β-Blockers	Glucagon 3–10 mg
Calcium channel blockers	Calcium gluconate 10% 10–30 mL IV
Cyanide	Amyl nitrite
	Sodium thiosulfate
	Sodium nitrite (3% solution)
	Vitamin B12
Digoxin	Digoxin Fab 5–10 vials
Isoniazid	Pyridoxine (vitamin B6) 70 mg/kg IV (maximum 5 gm)
Methanol, ethylene glycol	Ethanol Loading 8 mL/kg of 10% ethanol then 1–2 mL/kg/h of 10% ethanol
	Fomepizole Loading: 15 mg/kg in 100 mL IV over 30 min
	Maintenance: 10 mg/kg IV over 30 min every 12 h for 48 h
Narcotics	Naloxone 0.1–0.4 mg, may repeated
Tricyclic antidepressants	Sodium bicarbonate
	1–2 mEq/kg IV bolus followed by 2 mEq/kg per h IV infusion
iron	Desferrioxamine IV infusion dose of 15 mg/kg/h
methaemoglobinaemia	Methylene Blue 1–2 mg/kg (0.1–0.2 mL/kg of 1% solution) IV slowly over 5 min
local anaesthetics	Intravenous lipid emulsion 1–1.5 mL/kg 20% IV bolus over 1 min Repeat bolus at 3–5 min
	Then Infuse 0.25 mL/kg/min

Table 1. Antidote.

Clinical presentation of Acetaminophen toxicity divided into four stages:

- Stage I (first 24 h): Patients may present nausea, vomiting, malaise, anorexia, or may be asymptomatic. Also hypokalaemia and metabolic acidosis can be found in blood test.
- -Stage II (Days 2–3): patients develop nausea, vomiting, right upper quadrant abdominal pain and laboratory evidence of hepatotoxicity. Aminotransferases (AST and ALT) elevate into thousands.
- -Stage III (3–4 days) defined by maximum hepatotoxicity, Patients exhibit coma, encephalopathy, coagulopathy, renal failure, Jaundice, acute respiratory distress syndrome (ARDS), sepsis and cerebral oedema.
- -Stage IV (7–8 d): recovery or deterioration to multi-organ failure and death [12, 13].

http://dx.doi.org/10.5772/intechopen.77011

8.3. Treatment

After initial support of airway, breathing and circulation, the clinician should consider gastrointestinal (GI) decontamination by activated charcoal. The cornerstone of acetaminophen overdose is N-acetylcysteine (NAC). NAC serves as a precursor to glutathione and may also directly reduce NAPQI. Clinical data suggest that if therapy is initiated within 8 h of ingestion, NAC is completely effective in preventing hepatotoxicity. Although NAC decreases in efficacy after 8 h, the drug has a benefit at all points in time, even for patients with fulminant hepatic failure.

N-acetylcysteine should only be given to patients with hepatotoxicity or risk of developing hepatotoxicity. The Rumack-Matthew nomogram is a tool for determining potential hepatotoxicity based on Acetaminophen level and time after ingestion. The nomogram is used to determine the risk for APAP hepatotoxicity for patients who present within 24 h of an acute ingestion. Risk determination of hepatotoxicity becomes more difficult

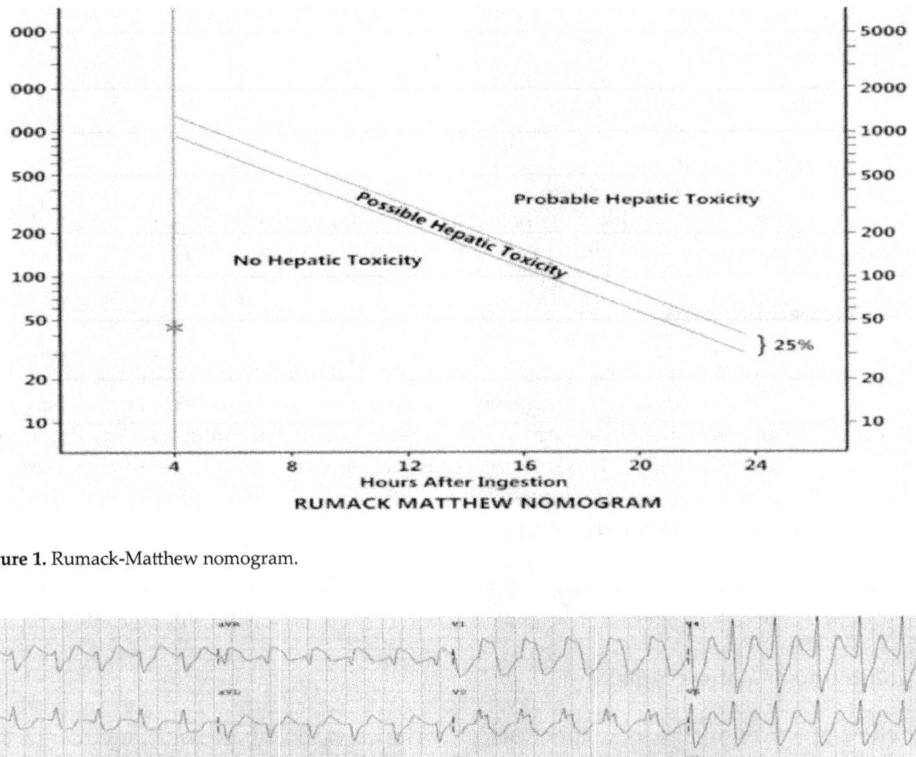

Figure 1. Rumack-Matthew nomogram.

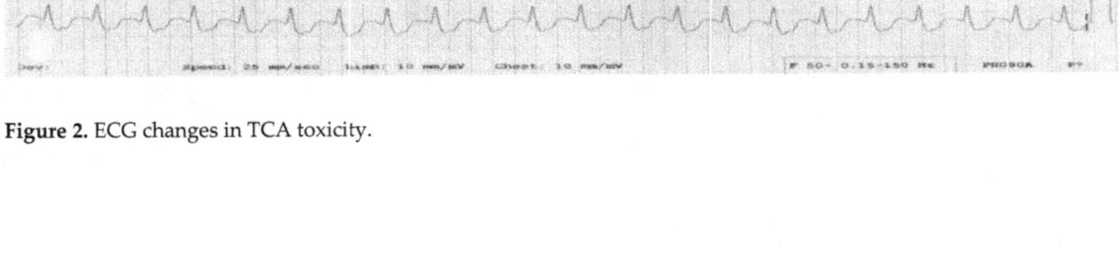

Figure 2. ECG changes in TCA toxicity.

when the nomogram is not applicable. Examples of such cases would be when the time of ingestion is unknown, when patients present more than 24 h after the ingestion and following ingestions that occur over many hours. In all of these cases NAC should be administered immediately. If aminotransferases (ALT, AST) are normal and APAP concentration is undetectable, the NAC may be discontinued. Otherwise, treatment with NAC should be continued.

N-acetylcysteine dose Oral 140 mg/kg loading dose 70 mg/kg q4 h × 17 doses or Intravenous 150 mg/kg loading dose 50 mg/kg over 4 h 100 mg/kg over 16 h [14–16] (**Figures 1** and **2**).

9. Cyclic antidepressants (CA) poisoning

Cyclic antidepressants were used to depression, but now their use has reduced greatly because of the presences of more safe agents. Cyclic antidepressants were most common antidepressants associated with overdose-related deaths in 2013 [17].

9.1. Mechanism of action

CA has multiple pharmacologic effects.

9.2. Antihistamine effects

Cyclic antidepressants are inhibiting postsynaptic histamine receptors, causing sedation, decrease level of conscious and coma.

9.3. Antimuscarinic effects

Antimuscarinic effects are divided to central and peripheral. Inhibition central acetylcholine receptors cause agitation, delirium, confusion, hallucinations, slurred speech, ataxia and coma. Inhibition Peripheral acetylcholine receptors inhibition cause dilated pupils, tachycardia, hyperthermia, hypertension, dry skin, ileus, urinary retention, increased muscle tone and tremor [18].

9.4. Inhibition of α-adrenergic receptors

This effects cause sedation, orthostatic hypotension, tachycardia and pupillary constriction, but because of the antimuscarinic effects, this action usually offsets pupillary dilatation [18].

9.5. Inhibition of amine reuptake

This effect produces mydriasis, diaphoresis, tachycardia, early hypertension, myoclonus and hyperreflexia.

9.6. Inhibition sodium channel block

This effect produces decreased conduction velocity, increases the duration of repolarization and depressed myocardial contractility which lead to heart blocks, bradycardia and widening of the QRS complex [19].

9.7. Inhibition potassium channel block

This effect produces QT interval prolongation and rarely torsades de pointes can be seen [19].

9.8. Clinical features

Symptoms occur typically within 2 h of ingestion, which varies from mild antimuscarinic symptoms to severe cardio-toxicity. Patient may present with drowsiness, confusion, slurred speech, ataxia, sinus tachycardia, urinary retention, myoclonus and hyperreflexia. Serious toxicity is almost seen within 6 h of ingestion and patient present with: coma, cardiac conduction delays, supraventricular tachycardia, hypotension, respiratory depression, ventricular tachycardia and seizures [20, 21].

9.9. ECG changes in cyclic antidepressant poisoning

- Sinus tachycardia, most common
- Right axis deviation of the terminal 40 milliseconds positive terminal R wave in lead aVR and a negative S wave in lead I)
- Prolongation of QRS,(risk of seizures increases if the QRS complex is >100 milliseconds)
- Prolongation QT, PR
- Brugada pattern is seen 10–15%

9.10. Treatment

Treatment starts with supportive management securing airway, bolus i.v fluid in case of hypotension, GI decontamination with activated charcoal within 1 h of ingestion.

Add vasopressors if hypotensive refractory to IV normal saline. Cardiac conduction abnormalities, ventricular dysrhythmias, or hypotension refractory to IV fluid are indicated to start blood alkalization by Sodium bicarbonate Keep blood pH 7.50–7.55. Seizures, treat with Benzodiazepines if seizure refractory use Phenobarbital 10–15 mg/kg, The medication contraindication in CA toxicity are: Class I antiarrhythmic (lidocaine, phenytoin, and flecainide), Class III antiarrhythmic (amiodarone, sotalol), B-blockers, Ca channel blockers, Physostigmine and Flumazenil [22, 23].

10. Salicylate (aspirin) poisoning

Aspirin is the most common analgesic antiplatelet therapy used in cardiovascular and cerebrovascular disease. Aspirin is over-the-counter drugs and widespread used lead to accidental and intentional toxicity [24].

10.1. Mechanism of action

Salicylate Inhibit cyclooxygenase leads to decreased synthesis of prostaglandins; prostacyclin and thromboxane. It also leads to platelet dysfunction and gastric mucosal injury. Salicylate Stimulate the chemoreceptor trigger zone in the medulla which causes nausea and vomiting. Also activate respiratory centre of the medulla leading to hyperventilation and respiratory alkalosis. Uncoupling of oxidative and Inhibit the Krebs which lead to metabolic acidosis [25].

10.2. Clinical features

Salicylate toxicity divided to **acute** and **chronic** toxicities.

10.3. Acute toxicity

Acute salicylate toxicity manifests initially through GI, CNS effects and metabolic effects. Gastric irritation, vomiting and nausea may predominate early in the course and are more predominant in the acute poisoning. Rising CNS salicylate concentrations produce tinnitus, diminished auditory acuity, vertigo and hyperventilation. As the poisoning continues, the CNS effects may progress to agitation, hallucinations, delirium, seizure and lethargy. The metabolic effects of salicylate toxicity cause uncoupling of oxidative phosphorylation leading to temperature elevation (an indicator of severe toxicity) and a large anion gap metabolic acidosis. Subsequent squeal of salicylate toxicity include renal failure, acute lung injury and platelet dysfunction.

10.4. Chronic toxicity

In contrast, chronic poisoning occurs over a longer period of time, when patients ingest more drug than they can eliminate over a prolonged period. These patients tend to be older and the overdose is unintentional. The initial presenting signs and symptoms include those of acute toxicity although with slower onset and lesser severity. Chronic toxicity may easily be confused in the elderly for sepsis, ketoacidosis, delirium, dementia, CHF or respiratory failure. Diagnostic delay in the chronically poisoned patient has been shown to cause increased morbidity and mortality.

10.5. Treatment

Stabilization of the airway, breathing and circulation are the first steps in management. Intubation may increases the severity of the aspirin toxicity, so it is better to be avoided, but if intubation is necessary patients need appropriately high minute ventilation sitting. In case of volume depleted and acidosis, start treatment with I. V fluid. Gastrointestinal decontamination with Activated charcoal may help in early ingestion. Whole bowel irrigation

http://dx.doi.org/10.5772/intechopen.77011

(WBI) is useful in case of massive ingestions or sustained preparation or enteric-coated. Sever Salicylate toxicity treated with serum Alkalinisation by sodium bicarbonate with a aim of a serum pH of ~7.5.Patients may need haemodialysis and the indications for haemodialysis are clinical deterioration, severe acid-base disturbance, altered mental status, and acute lung injury, failure of serum and urine alkalinisation and renal failure [26–28].

11. Opioids poisoning

Opioid abuse is a significant medical and social problem in the world. In the past 10 years, the number of abuses and deaths from opioid overdoses had been increased. Opioids are all substances related to opium. They have analgesic and sedative effects. Opiate is extracted from the poppy plants [29].

11.1. Mechanism of action

There are three main opioid receptors: μ (mu), κ (kappa), and δ (delta), and Opioids have agonists effect on this receptors. Stimulation of opioids receptors will cause miosis, respiratory depression, cough suppression, euphoria and decreased GI motility.

11.2. Clinical features

Classic signs of opioid intoxication toxidrome, depressed mental status, decreased respiratory rate miosis, (constricted) pupils. Other finding includes: decreased bowel sounds orthostatic hypotension, urinary retention and localized urticaria. Normal pupil examination can be seen, meperidine diphenoxylate, propoxyphene toxicity and co-ingestion of other toxin such as sympathomimetic or anticholinergic.

Same opioids have specific clinical feature (**Table 2**) [30, 32]:

Opioids agent	**Specific clinical feature**
Dextromethorphan	Serotonin toxicity; at high doses
Loperamide	QRS and QT prolongation; Wide-complex tachycardia
Meperidine	Seizure, normal pupils size
	Serotonin syndrome (in combination with other agents)
Methadone	long-acting;
	QT prolongation, Torsade de Pointes
Oxycodone	QT interval prolongation
Tramadol	Seizure
Heroin	Acute lung injury

Body packing: swallowing packets or containers of drug for the purposes of smuggling.
Body stuffing: swallowing of a smaller quantity of drug because of fear of arrest.

Table 2. Opioids with specific clinical feature.

11.3. Treatment

Secure Airway and maintain adequate oxygenation and ventilation by using bag-valve mask are the first important steps in treatment; serum glucose should be checked. After that administer naloxone 0.4 mg IV, in non-opioid-dependent with minimal respiratory depression abut if patient is opioid-dependent present with minimal respiratory depression, administer small dose of naloxone, 0.1 mg IV, because larger doses can induce opioid withdrawal symptoms. Patients presenting with apnea or near-apnea and cyanosis, start naloxone, 2 mg IV regardless of drug use history, can be repeated IV every 3 min [30–32].

12. Sympathomimetic (cocaine) poisoning

Cocaine is one of the most potent Sympathomimetic, extracted from the leaves of the coca by indigenous to South America; therapeutically, first time Cocaine was used in 1884 as a local anaesthetic for ophthalmologic procedures. In the United States Cocaine is one of the most common causes of acute drug-related emergency department visits.

12.1. Mechanism of action

Cocaine stimulates alpha and adrenergic receptors by increasing levels of norepinephrine, causing vasoconstriction in cardiovascular system, also inhibits neuronal serotonin reuptake which lead to euphoria. Cocaine blocks Sodium (Na+) channel causing QRS interval prolongation [33, 34].

12.2. Clinical features

Cocaine toxicity may cause sympathomimetic and vasoconstrictive effects on variety systems (cardiovascular, CNS …etc.).

Cardiovascular: patients with cocaine toxicity present with high blood pressure and dysrhythmias include tachycardia, such as sinus tachycardia, SVT, and AF. ECG changes include rightward shift of the terminal portion of the QRS complex and prolongation the QT interval. Patients may present with acute coronary syndromes (cocaine-associated acute coronary syndrome), aortic and coronary artery dissection, myocarditis and cardiomyopathy. CNS: patients with Cocaine present with a variety CNS clinical features including: agitation, seizures, and coma. Pulmonary: mainly seen in patients who smoke crack cocaine includes pulmonary haemorrhage, barotrauma, pneumonitis and asthma.

Gastrointestinal: Cocaine may cause intestinal ischemia, bowel necrosis and ischemic colitis, also increase risk for bleeding and ulcer perforation. Renal: acute kidney failure may occur because of rhabdomyolysis [35–37].

12.3. Treatment

Securing the airway and adequate breathing are initial steps in treatment. CNS manifestation (agitation, seizure) treated with sedation by Benzodiazepines, patient with Hyperthermia should be cooled rapidly, severe hypertension not responding to sedation can be treated with a sodium nitroprusside infusion or phentolamine; (avoid B-ac blockers). Cocaine toxicity with acute coronary syndrome are treated with aspirin and nitroglycerin also may add calcium channel blockers, wide-complex tachycardia with cocaine toxicity treated with serum alkalinisation by sodium bicarbonate, make sure serum Ph do not exceed 7.55. Intravenous lipid emulsion can be used in severe cocaine toxicity, with refractory cardiovascular instability or refractory wide-complex tachycardia [37].

13. Digitalis glycosides poisoning

Cardiac glycosides were used in treatment of heart failure since long time. Since 1785 glycosides found in plants like lily of the valley foxglove and oleander. Digoxin is most common digitalis drug used today for treatment of atrial fibrillation and congestive heart failure [38].

13.1. Mechanism of action

Digoxin inhibits Na + -K + -ATPase during repolarization which leading to increase in intracellular sodium and a decrease in intracellular potassium leading to increase in the intracellular concentration of calcium causing Positive inotropic, also increase automaticity and shorten the repolarization intervals of the atria and ventricles [39].

13.2. Clinical features

Digoxin toxicity divided to acute and chronic toxicities.

13.3. Acute toxicity

The cause of acute toxicity is usually intentional or accidental ingestion, symptoms usually abrupt in onset, patients present with nausea, vomiting, non-specific abdominal pain, headache and dizziness. Sever toxicity may cause confusion and coma, Bradydysrhythmia and atrioventricular block or supraventricular tachydysrhythmia and hyperkalaemia. Xanthopsia is a classic eye future in digoxin toxicity (viewing yellow-green halos around objects), but the most common finding is nonspecific changes in their colour vision. Serum digoxin level usually marked elevated [40, 41].

13.4. Chronic toxicity

Chronic toxicity is commonly and mainly seen in elderly patients and common causes are interaction with other medications (calcium channel antagonists, amiodarone, β-receptor antagonists, and diuretics) or renal insufficiency which causes decree the clearance of digoxin.

In contract of acute toxicity, where Gastrointestinal symptoms are prominent in chronic toxicity CNS symptoms (weakness, fatigue, confusion, or delirium) are more prominent. Ventricular dysrhythmias are commonly seen in chronic toxicity. Serum potassium level can be normal or decreased, also serum digoxin level usually minimally elevated [40, 41].

13.5. Treatment

General supportive care is an Initial step in treatment of digoxin toxicity; it includes securing airway and adequate ventilation and boluses of fluid IV in case of hypotension. Activated charcoal helps in early acute ingestion [42], Atropine can be given in case of Symptomatic bradycardia). Digoxin-specific antibody fragments (digoxin-Fab) are antidotes for digoxin. The indication to use (digoxin- Fab) includes Life-threatening dysrhythmias unresponsive to standard therapy and hyperkalaemia excess 6 mEq/L. [43] Digoxin-Fab doses are based on the total-body load of digoxin, which can be calculated from either the estimated dose ingested or the serum digoxin level, each vial of Digoxin-Fab reverses approximately 0.5 mg of ingested digoxin. If the amount of ingested digitalis is unknown, digoxin Fab 10 vials for adults empirically can be given. Hyperkalaemia is treated with insulin, dextrose, sodium bicarbonate. The use of calcium salts in digoxin induced hyperkalaemia is controversial because old literature shows increase incidence of ventricular dysrhythmias and increase mortality [44].

14. Beta-blockers poisoning

Beta adrenergic antagonists (beta blockers) are groups of medications which have been used in treatment of different cardiovascular, neurological and ophthalmological diseases more than 30 years, Bête blockers toxicity has significant morbidity and mortality [17].

14.1. Mechanism of action

Beta receptors are divided by location and action to beta 1, beta 2, and beta 3 (see the **Table 3**).

There are two groups of beta-blockers: selective and non-selective.

Competitive antagonism of the beta receptor decreases cellular levels of cyclic adenosine monophosphate (cAMP). Beta-1 selective blocker causing in depressed myocardial contractility,

	Location	Action	Antagonism
B1	Myocardium Kidney Eye	Increases inotropy Increases chronotropy Stimulates renin release	Decreases inotropy Decreases chronotropy Inhibits renin release
B2	Bronchial smooth muscle Skeletal muscle Liver Vascular	bronchodilation Relaxes uterus Increases force of contraction Stimulates glycogenolysis and gluconeogenesis Vasodilation	Causes bronchospasm Inhibits glycogenolysis and gluconeogenesis Minimal vasoconstriction
B3	Adipose tissue Skeletal muscle	Stimulates lipolysis Stimulates thermogenesis	Inhibits lipolysis Inhibits thermogenesis

Table 3. Beta receptor: Locations and actions.

http://dx.doi.org/10.5772/intechopen.77011

decreased automaticity in pacemaker cells, and decreased conduction through the AV node. Non- selective beta blockade results in systemic effects including bronchoconstriction, impaired gluconeogenesis and decreased insulin release. Same Beta blockers (e.g., propranolol) have high lipid solubility leading to rapid cross of the blood brain barrier into the central nervous system, causing a neurological manifestation such as seizures and delirium [45, 47].

14.2. Clinical features

The major system affected by β-blocker toxicity is the cardiovascular system; patients present with bradycardia and hypotensive. The cause of bradycardia is sinus node suppression or conduction abnormalities but ingestion of β-blockers with partial agonist activity may cause hypertension and tachycardia as early presentation. The β-blockers with sodium channel block affect may cause a wide-complex bradycardia.

Sotalol causes potassium channels block leading to prolonging the QT interval.

B-Blockers also have effect on CNS and pulmonary system. Neurologic features include delirium, coma and seizures with more lipophilic. B-blockers (propranolol) have more neurological manifestations. Bronchospasm and hypoglycaemia can be in β-blockers toxicity [47, 48].

14.3. Treatment

GI decontamination can be done by giving Activated charcoal within 1 h of ingestion and air way is the main aim treatment in beta-blocker toxicity focusing on restore perfusion to critical organ systems by increasing cardiac output by: fluid resuscitation and glucagon (3–10 mg), vasopressor (e.g., epinephrine) and high dose Insulin- glucose (insulin 1 unit/kg IV bolus). Intravenous lipid emulsion therapy may be used in case of sever toxicity and refractory to treatment. In case of refractory to pharmacologic therapy, haemodialysis, haemoperfusion, cardiac pacing, placement of intra-aortic balloon pumps can be used. Wide QRS-interval dysrhythmias due to sodium channel blockade treated with sodium bicarbonate 2–3 mEq/kg over 1–2 min [49, 50].

15. Calcium channel blocker poisoning

Calcium channel blockers (CCBs) are mainly used in the treatment of cardiovascular diseases such as hypertension, coronary artery disseise- CAD and cardiac arrhythmias Calcium channel blockers one most prescribed cardiovascular drugs and can be immediate-release or extended-release [17].

15.1. Mechanism of action

The calcium channel blockers (CCBs) can be divided into two major groups based upon their major physiologic effects: the dihydropyridines, group which mainly block the L-type calcium channels in the vasculature and the non-dihydropyridines, which selectively block L-type calcium channels in the myocardium such as verapamil. Dihydropyridine group toxicity causes arterial vasodilation and reflex tachycardia, whereas non-dihydropyridines toxicity cause peripheral vasodilation decreased cardiac inotropy, and bradycardia [46].

15.2. Clinical features

Cardiovascular system is the most affected system in CCBs toxicity. Patient present with hypotension and bradycardia or reflex tachycardia. Verapamil or diltiazem toxicity usually patients present with sinus bradycardia, on the hand dihydropyridine overdoses cause peripheral vasodilatation causing reflex tachycardia [55]. CCBs have not primary effect on pulmonary and CNS System; CNS symptoms (seizures, delirium, and coma) occur secondary to decrease organ perfusion. Cardiogenic pulmonary oedema and acute lung injury (non-cardiogenic pulmonary oedema) have also been reported in severe toxicity [48].

15.3. Treatment

First step in management is secure airway, stabilize ventilation and circulation.

Decontamination can be done by oral activated charcoal if patient present within 1 h of ingestion also the whole-bowel irrigation is useful in case of extended-release CCBs. Hypotension treated with IV fluid, Calcium chloride or calcium gluconate, glucagon (3–10 mg), if not responding start Vasopressors (e.g., norepinephrine). If symptoms refractory to vasopressor therapy start, high dose Insulin -glucose. If patient still not responding, lipid emulsion can be started. Finally, circulatory support measures, such as the placement of intra-aortic balloon pumps may be used in case of sever toxicity not responding to standard therapy [49–51].

16. Carbon monoxide poisoning

Carbon monoxide (CO) is an odourless, tasteless, colourless and non-irritating gas.

Potential sources of Carbon monoxide (CO) are automotive exhaust, fuelled heaters, Wood- or coal-burning stoves, Structure fires and gasoline-powered generators other than fires.

The incidence of co -poisoning increases during winter time because the use of space heaters, wood-burning stoves and charcoal burning for heat.

16.1. Mechanism of action

Carbon monoxide (CO) diffuses fast in the pulmonary capillary membrane and because of his rapid binding affinity (more than oxygen by 200 times), carbon monoxide bind to haemoglobin, that cause impaired releasing oxygen to tissue leading to shift the oxyhaemoglobin dissociation curve to the left [51].

16.2. Clinical features

Carbon monoxide poisoning have variable clinical picture depend on severity of exposure ranging from non-specific symptoms like headache, nausea and dizziness in mild to moderate cases to confusion, seizure and coma in severe cases patients may present with mild fever, tachycardia, tachypnoea and hypertension. Acute myocardial injury and life-threatening dysrhythmias are the most cardiovascular complications in case of severe Carbon monoxide poisoning. Delayed neuropsychiatric syndrome is long term neurological complication in

http://dx.doi.org/10.5772/intechopen.77011

severe cases characterized with different symptoms including cognitive deficiency, movement disorders and focal neurologic deficit. The standard pulse oximetry cannot differentiate carboxyhaemoglobin from oxyhaemoglobin, so it is unreliable in the diagnosis or screen carbon monoxide poisoning, so measuring carboxyhaemoglobin level in an arterial blood gas helps in diagnosis [52–55].

16.3. Treatment

After securing the airway, the most important step in treatment is oxygen 100% via non-rebreathing mask or intubation and mechanically ventilation with 100% oxygen if the patient is comatose and cannot secure his air way, half-life of carboxyhaemoglobin in room air 250–320 min while via non-rebreathing with 100% oxygen decreased to 90 min. Hyperbaric oxygen therapy could be considered in certain cases, the indication for Hyperbaric oxygen includes Pregnancy with carboxyhaemoglobin level > 15%, Carboxyhaemoglobin >25%, evidence of acute myocardial ischemia, and severe metabolic acidosis [56].

17. Iron toxicity

Iron tablets are usually available in homes with small children and young women especially pregnant women. Because of its colour, sugar taste and appearance like a candy make iron tablet more attractive for accidental ingestion for children [57].

17.1. Mechanism of action

Iron exerts a direct corrosive effect on the gastrointestinal tract at high plasma concentrations; it also possesses cytotoxic actions, particularly on the liver, leading to hepatocellular necrosis. Additionally, iron has a direct cardio- toxic effect acting as a negative inotrope and inhibits thrombin leading to a coagulopathy independent of hepatotoxicity. The direct corrosive effects and cellular toxicity contribute to metabolic acidosis [58].

17.2. Clinical features

Serious iron poisoning usually causes symptoms within 6 h of the overdose and if the ingested elemental iron more than 20 mg/kg body, the symptoms of iron poisoning typically occur in 5 stages:

Stage 1 (within 6 h after the overdose): Symptoms include vomiting, vomiting blood, diarrhoea, abdominal pain, irritability and drowsiness. If poisoning is very serious, rapid breathing, a rapid heart rate, coma, unconsciousness, seizures, and low blood pressure may develop.

Stage 2 (6–48 h after the overdose): condition can appear to improve (there is often a latent phase with minimal symptoms which may last up to 24 h and may be misinterpreted as an apparent recovery).

Stage 3 (12–48 h after the overdose): Very low blood pressure (shock), fever, bleeding, jaundice, liver failure, metabolic acidosis and seizures can develop.

Stage 4 (2–5 days after the overdose): The liver fails and people may die from shock, bleeding, and blood-clotting abnormalities. Sugar levels in the blood can decrease. Confusion and sluggishness (lethargy) or coma may develop.

Stage 5 (2–5 weeks after the overdose): The stomach or intestines can become blocked by scars [59, 60].

17.3. Treatment

First step stabilize the air way, breathing and circulation. An abdominal x-ray may be helpful to confirm the presence of iron tablets. Consider GI decontamination by whole bowel irrigation if the patient is stable and has no contraindications, especially for large ingestions of modified release products, providing the airway can be protected. Activated charcoal does not bind iron. Asymptomatic patients need observation for 6 h and serum iron levels less than 300–350 mcg/dL may be discharged.

Chelation therapy with deferoxamine is indicated for patients with serum iron levels >350 mcg/dL and have evidence of toxicity, or levels of >500 mcg/dL regardless of signs or symptoms. In patients with significant clinical manifestations of toxicity persistent emesis, metabolic acidosis, chelation therapy should not be delayed while one awaits serum iron levels. Haemodialysis does not remove iron effectively but should be considered on a supportive basis for acute renal failure as this will facilitate removal of the iron-deferoxamine complex [61, 62].

18. Toxic alcohol poisoning

The term toxic alcohol has generally referred to isopropanol, methanol, and ethylene glycol (EG). Poisoning involving toxic alcohols are relatively uncommon, but remain important causes of suicide or epidemic poisonings; Mortality and morbidity of toxic alcohols are high if prompt diagnosis and treatment are not initiated rapidly [63, 64].

18.1. .Mechanism of action and clinical features

Methanol also called methyl alcohol is found in paint removers or photocopying fluid, de-icing products and windshield wiper fluid. Methanol metabolism in the liver by alcohol dehydrogenase to formaldehyde. Aldehyde dehydrogenase then rapidly converts formaldehyde to formic acid with no appreciable accumulation of formaldehyde in the blood.

The formic acid inhibits cytochrome c in the mitochondria, shifting the cell to anaerobic glycolysis, leading to lactic acid accumulation. The clinical features of methanol poisoning are the triad of severe anion gap metabolic acidosis, visual changes, and mental status depression. Other methanol intoxication symptoms include headache, light-headedness, nausea, vomiting, abdominal pain and dyspnoea. Methanol may produce pancreatitis by direct toxic effect on the pancreas.

Ethylene glycol is found in radiator antifreeze, metal cleaners, and degreasing agents. It has no smell or colour and tastes sweet. Ethylene glycol is metabolized in the liver to glycolaldehyde

http://dx.doi.org/10.5772/intechopen.77011

by alcohol dehydrogenase. Glycolaldehyde is then converted to glycolic acid which is then converted to oxalic acid. Oxalic acid combines with serum calcium to form the classic calcium oxalate crystals found in the urine of patients who have consumed ethylene glycol.

Ethylene glycol causes an elevated anion gap metabolic acidosis. The neurologic effects of ethylene glycol are coma, seizures, meningism, muscle spasms, and paralysis of the extraocular muscles. It can also affect the heart and lungs, causing tachycardia, hyperventilation, ARDS, and heart failure. Hypocalcaemia and resulting QT prolongation are due to serum calcium combining with oxalic acid. Lastly, kidney failure is due to these calcium crystals depositing into renal tubules.

Isopropyl alcohol is found in solvents and disinfectants. It is also found in mouthwashes, lotions, as well as rubbing alcohol and hand sanitizers. It is also hepatically metabolized by alcohol dehydrogenase to acetone. Isopropanol produces an increased osmole gap; however, it normally does not produce a metabolic acidosis unless concomitant hypotension causes lactic acidosis. It can cause haemorrhagic gastritis and profound inebriation with cerebellar signs and coma [64–70].

18.2. Investigations

An osmolar gap more than 10 mOsm/kg is suggestive of ethylene glycol, methanol, isopropanol, ethylene oxide, or acetone toxicity. A high anion gap metabolic acidosis may be revealed at later stages of methanol and ethylene glycol poisoning. Hypoglycaemia may be detected with isopropanol, while hyperglycaemia and hypocalcaemia may be detected in methanol and ethylene glycol poisonings, respectively. Hyperkalaemia due to acidosis is observed in methanol and ethylene glycol poisoning, whereas hypokalaemia due to vomiting may occur in ethanol intoxication.

Urine calcium oxalate crystals can be seen in ethylene glycol intoxication. These findings should be evaluated together with the other manifestations and observations [71, 72].

18.3. Treatment

Any patient with serious poisoning may present in a critical condition. As with all poisoned patients, initial stabilization must be instituted before other possible treatments can be employed Initial evaluation should be focused on the improvement of vital signs: airway, respiration and circulation.

Consider toxic alcohol poisoning in a patient with an unexplained elevated anion gap metabolic acidosis and elevated osmolar gap.

Fomepizole competitively inhibits alcohol dehydrogenase, which is involved in the metabolism of all alcohols, including ethanol. It is given to prevent the build-up of toxic metabolites from ethylene glycol (glycolic acid, glyoxylic acid, and oxalic acid) and methanol (formic acid) whose deposition in tissues can cause irreparable damage.

Fomepizole is indicated for methanol or ethylene glycol ingestion resulting in a metabolic acidosis with an elevated osmolar gap and a serum Methanol or ethylene glycol level of at least 20 mg/dL.

Haemodialysis is indicated for toxic alcohol poisoning with an elevated osmolar gap and/or severe metabolic acidosis refractory to standard therapy, refractory hypotension, or end organ damage (i.e. acute renal failure. Vitamin Supplementation: Give folic or folinic acid to patients with methanol toxicity to divert metabolism away from formic acid to carbon dioxide and water. Give folic acid, pyridoxine, and thiamine to patients with EG toxicity to divert metabolism to nontoxic metabolites [73–76].

19. Organophosphates poisoning

Organophosphates (OP) are used in insecticides for domestic and agricultural use. They are also the main toxins in nerve gases like Sarin. OP pesticide self-poisoning is a major clinical and public-health problem across much of rural Asia [77].

19.1. Mechanism of action

The most serious poisoning of OP occurs by ingestion; cutaneous absorption and inhalation of sprays rarely cause serious toxicity. OP is extremely toxic pesticides, which produce acetylcholine excess with muscarinic, nicotinic and CNS effects.

19.2. Clinical features

Patients present with degrees of cholinergic crisis, usually within 4 h of ingestion or exposure. Specific manifestations include: Muscarinic manifestations like bronchospasm, vomiting, pinpoint pupils, bradycardia and hypotension, excessive sweating, lacrimation, salivation, profuse diarrhoea and urination (**Table 4**).

Over-stimulation of nicotinic receptors causes tachycardia, hypertension and sweating. Accumulation of acetylcholine at the neuromuscular junction causes initial stimulation followed by depolarization and paralysis. This appears first as fasciculations, cramps and muscle weakness. Central nervous system (CNS) effects include delirium, coma and seizures. Most deaths are due to respiratory failure. Toxicity from gradual, cumulative exposure may be much more subtle. These patients commonly exhibit vague confusion or other central nervous system complaints; mild visual disturbances; or chronic abdominal cramping, nausea, and diarrhoea. A unique effect of organophosphorus insecticides results from "aging," the irreversible conformational change that occurs when the organophosphorus agent is bound to the

Diarrhoea
Urination
Miosis
Bronchospasm
Emesis
Lacrimation
Salivation

Table 4. DUMBELS mnemonic for signs of cholinergic excess.

cholinesterase enzyme for a prolonged time, causing clinical effects to persist for a prolonged time. On average, some aging for commercial organophosphorus agents will occur by 48 h but may take longer. The intermediate syndrome is distinct from OP in the following ways: start within 24–96 h after recovery from acute cholinergic crisis, cranial nerves INNERVATED muscle and proximal muscles weakness, and rapid clinical recovery over 4–18 days. Any patient with a clinically apparent cholinergic syndrome should be treated empirically without waiting for laboratory confirmation of decreased cholinesterase activity [78].

19.3. Treatment

Medical management of OP pesticide poisoning demands close observation, timely institution of antidote in adequate doses and duration and good supportive. The Treating staff should wear protective clothing. The patient's clothes should be removed and destroyed and the patient should be showered in a designated decontamination area.

Treatment includes: resuscitation of patients giving oxygen, a muscarinic antagonist (usually atropine), fluids and an acetylcholinesterase reactivator (an oxime that reactivates acetylcholinesterase by removal of the phosphate group).

Respiratory support is given as necessary. Patients must be carefully observed after stabilization for changes in atropine needs, worsening respiratory function because of intermediate syndrome, and recurrent cholinergic features occurring with fat-soluble OP [79].

20. Conclusion

Poisoned patient in emergency department have unique Approach because of difficulties in obtain history, poisoned patients need careful physical examination looking for toxidromes or sign of illegal drugs abuse. Intoxicated patient's management started with resuscitation and stabilization of air way, breathing and circulation. Consider decontamination in early time post ingestion. Most of the patient need laboratory test includes full cell count and electrolytes and kidney functions, specific drug level. Paracetamol level must be send for every present with history intestinal over dose. Symptomatic treatment is cornerstone treatment for post intoxicated patient also antidotes need for specific substances in specific conditions. Finally physicians in emergency department need to call the local poisoning centre to help them in management.

Author details

Ehab Said Aki*, Waleed Awad Salem and Jalal Alessai

*Address all correspondence to: akiehab2004@gmail.com

Hamad Medical Corporation, Doha, Qatar

References

[1] Warner M, Chen LH, Makuc DM, et al. Drug Poisoning Deaths in the United States, 1980-2008. NCHS Data Brief, no. 81. Hyattsville, MD: National Center for Health Statistics; 2011

[2] Liu Q, Zhou L, Zheng N, et al. Poisoning deaths in China: Type and prevalence detected at the Tongji Forensic Medical Center in Hubei. Forensic Science International. 2009;**193**:88

[3] Erickson TB, Thompson TM, Lu JJ. The approach to the patient with an unknown overdose. Emergency Medicine Clinics of North America. 2007;**25**:249

[4] Greene S. General management of poisoned patients. In: Tintinalli JE et al., editors. Tintinalli's Emergency Medicine: A Comprehensive Study Guide. 8e ed. New York, NY: McGraw-Hill; 2016

[5] Mofenson HC, Greensher J. The nontoxic ingestion. Paediatric Clinics of North America. 1970;**17**(3):583-590

[6] Manoguerra AS, Cobaugh DJ. Guidelines for the Management of Poisoning Consensus Panel: Guideline on the use of ipecac syrup in the out-of-hospital management of ingested poisons. Clinical Toxicology (Philadelphia, Pa.). 2005;**43**:1

[7] Adams BK, Mann MD, Aboo A, et al. Prolonged gastric emptying half-time and gastric hypomotility after drug overdose. The American Journal of Emergency Medicine. 2004;**22**:548

[8] Position paper: Whole bowel irrigation. Journal of Toxicology. Clinical Toxicology. 2004;**42**:843

[9] Bunchorntavakul C, Reddy KR. Acetaminophen-related hepatotoxicity. Clinics in Liver Disease. 2013;**17**:587

[10] Watson WA, Litovitz TL, Klein-Schwartz W, et al. 2003 Annual report of the American association of poison control centers toxic exposure surveillance system. The American Journal of Emergency Medicine. 2004;**22**:335

[11] Manyike PT, Kharasch ED, Kalhorn TF, Slattery JT. Contribution of CYP2E1 and CYP3A to acetaminophen reactive metabolite formation. Clinical Pharmacology and Therapeutics. 2000;**67**:275

[12] Fontana RJ. Acute liver failure including acetaminophen overdose. The Medical Clinics of North America. 2008;**92**:761

[13] Waring WS, Stephen AF, Malkowska AM, Robinson OD. Acute acetaminophen overdose is associated with dose-dependent hypokalaemia: A prospective study of 331 patients. Basic & Clinical Pharmacology & Toxicology. 2008;**102**:325

[14] Bernal W et al. Blood lactate as an early predictor outcome in paracetamol-induced acute liver failure: A cohort study. Lancet. 2002;**359**:558-563

[15] Harrison PM, Wendon JA, Gimson AES, et al. Improvement by acetylcysteine of hemodynamic and oxygen transport in fulminant hepatic failure. The New England Journal of Medicine. 1991;**324**:1852-1857

[16] Rumack-Matthew H. Acetaminophen poisoning and toxicity. Pediatrics. 1975;**55**:871

[17] Mowry JB, Spyker DA, Cantilena LR, McMillan H, Ford M. Annual report of the American association of poison control centers' national poison data system (NPDS): 31th annual report. Clinical Toxicology (Philadelphia, Pa.). 2013;**52**:1032-2014

[18] Furukawa TA, McGuire H, Barbui C. Meta-analysis of effects and side effects of low dosage tricyclic antidepressants in depression: Systematic review. BMJ. 2002;**325**:991

[19] Fanoe S, Kristensen D, Fink-Jensen A, et al. Risk of arrhythmia induced by psychotropic medications: A proposal for clinical management. European Heart Journal. 2014;**35**:1306

[20] White N, Litovitz T, Clancy C. Suicidal antidepressant overdoses: A comparative analysis by antidepressant type. Journal of Medical Toxicology. 2008;**4**:238

[21] Bateman DN. Tricyclic antidepressant poisoning, central nervous system effects and management. Toxicological Reviews. 2005;**24**:181

[22] Teece S, Hogg L. Towards evidence based emergency medicine: Best BETs from the Manchester Royal Infirmary. glucagon in tricyclic overdose. Emergency Medicine Journal. 2003;**20**:264

[23] LoVecchio F. Cyclic antidepressants. In: Tintinalli's Emergency Medicine: A Comprehensive Study Guide. 8e ed. New York, NY: McGraw-Hill; 2016

[24] Herres J, Ryan D, Salzman M. Delayed salicylate toxicity with undetectable initial levels after large-dose aspirin ingestion. American Journal of Emergency Medicine. 2009, 1173;**27**:e1

[25] O'Malley GF. Emergency department management of the salicylate-poisoned patient. Emergency Medicine Clinics of North America. 2007;**25**:333

[26] Greenberg MI, Hendrickson RG, Hofman M. Deleterious effects of endotracheal intubation in salicylate poisoning. Annals of Emergency Medicine. 2003;**41**:583

[27] Thanacoody R, Caravati EM, Troutman B, et al. Position paper update: Whole bowel irrigation for gastrointestinal decontamination of overdose patients. Clinical Toxicology (Philadelphia, Pa.). 2015;**53**:5

[28] Juurlink DN, Gosselin S, Kielstein JT, et al. Extracorporeal treatment for Salicylate poisoning: Systematic review and recommendations from the EXTRIP workgroup. Annals of Emergency Medicine. 2015;**66**:165

[29] Watson WA, Litovitz TL, Rodgers GCJ, et al. Annual report of the American association of poison control centers toxic exposure surveillance system. American Journal of Emergency Medicine. 2004, 2005;**23**:589

[30] Sporer KA. Acute heroin overdose. Annals of Internal Medicine. 1999;**130**:584

[31] Dowling J, Isbister GK, Kirkpatrick CM, Naidoo D, Graudins A. Population pharmacokinetics of intravenous, intramuscular, and intranasal naloxone in human volunteers. Therapeutic Drug Monitoring. 2008;**30**:490

[32] Burillo-Putze G, Opioids MO. Tintinalli's Emergency Medicine: A Comprehensive Study Guide. 8e ed. New York, NY: McGraw-Hill; 2016

[33] Hoffman RS, Kaplan JL, Hung OL, Goldfrank LR. Ecgonine methyl ester protects against cocaine lethality in mice. Journal of Toxicology. Clinical Toxicology. 2004;**42**:349

[34] Ritz MC, Lamb RJ, Goldberg SR, Kuhar MJ. Cocaine receptors on dopamine transporters are related to self-administration of cocaine. Science. 1987;**237**:1219

[35] Lange RA, Cigarroa RG, Flores ED, et al. Potentiation of cocaine-induced coronary vasoconstriction by beta-adrenergic blockade. Annals of Internal Medicine. 1990;**112**:897

[36] Osborn HH, Tang M, Bradley K, et al. New onset bronchospasm or recrudescence of asthma associated with cocaine abuse. Academic Emergency Medicine. 1997;**4**:689

[37] Prosser JM, Perrone J. Cocaine and amphetamines. In: Tintinalli's Emergency Medicine: A Comprehensive Study Guide. 8e ed. New York, NY: McGraw-Hill; 2016

[38] Eichhorn EJ, Gheorghiade M. Digoxin. Progress in Cardiovascular Diseases. 2002; **44**:251-266

[39] Smith TW. Digitalis. Mechanisms of action and clinical use. The New England Journal of Medicine. 1988;**318**:358

[40] Kanji S, MacLean RD. Cardiac glycoside toxicity: More than 200 years and counting. Critical Care Clinics. 2012;**28**:527

[41] Bhatia SJ. Digitalis toxicity—Turning over a new leaf? The Western Journal of Medicine. 1986;**145**:74

[42] Roberts DM, Buckley NA. Antidotes for acute cardenolide (cardiac glycoside) poisoning. Cochrane Database of Systematic Reviews. 2006;**4**:CD005490

[43] Antman EM, Wenger TL, Butler VPJ, Haber E, Smith TW. Treatment of 150 cases of life-threatening digitalis intoxication with digoxin-specific Fab antibody fragments. Final report of a multicentre study. Circulation. 1990;**81**:1744

[44] Hack JB, Woody JH, Lewis DE, Brewer K, Meggs WJ. The effect of calcium chloride in treating hyperkalemia due to acute digoxin toxicity in a porcine model. Journal of Toxicology. Clinical Toxicology. 2004;**42**:337. [PubMed: 15461240]

[45] Vucinić S, Joksović D, Jovanović D, et al. Factors influencing the degree and outcome of acute beta-blockers poisoning. Vojnosanitetski Pregled. 2000;**57**:619

[46] Samuels TL, Uncles DR, Willers JW, et al. Logging the potential for intravenous lipid emulsion in propranolol and other lipophilic drug overdoses. Anaesthesia. 2011;**66**:221

[47] DeWitt CR, Waksman JC. Pharmacology, pathophysiology, and management of calcium channel blocker and beta-blocker toxicity. Toxicological Reviews. 2004;**23**:223

[48] Kerns W. Management of beta-adrenergic blocker and calcium channel antagonist toxicity. Emergency Medicine Clinics of North America. 2007;**25**:309

[49] Wax PM, Erdman AR, Chyka PA, et al. Beta-blocker ingestion: An evidence-based consensus guideline for out-of-hospital management. Clinical Toxicology (Philadelphia, Pa.). 2005;**43**:131

[50] Jang DH, Spyres MB, Fox L, Manini AF. Toxin-induced cardiovascular failure. Emergency Medicine Clinics of North America. 2014;**32**:79

[51] Hardy KR, Thom SR. Pathophysiology and treatment of carbon monoxide poisoning. Journal of Toxicology. Clinical Toxicology. 1994;**32**:613

[52] Kao LW, Nañagas KA. Carbon monoxide poisoning. Emergency Medicine Clinics of North America. 2004;**22**:985

[53] Thom SR, Taber RL, Mendiguren II, et al. Delayed neuropsychologic sequelae after carbon monoxide poisoning: Prevention by treatment with hyperbaric oxygen. Annals of Emergency Medicine. 1995;**25**:474

[54] Henry CR, Satran D, Lindgren B, et al. Myocardial injury and long-term mortality following moderate to severe carbon monoxide poisoning. JAMA. 2006;**295**:398

[55] Bozeman WP, Myers RA, Barish RA. Confirmation of the pulse oximetry gap in carbon monoxide poisoning. Annals of Emergency Medicine. 1997;**30**:608

[56] Ziser A, Shupak A, Halpern P, et al. Delayed hyperbaric oxygen treatment for acute carbon monoxide poisoning. British Medical Journal (Clinical Research Ed.). 1984;**289**:960

[57] Morris CC. Paediatrics iron poisonings in the United States. Southern Medical Journal. 2000;**93**:352

[58] Anderson GJ, Wang F. Essential but toxic: Controlling the flux of iron in the body. Clinical and Experimental Pharmacology & Physiology. 2012;**39**:719

[59] Singhi SC, Baranwal AK, Jayashree M. Acute iron poisoning: Clinical picture, intensive care needs and outcome. Indian Paediatric. 2003;**40**:1177

[60] Robertson A, Tenenbein M. Hepatotoxicity in acute iron poisoning. Human & Experimental Toxicology. 2005;**24**:559

[61] Manoguerra AS, Erdman AR, Booze LL, et al. Iron ingestion: An evidence-based consensus guideline for out-of-hospital management. Clinical Toxicology (Philadelphia, Pa.). 2005;**43**:553

[62] Baranwal AK, Singhi SC. Acute iron poisoning: management guidelines. Indian Podiatric. 2003;**40**:534

[63] Jammalamadaka D, Raissi S. Ethylene glycol, methanol and isopropyl alcohol intoxication. The American Journal of the Medical Sciences. 2010;**339**:276-281

[64] Burkhart KK, Kulig KW. The other alcohols—Methanol, ethylene glycol, and isopropanol. Emergency Medicine Clinics of North America. 1990;**8**:913-928

[65] Barceloux DG, Bond GR, Krenzelok EP, et al. American academy of clinical toxicology practice guidelines on the treatment of methanol poisoning. Clinical Toxicology. 2002;**40**:415-446

[66] Onder F, Ilker S, Kansu T, et al. Acute blindness and putaminal necrosis in methanol intoxication. International Ophthalmology. 1999;**22**:81-84

[67] Hantson P, Mahieu P. Pancreatic injury following acute methanol poisoning. Clinical Toxicology. 2000;**38**:297-303

[68] Eder AF, McGrath CM, et al. Methylene glycol poisoning: Toxicokinetic and analytical factors affecting laboratory diagnosis Shaw. Clinical Chemistry. 1998;**44**(1):168-177

[69] Wolfson AB et al. Ethylene glycol. In: Burns MJ, editor. Harwood-Nuss' Clinical Practice of Emergency Medicine. Philadelphia: Lippincott Williams and Wilkins Co; 2005. pp. 1454-1458

[70] Jacobsen D, Bredesen JE, Eide I, et al. Anion and osmolal gaps in the diagnosis of methanol and ethylene glycol poisoning. Acta Medica Scandinavica. 1982;**22**:17-20

[71] Hassanian-Moghaddam H, Pajoumand A, Dadgar SM, Shadnia S. Prognostic factors in methanol poisoning. Human & Experimental Toxicology. 2007;**26**:583-586

[72] Wiener SW. Toxic alcohols. In: Nelson LS et al., editors. Goldfrank's Toxicologic Emergencies. 10th ed. McGrawHill; 2015. pp. 1346-1358

[73] Mégarbane B, Borron SW, Baud FJ. Intensive Care Medicine. 2005;**31**:189

[74] Lepik KJ et al. Adverse drug events associated with the antidotes for methanol and ethylene glycol poisoning: A comparison of ethanol and fomepizole. Annals of Emergency Medicine. 2009;**53**(4):439-450

[75] Kraut JA, Kurtz I. Toxic alcohol ingestions: Clinical features, diagnosis, and management. Clinical Journal of the American Society of Nephrology. January 2008;**3**(1):208-225

[76] Emmett M, Palmer BF. Serum osmolal gap. In: Forman JP, editor. UpToDate. Waltham, MA: UpToDate; 2016

[77] Hulse EJ, Davies JOJ, Simpson AJ, et al. Respiratory complications of organophosphorus nerve agent and insecticide poisoning. American Journal of Respiratory and Critical Care Medicine. 2014;**190**(12):1342-1354

[78] Wayne R. Diagnosis and treatment of poisoning due to pesticides. In: Hayes' Handbook of Pesticide Toxicology. 3rd ed. p. 2010

[79] Eddleston M, Singh S, Buckley N. Organophosphorus poisoning (acute). Clinical Evidence. 2005;**13**:1744-1755

Chapter 12

Problem of Burns in Children: Opportunities for Health Improvement

Agata Maria Kawalec

Additional information is available at the end of the chapter

http://dx.doi.org/10.5772/intechopen.74490

Abstract

Burns are one of the most devastating types of trauma in medicine. Children under 5 years of age are a high-risk group to burns. The most common type is thermal burn caused by hot fluids (scald). Most childhood burns occur at home under parental supervision. These are preventable injuries. The chapter presents results of my studies about risk factors of burns in children and possibilities of health improvement. Simple changes in children's environment and increasing awareness of caregivers can lead to a decrease in the number of this type of injuries. Moreover, the first aid given to burnt children soon after the injury usually is not adequate (no cooling thermal burns and no analgesia). Health improvement can be obtained by reducing the number of burns, the correct first aid given after the injury, and the organization of specialized health-care centers and rehabilitation services for victims of burns.

Keywords: children, burns, scalds, thermal burns, trauma

1. Introduction

Burns are often called one of the most devastating types of trauma in medicine because their consequences have physical and mental dimensions.

Severe burns can cause death. Physical consequences of nonfatal burns include scars, contractures, and keloids. The victims suffer due to disfigurement and disability often leading to stigma and rejection by the society. Among mental consequences of burns are, for example, low self-esteem, depression, or anxiety.

Burns are type of trauma that can be caused by thermal energy, chemical agents, electricity, or radiation. According to the World Health Organization, burn is an injury to the skin or other organic tissues primarily caused by heat or due to radiation, radioactivity, electricity, friction, or contact with chemicals.

According to Juan P. Barret, trauma can be defined as bodily injury severe enough to pose a threat to life, limbs, tissues, and organs, but burn injury is different, because unlike other traumas, it can be quantified as to the exact percentage of body injured and can be viewed as a paradigm of injury from which many lessons can be learned about critical illness involving multiple organ systems [1].

2. Epidemiology of burns

According to the statistics of the World Health Organization, 180,000 deaths every year are caused by burns [2]. Majority of them occur in low- and middle-income countries. It is estimated that almost two thirds occur in the African and South-East Asia regions. The highest fire-related mortality rates are in Southeast Asia, 11.6 deaths per 100,000 population per year; in the Eastern Mediterranean, 6.4 deaths per 100,000 population per year; and in Africa, 6.1 deaths per 100,000 population per year [3].

Among pediatric population the rate of deaths from burns is over seven times higher in low- and middle-income countries than in high-income countries. Lowest mortality rates due to burns in high-income countries are the successful result of preventive interventions of many kinds, such as promotion of the use of smoke detectors, the lowering of temperatures of hot water heaters, the installation of sprinkler systems, the promotion of flame-retardant children's sleepwear, and the development of safer buildings and household fuels [3].

The epidemiology of burns differs in different age groups and depends on sex [3]. For example, in low- and middle-income countries, fire-related burns are the sixth leading cause of death among 5–14-year-old victims and the eighth leading cause death among 15–29-year-old victims [3].

In low- and middle-income countries, women (especially young) are at higher risk of burns [3]. However in high-income countries, men are at higher risk of burns.

In pediatric population, it is estimated that worldwide approximately 1% of all children sustain a burn injury each year [4].

The results of our studies conducted in Lower Silesia (the region of Poland) among children with burns indicate that boys are at higher risk of burn injury [5, 6].

The analysis of mechanism of trauma revealed that the most common type of injury in children treated in ambulatory conditions by general practitioners (GP) and requiring hospitalization due to burns in Lower Silesia was thermal burns [5, 6]. The second reason for hospitalization and ambulatory treatment were chemical burns [5]. In the studied population, there were no cases of burns caused by radiation [5, 6].

Among the pediatric patients hospitalized due to thermal injury in Lower Silesia, 2010–2012, burns were usually located in the upper limbs [5]. Trunk and lower limbs were also frequently affected [5].

The detailed analysis of the thermal burns of upper limbs revealed that the hand and wrist were more often affected than forearm, arm, and shoulder. However, the detailed analysis of the thermal burns of lower limbs revealed that the injury affected more often the hip, tight, knee, and lower leg than ankle and feet [5].

Most of patients under 18 years old treated by GP due to burns in Lower Silesia of children were under 2 years old [6]. Moreover, in the studied population, the percentage of children hospitalized due to burns in Lower Silesia in 2010 according to individual age groups in age group under 2 years old was 0.5%, in children from 3 to 6 years old was 0.12%, in children from 7 to 12 years old was 0.06%, in children from 13 to 15 years old was 0.07%, and in children from 16 to 18 years old was 0.06% [5]. Similarly in the studied population, percentage of children hospitalized due to burns in Lower Silesia in 2011 according to individual age groups in age group under 2 years old was 0.54%, in children from 3 to 6 years old was 0.13%, in children from 7 to 12 years old was 0.06%, in children from 13 to 15 years old was 0.07%, and in children from 16 to 18 years old was 0.08% [5].

The chemical injuries were less common in pediatric population of Lower Silesia in the analyzed period of time. However, it was noticed that this type of burns more frequently affects the upper gastrointestinal tract than thermal burns [5, 6].

The obtained results are coherent with other studies realized in Polish pediatric population [7].

3. Classifications of burns

There are many ways in which burn injury can be classified.

Apart from the mechanism of injury, usually four criteria are taken into account: depth of injury, percent of body surface area involved, location of the burn, and association with other injuries [4].

3.1. Etiologic factor of injury

According to the etiological factor (factor that caused the burn injury), we can distinguish thermal, electrical, and chemical injury and burns caused by radiation.

The most common types of burns in children are thermal burns. Thermal injuries are caused by heat. They can be the result of hot liquids (scalds), hot solids (contact burns), and flames (flame burns). In pediatric population, especially in children under 2 years old, the most common type of burns is scalds.

3.2. Location of injury

Anatomic location is important in triage decision [4]. Burns can affect all parts of the body: head, neck, trunk, upper and lower extremities, perineum, and upper anterior abdominal wall (**Figures 1–3**).

International Classification of the Disease (ICD) is used by physicians, nurses, health-care providers, and researchers to classify the diseases and other health-care problems. It facilitated the comparison of date between different regions and is widely used for epidemiological purposes.

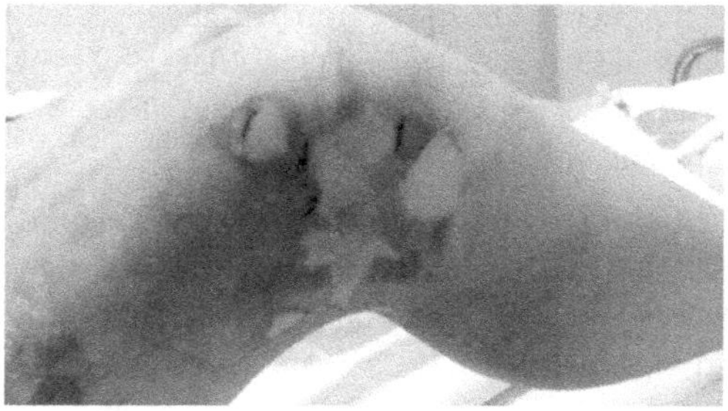

Figure 1. The child with the thermal burn of the knee (partial thickness burn).

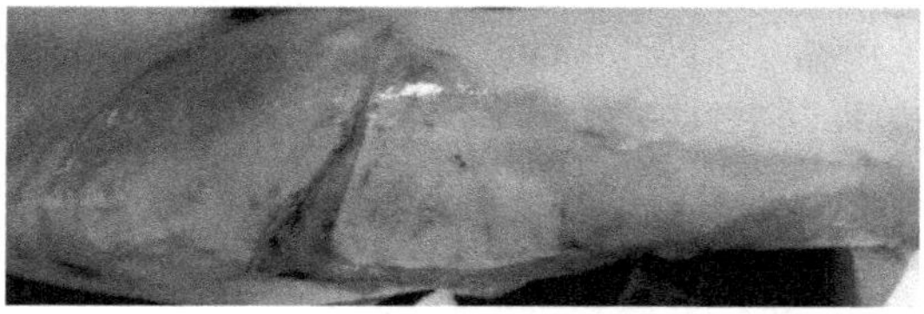

Figure 2. The child with the thermal burn of the lower extremity (partial thickness burn).

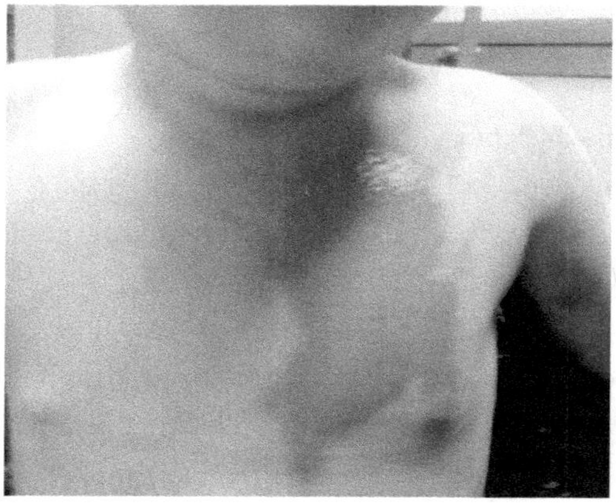

Figure 3. The child with the thermal burn (superficial) of the trunk caused by hot water (scald).

In the ICD-11 burns are divided into burns of external body surface, specified by site; burns of the eye or internal organs; and burns of multiple or unspecified body regions. In the ICD-10 the group of burns of external surface included burns and corrosions of all depth divided into burns and corrosions of head and neck (T20); burns and corrosions of trunk (T21); burns and corrosions of shoulder and upper limb, except the wrist and hand (T22); burns and corrosions of the wrist and hand (T23); burns and corrosions of the hip and lower limb, except the ankle and foot (T24); and burns and corrosions of the ankle and foot (T25) [8].

Burns involve also inhalation injuries. Inhalation injuries should be suspected in patients with facial burns, singed nasal hairs, and carbonaceous sputum [4].

The location is important in assessment of the risk of disability—the greatest is in the case of patients with affected face, eyes, feet, perineum, and hands [4].

3.3. Depth of burns

The skin is composed of two layers: epidermis and dermis. The epidermis is composed of stratified squamous epithelium, which acts as a barrier to infectious agents and also prevents fluid loss from the body [9].

As children's skin is thinner than adult's skin, exposure to the same agent will cause deeper burns in an infant compared to adults. For example, water at 60°C will cause a full-thickness burn in less than 1 s in an infant and 20 s in an adult [10].

At the emergency department, it is difficult to describe the thickness of burn injury because the appearance of burn wound evolves during first 24–48 h [9].

Usually in one pediatric patient, we observe burns of different depth.

According to depth of the skin affected, burns can be divided into superficial, partial-thickness, and full-thickness burns [9].

Superficial burns involve only the epidermal layer; the skin is erythematosus.

In partial-thickness burns, the whole epidermis and part of the dermis are affected. Most of authors distinguish superficial partial-thickness burns and deep partial-thickness burns. In the superficial partial-thickness burns, the papillary layer of the dermis is affected, and the erythema of the skin and blistering are observed. In the deep partial-thickness burns, the reticular layer of the dermis is affected, and the skin looks paler and has a speckled appearance due to thrombosis of superficial vessels. The deep partial-thickness burns are less painful than the superficial partial-thickness burns.

In the full-thickness burns, the epidermis and dermis with epidermal appendages are affected [9]. This type of burns is usually the result of flame, prolonged contact with hot objects, and hot oil [9].

In some old literatures, the classification involves first, second, third, and fourth degrees. The first degree corresponds with the superficial burns. The second degree A corresponds with the superficial partial-thickness burns; the second degree B corresponds with the deep partial-thickness burns. The third degree corresponds with the full-thickness burns. The fourth degree burns involve full depth of the skin and underlying fascia, muscles, or even bones [4].

3.4. Surface of burns

The extension of burn injury is expressed as percentage of total body surface area. There are several methods used to count the surface of burn.

In the teenagers and adults, the extent of the skin involved is estimated on the basis of "rule of nines." That means the surface of each upper extremity is 9% of total body surface area, each lower extremity is 18% of total body surface area, the anterior part of the trunk is 18% of the total body surface area, the posterior surface of the trunk is 18% of the total body surface area, the head is 9% of the total body surface area, and the perineum is 1% of the total body surface area [4]. There is a modified rule of nines for infants and children (**Figure 4**).

According to "rule of palm," the inner surface of the patient's palm is approximately 1% of total body surface area.

In younger children the Lund and Bowder charts are used to estimate the extension of burn wound [4].

According to extent of body surface involved, ICD-10 classified burns into burns involving less than 10% of body surface (T31.0), burns involving 10–19% of body surface (T31.1), burns involving 20–29% of body surface (T31.2), burns involving 30–39% of body surface (T31.3), burns involving 40–49% of body surface (T31.4), burns involving 50–59% of body surface (T31.5), burns involving 60–69% of body surface (T31.6), burns involving 70–79% of body surface (T31.7), burns involving 80–89% of body surface (T31.8), and burns involving 90% or more of body surface (T31.9) [8].

The extension of burn injury plays a crucial role in the process of decision-making about hospitalization of the patient. It is also important to count the amount of intravenous fluids that should be given to the patient.

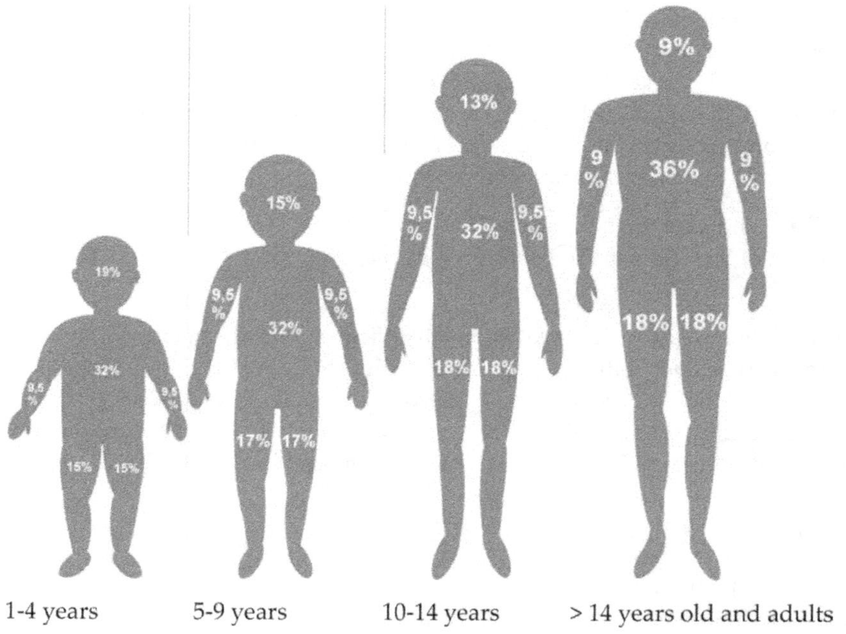

Figure 4. Modified rule of nines in children in different age groups.

3.5. Jackson's zones of injury

According to Jackson it is possible to classify thermal burns into three zones of injury: the inner, the intermediate, and the outer zone. The inner zone is the zone of coagulative necrosis. The intermediate zone is the zone of stasis, while the outer zone is the zone of hyperemia [11].

4. Pathophysiological effects of burn injury

Pathophysiological effects of burn injury can be divided into local and systemic [11].

The local effects include release of inflammatory mediators from the capillary walls, white blood cells, and platelets. These inflammatory mediators result in vasodilatation and increased vessel permeability that leads to fluid loss from the circulation into the interstitial space [11].

Systemic effects occur in extended burns (usually in those that burned surface area exceeds 20% of total body surface area) and include hypovolemia, immunosuppression, catabolism, loss of the protective function of the gut, and pulmonary edema [11].

A major burn injury leads to fluid and electrolyte imbalance with systemic intravascular losses of water, sodium, albumin, and red blood cells. If the intravascular volume is not rapidly restored, the shock develops [1]. Moreover, burns can lead to malnutrition and organ dysfunction due to metabolic disturbances (hypermetabolism and muscle catabolism) [1].

5. Causes of burns

The burns according to the cause of the injury can be divided into accidental and nonaccidental.

Most of burns in children are caused by the accident [12].

There are several features that can make a health-care provider to suspect nonaccidental injury.

Among them is delay in seeking medical help by parents. It is very important to write down all the details of mechanism of the injury provided by caregivers, because sometimes caregivers change the history of trauma with time. The non-accidental injury is suspected when the mechanism of injury given by parents is not coherent with the burn wound found in child and also when the history of trauma is not consistent with the developmental stage of the child. In older children the abnormal behavior, such as avoiding eye contact, can be observed.

Characteristic for nonaccidental burns are burn wound caused by cigarettes. Also the so-called glove or sock burns are typical for nonaccidental injury. In many children with nonaccidental burns, additional sings of trauma can be found, for example, bruises, fractures, etc.

According to Adronicus et al., there were no differences between the groups in age or mortality between children with accidental and nonaccidental burn injuries. The authors found that in the group of children with nonaccidental injuries, burns involving both hands or both legs were more common; these patients were more likely to require skin grafting and treatment in the intensive care unit [12]. Moreover the abused/neglected children were more likely to come from single parent families [12].

6. First aid in burns

The appropriate first aid after burn injury is very important in reduction of burn depth, which means that it influences the requirement for surgical treatment, can shorten the hospitalization time, and results in better esthetic scar.

According to WHO, the person who gives the first aid to the burned child should stop the burning process by removing clothing and irrigating the burns; extinguishing flames by allowing the patient to roll on the ground, or by applying a blanket, or by using water or other fire-extinguishing liquids; use cool running water to reduce the temperature of the burn; in chemical burns, remove or dilute the chemical agent by irrigating with large volumes of water; and wrap the patient in a clean cloth or sheet and transport to the nearest appropriate facility for medical care [2].

WHO also pays attention on the actions that the person who gives the first aid to the burned child should not do; for example, do not start first aid before ensuring your own safety (switch off electrical current, wear gloves for chemicals, etc.); do not apply paste, oil, haldi (turmeric), or raw cotton to the burn; do not apply ice because it deepens the injury; avoid prolonged cooling with water because it will lead to hypothermia; do not open blisters until topical antimicrobials can be applied, such as by a health-care provider; do not apply any material directly to the wound as it might become infected; and avoid application of topical medication until the patient has been placed under appropriate medical care [2].

The person who gives first aid to the child after the burn injury is usually the person that was present during the accident—in most of cases—the parent. Unfortunately, the own results indicate that parents do not provide first aid to burned children correctly. The most common mistakes were no cooling the burn wound and no analgesics used [13].

The aim of prehospital care is stabilizing ABCDEs (airway, breathing, circulation, disabilities, and environment control), preventing ongoing burn injury and provision of analgesia, covering area involved, and rapid transfer to emergency department [9].

It is worth to underline that also first aid provided by medical stuff in the place of the injury is not correct. The situation seems surprising, because in Poland young doctors are trained in first aid (including first aid in burns) during studies.

Nessler et al. conducted the pilot study (the anonymous questionnaire) among young doctors in Malopolska region (Poland) to evaluate the knowledge of burn first aid, because many patients admitted to burn centers in Poland receive inadequate treatment just after burn injury. The questionnaire verified the respondents' knowledge about appropriate first aid provided several minutes after burn trauma and included questions about possibilities of actions after burn trauma in cases of burned patients. The obtained results were alarming, which revealed that the knowledge of burn first aid among young doctors is not satisfactory—none of the respondents answered correctly to all the questions. Only in 75% respondents knew that burn wound require cooling with running water, whereas only 25% respondents knew how to react after chemical injury [14].

It seems that more attention should be paid on education of caregivers of small children and medical stuff about first aid in burns.

7. Treatment of burns

Care for burned pediatric patient is a challenge for medical and paramedical staff. Treatment of burns is multidisciplinary. According to Juan P. Barret and David N. Herndon, in the burn team, apart from surgeons who specialize in the treatment of burns (general, pediatric, and plastic surgeons), should work also nurses (experienced with care for burned patients), intensive care professionals, scrub and anesthesia nurses, case managers (acute and reconstructive), anesthesiologists, respiratory therapists, rehabilitation therapists, dietitians, psychosocial experts, social workers, volunteers, microbiologists, research personnel, quality control personnel, and workers of support services [1].

The triage decision is based on the extent of burn, body surface area involved, type of burn, associated injuries, any complicating medical or social problems, and availability of ambulatory management [4].

In addition to what has been mentioned above, the criteria that are taken into account to decide if the patient requires hospitalization or referral to the center of burns are anatomic location of the injury and age of the patient.

The most important aspect in pediatric population is age—all the children younger than 1 year old should be hospitalized. Moreover all patients with third-degree burns should be treated in the hospital. Apart from depth of the injury, also extension of burn is taken into account. Hospitalization should be considered in children from families with lower socioeconomic status. Pediatric patients with burns on the face, hands, feet, genitalia, perineum, and joints; all patients with inhalation injuries and electrical or chemical burns; and also patients with associated injury should be hospitalized. Moreover, each patient with suspected nonaccidental injury should be admitted to the hospital. In Poland children with burns are hospitalized in departments of pediatric surgery (with personnel educated about care of burnt patients) or burn centers (children with major burns).

It is possible to classify burn injury according to the severity into minor, moderate, and major [1]. Patients with moderate and major burns require hospital treatment. Minor burns are burns covering less than 15% total body surface area in adults and less than 10% total body surface area in children; less than 3% total body surface area is full-thickness burn; they do not involve the head, feet, hands, or perineum [1]. Moderate burns are burns covering 15–25% total body surface area in adults and 10–15% total body surface area in children, full-thickness burns 3–10% total body surface area, and superficial partial-thickness burns of the head, hands, feet, or perineum [1]. Each case of suspected child abuse is classified as moderate burn [1]. Moreover, in this group, all patients have burn injury and concomitant trauma, significant preexisting disease, and extreme age (neonate and infants). Major burns cover more than 25% total body surface area in adults and more than 15% total body surface area in children [1]. In this group are full-thickness burns of more than 10% total body surface area, deep burns of the head, hands, feet, and perineum, inhalation injuries, chemical burns, and electrical burns [1].

Initial treatment follows the ABCDEs of resuscitation. The aim is to stabilize the airway, breathing, and circulation [9].

Airway management should also include assessment for the presence of airway or inhalation injury [4]. In the cases of suspected airway burns, early intubation can be considered [9]. Children with stridor due to upper airway compromise also require urgent intubation [9]. Potential indications for ventilation are excessive burns that cover over 60–70% of total body surface area, full-thickness circumferential chest burns, and severe inhalation lung injury causing pulmonary edema and hypoxemia [9].

All children with burns over 20% of total body surface area should have intravenous access (peripheral access through non-burnt skin is preferred) [9]. Fluid resuscitation rates should be calculated using the time of burn, patient's body mass, and the surface of burn with the use, for example, of Parkland formula [9]. To determine the adequacy of fluid replacement, monitoring of urinary output is useful [9]. Some patients require nasogastric tube. Important issue in care of burned patient is analgesia.

The treatment of burns can be conservative and operative. Fortunately, most of children do not require surgical treatment, which is reserved for patients with deep (third degree) burns. Conservative treatment is indicated in children with superficial, partial-thickness burns.

Among the most often realized surgical procedures are escharotomy (rare), excision of the dead tissue, and skin grafting [1]. Escharotomy is indicated in patients with circumferential burns on the chest or limbs. The aim of escharotomy is to release the constrictive eschar. The burned skin should be released by incisions with electrocautery within the lines of escharotomy. Early excision of necrotic tissues and grafting is indicated in patients with full-thickness burns. In Poland burn wounds are covered with autografts (donor site is usually tight, less often scalp or back). Skin grafts can be split-skin grafts and full-thickness skin grafts. Most pediatric patients require split-skin grafts. Full-thickness skin grafts can be necessary in specific areas, such as the face (lips, eyelids, nose), hand/fingers, toes, and genitalia. In cases of extensive burns, it is possible to use meshed skin grafts.

Burn wound dressings play crucial role in the care for patient with burns. Burn dressing should protect the burn wound from further harm, such as desiccation, mechanical trauma, and infection. Moreover, they can facilitate the process of healing and relief pain [10]. The current literature is still inconclusive with regard to the gold standard burn dressing for the pediatric population [15]. In Poland burn wound is usually treated with silver sulfadiazine. However, it is commonly known that the ideal dressing for children should alleviate pain, decrease length of hospital stay, and minimize the risk of complications [15].

8. Consequences of burns

The consequences of burns are mostly related with the loss of skin functions. The skin is the largest organ in the body and plays a crucial role in regulating body's temperature by preventing heat loss to the environment. It also prevents water loss from the body and acts as a barrier to infective organisms [9].

It is important to underline the fact that children have a greater ratio of surface area to volume of the body, increased metabolic rate, increased heat loss (less fat and shivering), and increased evaporative water loss [10].

Possible complications of burns include variety of problems, for example, sepsis, hypovolemia, hypothermia, carbon monoxide poisoning, cyanide poisoning, gastric ulcers, cardiac dysfunction, hypermetabolic state, renal failure, transient antidiuresis, and anemia [4]. Another possible complication is laryngeal edema that can be treated with endotracheal intubation and tracheostomy [4]. Moreover, due to edema, compartment syndrome can develop, which means that the patient requires escharotomy [4]. Escharotomy technique involves making longitudinal incisions in segments with inelastic circumferential burns, usually of full thickness [1]. Possible contractures should be treated with physical therapy. Due to the risk of psychological trauma, it is important to provide to burn patients psychological rehabilitation [4]. The possible complications from respiratory system include pulmonary infiltrates, pulmonary edema, pneumonia, and bronchospasm [4]. Inhalation injuries may result in bronchospasm, airway inflammation, and impaired pulmonary function [4]. Moreover, they can result in difficulties in eating and drinking [4].

Among long-term consequences of burns in children are physical scarring and emotional impact of disfiguring burns [4].

9. Risk factors of burns in children: social, economic, and environmental issues related with burns in children

The risk of burn is the highest in children under 2 years old and in boys [5, 6]. Most of burns occur at home, when the child is under the supervision of parent. Appropriate supervision seems even more important than safe environment in prevention of burns in children [16].

Most of burns in children less than 2 years old occur when their mother or father is in the same room. The researchers found that family characteristics play a crucial role in increasing the likelihood of the injury. Lower maternal education, young age of mother and unemployment, and lone parenthood are identified risk factors of burns in children [17].

It is worth to underline that economic situation of the family is also important, because differences in the income result in differences in living conditions. The home environment plays an important role in the risk of burn injury among children.

Among effective strategies that reduce number of flame burns in pediatric population are installation of smoke alarms and smoke detectors [16].

According to the WHO, the possible modifications of the environment that can reduce the number of thermal injuries among children are improved heating and lighting equipment at homes [16].

The own review of the studies about environmental risk factors of burns in children indicates that effective strategy in prevention of scalds in pediatric population is lowering the temperature in the water heaters [17]. Moreover, several studies identified the lack of hot water supply in the household as a risk factor of scalds in children [17].

The arrangement of the apartment that decreases the likelihood of childhood injury includes limited access to the cooking area (and hot fluids). The own review of the studies about environmental risk factors of burns in children indicates that most burn accidents occur in the kitchen [17]. Kitchen without door was found to increase risk of burn injury [17]. The WHO also pays attention to the arrangement of the apartment and separation of cooking area from living area [16].

10. Opportunities for health improvement

Burns are preventable, so prevention strategies should address the hazards for specific burn injuries, education for vulnerable populations and training of communities in first aid. According to the European Report on Child Injury Prevention, there are many cost-effective strategies to prevent burns in children, for example, combination of approaches—involving legislation, engineering, environmental modification, and education [16].

Simple changes in the children's environment and increasing awareness of caregivers can lead to decrease in the number of this type of injuries.

11. Conclusions

To sum up, burns are injuries that affect approximately 1% of all children per year. Their consequences can have physical and mental dimension. Serious burns can lead to death.

Most of these injuries are preventable. Simple changes in the children's environment and increasing awareness of caregivers can lead to decrease in the number of burns in children. Moreover, the first aid given to burn children soon after the injury usually is not adequate (no cooling thermal burns and no analgesia). It is important to underline that also medical staff is not always well educated in providing first aid to burned patients.

Thus, education (medical stuff, paramedical stuff, and caregivers) about first aid in burns and increasing awareness of caregivers about the unsafe behaviors (such as leaving the mug with hot tea at the edge of the table, where the child can easily reach), avoiding the situations that puts child at risk of burn, seems to be one of the most important parts of prevention.

Moreover, legislation interventions such as laws to enforce smoke detectors, smoke alarms installation, or regulation of hot water at homes are promising strategies to reduce the number of burned children.

Health improvement can be also obtained by reducing number of pediatric patients with burns, correct first aid given after the injury, and organization of specialized health-care centers and rehabilitation services for victims of burns.

Conflict of interest

I confirm there are no conflicts of interest.

Acronyms and abbreviations

ABCDE	airway, breathing, circulation, disabilities, and environment control
ICD	The International Classification of Diseases
TBSA	total body surface area
WHO	World Health Organization

Author details

Agata Maria Kawalec

Address all correspondence to: agata_kawalec@wp.pl

Department of Hygiene, Wroclaw Medical University, Wroclaw, Poland

References

[1] Barret-Nerin J, Herndon DN. Principles and Practice of Burn Surgery. Marcel Dekker; 2004. p. 412

[2] World Health Organization. Burns. Fact sheet. Updated August 2017. Available from: http://www.who.int/mediacentre/factsheets/fs365/en/ [Accessed: 2018-01-08]

[3] Mock C, Peck M, Peden M, Krug E, editors. A WHO Plan for Burn Prevention and Care. Geneva: World Health Organization; 2008. p. 24

[4] Lee KJ, Marcdante K. Burns. In: Marcdante K, Kliegman RM, Jenson HB, Behrman RE, editors. Nelson Essentials of Paediatrics, 6th ed. Philadelphia: Saunders Elsevier; 2011. pp. 156-158

[5] Kawalec A, Pawlas K. Struktura oparzeń wśród dzieci na Dolnym Śląsku (Polska). Structure of burns in children in Lower Silesia (Poland) in 2010-2012. Problemy Higieny i Epidemiologii. 2014;**95**(2):394-399

[6] Kawalec A, Kawalec A, Pawlas K. Struktura oparzeń wśród dzieci na Dolnym Śląsku (Polska). Część II [Structure of burns in children in Lower Silesia (Poland) between 2010-2012. Part II]. Problemy Higieny i Epidemiologii. 2014;**95**(3):744-747

[7] Matuszczak E, Dębek W, Chomicz A, Dzienis-Koronkiewicz E, Oksiuta M, Hermanowicz A. Analiza etiologii i epidemiologii oraz ocena wyników leczenia oparzeń u dzieci. Pediatria Polska. 2011;**86**(3):254-259

[8] Zaniewski J, editor. Leksykon diagnoz medycznych. Warszawa: Poltext; 2005. p. 1095

[9] Barnett PLJ. Burns. In: Cameron P, Jelinek G, Everitt I, Browne G, Raftos J, editors. Textbook of Paediatric Emergency Medicine. 2nd ed. Edinburgh: Churchill Livingstone Elsevier; 2012. pp. 73-38. ISBN: 9780702033681

[10] Chiu TW, Burd A. Key Topics in Plastic and Reconstructive Surgery. London: Taylor & Francis; 2005. p. 192

[11] Richards AM. Key Notes on Plastic Surgery. Oxford: Blackwell Science; 2002. p. 313

[12] Andronicus M, Oates RK, Peat J, Spalding S, Martin H. Non-accidental burns in children. Burns. 1998;**24**(6):552-558. DOI: 10.1016/S0305-4179(98)00062-X

[13] Kawalec A. Czynniki środowiskowe ryzyka oparzeń u dzieci z uwzględnieniem profilaktyki [Thesis]. Wrocław: Wroclaw Medical University; 2016

[14] Nessler K, Nessler M, Krztoń-Królewiecka A, Chrapusta A, Windak A. The knowledge about burn first aid among young physicians in Malopolska Region—Pilot study. Chirurgia plastyczna i oparzenia. 2014;**2**(1):7-13. DOI: 10.15374/ChPiO2014013

[15] Fan C, Pek CH, Por YC, Lim GJS. Biobrane dressing for paediatric burns in Singapore: A retrospective review. Singapore Medical Journal. 2018;**1**:1-16. DOI: 10.11622/smedj.2017116

[16] Sethi D, Towner E, Vincenten J, Segui-Gomez M, Racioppi F. European Report on Child Injury Prevention. Rome: World Health Organization; 2008. p. 24

[17] Kawalec A. Environmental factors of burns in children—Review. Medycyna Środowiskowa - Environmental Medicine. 2015;**18**(3):40-46

Section 3

Academic Approach

Chapter 13

New Horizons in Emergency Medicine Teaching and Training

Shahzad Anjum

Additional information is available at the end of the chapter

http://dx.doi.org/10.5772/intechopen.75162

Abstract

Emergency medicine (EM) is a unique field where the logistics of work environment is the biggest challenge for any organized traditional teaching and training. The shift pattern of work, absence of availability of real-time situations in controlled environment, availability of teaching faculty 24/7 and quality control of teaching and training are the major challenges that need to be considered. It requires lot of organizational, departmental as well as operational support to run a successful teaching program where all the important aspects of teaching and training are considered. In the emergency teaching and training, issues of supervision are of prime importance. The fear of complaints and litigations is enormous. Meeting the six core competencies of Accreditation Council for Graduate Medical Education (ACGME) and achieving the milestones before the residents are signed off are the goals and objectives of any good teaching program. In this chapter, we discuss the important modifications in teaching methods, which can fulfill the important requirements and demands of this unique field which is full of challenges. We also discuss the different models of teaching and training which are different from standard traditional didactic teaching which can be adopted and may help in achieving emergency medicine core knowledge, competencies and skills.

Keywords: emergency medicine, teaching and training, didactic teaching, achieving goals of training, mentorship

1. Introduction

Teaching and training in emergency medicine (EM) is one of the biggest challenges considering the dynamics of this field. The nature of work, the pattern of shift duties and pressure of working environment is one of the biggest challenges in getting quality training and teaching.

All these problems can be addressed if proper guidance is provided to the trainers and the candidates, and there is an efficient system of assessing both the candidates and trainers.

2. Core of emergency medicine teaching: new horizons

Objective- and goal-oriented teaching and training are the core of modernized teaching and training. Achieving these objectives by training the trainers is the key. All these objectives will be achieved if we focus on the quality of trainers by educating them what to teach, how to teach, how to assess and how to assure achieving different milestones.

The objective of quality teaching and training program is to achieve the minimum, identifiable, and quantifiable results which can be compared to any international benchmark. It is very important to define these benchmarks at the start of any program so that everyone is aware of the expectations. In the USA, the residency teaching and training program follows the Accreditation council of Graduate Medical Education standards. The six core competencies of teaching and training are the tools used to evaluate and assess the candidates. These six core competencies include medical knowledge, patient care, professionalism, intercommunication skills, system-based practice and problem-based learning. Achieving all these competencies assures that all the important domains are met before the candidates are finally signed off from the program.

The assessment is done by looking at the milestones which are achieved in each competency mentioned earlier. Milestones are used to assess residents progress and achievement of required skill and competency over period of time. The milestones are identified in each of six core competencies. The performance in each milestone in any given core competency describes the residents' level. Each milestone is assessed individually to look at the level achieved by the resident to identify the areas which need extra support.

2.1. Important stakeholders in teaching and training

For a successful program, it is important that the stakeholders are identified. This helps in defining the roles and responsibilities of all the stakeholders. In any good teaching program, following are the stakeholders who play important roles:

1. Candidates
2. Faculty (Dedicated and nondedicated)
3. Department

Selection of focused and committed candidates is the first requirement for any successful program. Selected residents must be given the clear goals and objectives at the start of the program. The dedicated faculty is the core faculty who should lead and participate in important committees and groups to take necessary decisions and actions related to the candidates. The nondedicated faculty includes all other clinical staffs who are working in the department and responsible for the residents' teaching and training at the shop floor.

http://dx.doi.org/10.5772/intechopen.75162

All the stakeholders need to be educated to know their roles and responsibilities. Identifying the objectives and targets makes it easy to have a self-check.

2.1.1. Candidates

Candidate selection is done in consideration of dynamics of emergency medicine specialty. During selection, the panel should make sure that candidates understand the specialty requirements and demands. Selecting the candidates whose personality can cope with the nature of emergency medicine specialty is the principle of selection criteria. Selected candidates should be accommodative, flexible, tolerating, committed, dedicated with clear vision to stay and perform with all the challenges of this field.

After selection, it is important to educate the candidates about the program requirement objectives of each year of training. Proper counseling is needed to educate them to understand the program requirements. They must be given the clear targets at the start of each academic year and assessed at the end of the academic year to look for targets and milestones achieved.

2.1.2. Trainers: core faculty and faculty

The faculty members are the pillars of any training program. They are the ones who assure the quality of candidates and the program. Selection of suitable faculty members is one of the most important and difficult task. The faculty members can be broadly divided into two groups. One group includes core faculty members who are the most experienced members in the group and are responsible for important decisions taken in the program. The other group includes faculty members who are responsible for support at shop floor and continuous feedback and assessment of residents.

2.1.2.1. Core faculty members

They are the most experienced members in the group who are selected based on their performance, commitment, excellent portfolio and dedication to the program. The selection must be done after following robust rules and criteria and should include input from the department, candidates as well as their achievements. Core faculty members are involved in important committees and groups and must be given the leadership roles and responsibilities. They must be given tasks to work autonomously but at the same time be accountable to Program Director. Their number should be enough to make sure that they are not overwhelmed with work and they fulfill the program requirements. The number of trainees defines the number of core faculty needed. For every 5–6 candidates, there must be one core faculty member. They must be responsible for the close monitoring of trainee physicians.

2.1.2.2. Faculty members

In a training institution, every member of clinical team is considered the faculty member by default. They are expected to teach, train and assess trainee and provide them all the support required. In a tertiary care setup, this is a fundamental requirement and all the staff is bound to follow this. On the one hand, the faculty members are expected to do bedside training of trainee physician, and on the other hand, it is made sure that the faculty members are trained to train. They are capable, competent and committed. There must be a quality check on what they teach and this requires constant faculty development programs to educate them.

2.1.3. Department/training institution

The training department is one of the most important stakeholders in the program because it provides the ideal environment for teaching and training. Continuous and unlimited departmental support is a key for successful training program. All the faculty members are encouraged for professional training support and help. The department provides enough protected time to teaching core faculty to support the program. Department also provides important courses and training to faculty to run the quality program. They also provide environment for continuous medical education in the form of grand rounds, mortality and morbidity (M&M) conferences and journal clubs (JC).

2.2. Hierarchy, committees and role assignment

To run a successful program, there must be a defined hierarchy to make everyone accountable for their roles and job.

The Program Director is the overall responsible member for the whole program. The selection of Program Director is done considering the seniority, experience in education and training and the suitable portfolio for the job. The selection should be done by considering the training background, achievements in the field and performance. Program Director should delegate important tasks to all the members and make sure that they are done timely and efficiently. Different aspects of program are run and monitored by important committees. The purpose of the committees is to focus on important domains of the teaching and training.

The important domains to be addressed are education and training, program evaluation and trainees' clinical competencies. Each committee works autonomously under the leadership of a lead core faculty who report to Program Director.

2.2.1. Education group

There must be a dedicated core faculty to lead the education group to nurture the requirements of the education. The responsibility of this group should be to do curriculum mapping to international curriculum and improve it. The teaching planner must be prepared in such a way that all the important core topics are covered and important skills are taught. They must do frequent assessments to look for trainees' performance and knowledge of the subject. They choose suitable mentors who are given responsibilities of their mentee. The mentors supervise 2–3 mentees and all the important messages are delivered to residents through their mentors. Mentors should frequently hold meetings with the mentee for detailed assessment of candidates, which includes case logs, procedures, work-based assessment, medical knowledge, behavior and attitude. They are responsible for the assessment of medical knowledge by conducting exams.

2.2.2. *Program evaluation*

The lead core faculty of this group assures the program quality, faculty performance, trainee performance and quality of graduates. Multiple tools can be used to measure this against a standard benchmark. It must be done by maintaining the confidentiality so that the best feedback is taken. Program quality evaluation covers all the aspects of the program including candidate's orientation to the program when they join, program design, educational format, work environment, system of evaluations, research, departmental support, resources, infrastructure, faculty support and the support of core faculty and Program Director. This is done by both residents and faculty members. The lead of the committee should maintain the confidentiality, and the result is relayed to the Program Director to take necessary actions.

The group also ensures that residents are evaluated through a robust system where all the six core competencies are assessed. Trainees work-based assessments are done. This includes case-based discussion, Mini-Cex, direct observation of procedural skills (DOPS), standardized direct observational assessment tool (SDOT), formative assessment, summative assessment, biannual evaluation and 360 evaluation.

All these evaluation helps in assessing the overall teaching environment as well as the performance. It will cover all the important stakeholders (candidates, trainers and training site) and important parameters like contents, quality, performance, professionalism, behavior and attitude. It will also look at policies and protocols followed and outcome of the product.

2.2.3. *Trainees' clinical competency*

The lead for clinical competency group is responsible for keeping a quality check on the milestones achieved, professionalism, performance, medical knowledge, patient care, system-based practice, problem-based learning and communication skills.

The committee report decides for final signing off of trainee at the end of each year of training. The promotion to next stage is not done if trainee fails to achieve the minimum standards.

2.3. Mentors and mentee

Mentor mentee program is one of the best ways of monitoring the resident's performance [1]. The selection of mentors should depend on competency, teaching skills, willingness to teach and train and expertise in evaluating the trainee. The number of mentors should be kept minimum. Ideally, each mentor should not supervise more than 3–4 mentees. The core faculty should further supervise 3–4 mentors as chief mentors so that there is a proper guidance of mentors as well as mentees. The chief mentors will make sure that uniform message is passed down to each mentor level. The chief mentors will make sure that all the mentors are following the same standards and protocols.

There must be 4 monthly feedbacks about the mentors and mentees. The mentors should evaluate mentees to look for their performance including work-based assessment, educational day attendance, logbook record, professionalism, 360 evaluations as well as exam preparation [2].

The mentee should also do 4 monthly evaluations of their mentors, which include availability of mentors whenever needed, their attitude, behavior, willingness to teach, bedside teaching and their support to residents in preparing for lectures and exams.

2.4. Faculty development programs and continued medical education

Teaching and training of residents need lot of faculty training and development. To have a good teaching and training program, there must be a system where the trainer must be trained and guided. Trainers need professional support and guidance to understand the requirements of the program and the candidates. They should be given expertise to know the milestones in the program and system to assess them. There should be harmony in the evaluation system so that all evaluate candidates on the same parameters. The important milestones are tested and candidates are scored. Those who are weak and are not achieving the minimum required milestones must be highlighted through a fair system and then referred to the senior core faculty for proper counseling and mitigation.

The faculty should also be provided all important courses and trainings which are needed by them for proper teaching of trainee physician. In a tertiary care setup where there is a rapid staff turnover, there is a strong need of having a good faculty development programs so that the new faculty members are given guidance and orientation to the program.

Program requirements are assessed by the senior management, and all the arrangements need to be done to provide important training courses and workshops to the trainers. The faculty is also encouraged to improve their scholarly activities and educational portfolio. It has to be assessed regularly so that necessary actions are taken if there is any deficiency in their scholarly portfolio.

2.5. Tools for assessment

For a quality education program, there must be a robust way of evaluating the candidates. Different tools must be created to assess each aspect of the program. The tools must include forms, questionnaire and surveys to assess the program quality, faculty, residents, mentors, mentee and evaluation of clinical skills and medical knowledge. Following are the different types of evaluating tools to assess the program in detail:

1. Program Evaluation Form: See **Table 1**
2. Mentors Evaluation by mentee: See **Table 2**
3. Mentee Evaluation by mentor: see **Table 3**
4. Work Based Assessment: the Work Based Assessment is one of the best ways to do detailed trainee assessment. It rely more on how the trainer is trained to do this assessment. The responsibility of evaluation lies on the trainer, and this cannot be done unless the trainer has the expertise and experience of doing this. It needs good faculty development programs which again is the responsibility of teaching institution. Thus, the responsibility of training is shared by all the three stakeholders, which form triangle of learning

http://dx.doi.org/10.5772/intechopen.75162

A. Induction and introduction of EMRTP according to residency year	**1**	**2**	**3**	**4**	**5**
A1.You are given proper guidance for your whole year of training.					
A2.You are given proper goals, objectives to be achieved during your residency year.					
A3.You are given proper orientation and introduction about the departments, facilities, teaching faculty, educational materials.					
Your overall rating for the Induction and Introduction module	Not Satisfactory (please comment why it is not satisfactory and what can be done to improve it)			Satisfactory	

Additional comments:

B. Over all Program design	**1**	**2**	**3**	**4**	**5**
B1.EMRTP has well defined goals and objectives					
B2.The Program is well structured and organized					
B3.The faculty and residents are aware of these goals.					
B4. The program has the means to achieve its goals and objectives					
B5.The Program incorporates core competencies into all levels of its training and evaluation					
B6.Program complies with duty hour policy for residents					
Your overall rating of this module:	Unsatisfactory			Satisfactory	

Additional comments

C. Educational format and rating	**1**	**2**	**3**	**4**	**5**
C1.The program provides ample opportunity (time and resources) for se006Cf-directed learning					
C2.The format is easy to understand and learn					
C3.The format is addressing the requirements of the candidate					
C4.The format is based on scientific and professional needs.					
C5.The bed side teaching is appropriate in terms of quality and quantity					
C6.The Tuesday activities are very helpful and informative for learning and improving					
C7. The journal clubs are very useful in developing residents' awareness of EBM and research					
C8.The additional courses and workshops are very good and helpful in terms of quality and numbers.					
Overall rating of this module:	Unsatisfactory			Satisfactory	

Additional comments

D. Work environment	**1**	**2**	**3**	**4**	**5**
D1. Your training sites are adequate in terms of number and educational contents?					
D2.The EM patient population case mix is adequate in number and variety.					
D3.You are fairly exposed to the critical cases in the ED.					
D4.Your clinical work is continuously supervised and proper teaching is assured					
D5. The supervisors and consultants guide you and teach you in most cases you see in the ED					
D6. You have ample opportunity to develop procedural, teaching and leadership skills.					
D7.You are provided with progressive responsibilities appropriate to their PGY level of training.					
D8. There is adequate number of medical staff to meet the demand for service needs of the ED					
D9. At shop floor, you can get help of seniors and Faculty whenever its required					
D10. There is presence of Consultants and faculty 24/7 at the shop floor					
How you Overall rate this module	Unsatisfactory		Satisfactory		
Additional comments					

E. Evaluation	**1**	**2**	**3**	**4**	**5**
E1.My Formative evaluation have been useful and constructive					
E2.My summative evaluation has been useful and constructive					
E3.My Summative evaluation has been comprehensive in assessing all the 6 core competencies					
E4.My evaluation process has been conducted in a fair and reasonable manner and my deficiencies are discussed for my improvement.					
E5. I am given the chance to discuss my deficiencies to improve					
E6.I am regularly given proper feed backs by mentor and PD/APD on my progress.					
E7. I am given full support and help to make me eligible to sit for the board exam					
How you Overall rate this module	Unsatisfactory		Satisfactory		
Additional comments					

F. Research	**1**	**2**	**3**	**4**	**5**
F1.I have been given ample opportunity to develop understanding and interest in EM research					
F2.I have received guidance and encouragement in research activities					
How you overall rate this module	Unsatisfactory		Satisfactory		
Additional comments					

http://dx.doi.org/10.5772/intechopen.75162

G. Departmental and interdepartmental support/relations	**1**	**2**	**3**	**4**	**5**
G1.Relationship with other dept. is optimum					
G2.Other dept. co-operates in getting the required standards of teaching during rotations.					
G3. Other departments teach the required curriculum during rotations					
G4.Support of ED department staff is optimum during training					
G5.Other departments support your attendance during Tuesday activity.					
How you Overall rate this module	Unsatisfactory			Satisfactory	
Additional comments					

H. Resources, infrastructure	**1**	**2**	**3**	**4**	**5**
H1.ED infrastructure provides adequate and ample space and facilities for educational needs.					
H2.HMC infrastructure provides adequate and ample space and facilities for educational need.					
Your overall rating of this module:	Unsatisfactory			Satisfactory	
Additional comments					

I. Faculty/Mentor role	**1**	**2**	**3**	**4**	**5**
I1.There is adequate EM faculty in terms of number and availability for my educational need					
I2.The Faculty is given ample opportunity to supervise trainees in developing their clinical skills, professional, teaching, leadership, and management skills					
I3.The faculty actively participates in bedside teaching of residents					
I4.Faculty actively participates in the Tuesday activity.					
I5. The faculty gives regular feedbacks to the residents about their progress					
Your overall rating of this module	Unsatisfactory			Satisfactory	
Additional comments:					

J. Program Director	**1**	**2**	**3**	**4**	**5**
J1. PD gives feedback about your progress and deficiencies					
J2.PD addresses all the issues and problems which are relayed to him					
J3.PD plays effective role in dealing with educational and teaching issues					
J4.PD plays effective role in dealing with issues of services, Rota, education, faculty and rotation issues in other departments					
J5. The PD is approachable and respond to you whenever contacted.					
J6. The PD is Helpful and understands your problems.					
J7. The PD discuss with you to sort out your problems.					
Your overall rating of this module:	Unsatisfactory			Satisfactory	
Additional comments					

Associate Program Director	Strongly disagree	Disagree	Unable to comment	Agree	Strongly agree
K1.APD gives regular feedback about your progress and deficiencies					
K2.APD addresses all the issues and problems which are relayed to him					
K3.APD plays effective role in dealing with educational and teaching issues					
K4.APD plays effective role in dealing with issues of services, Rota, education, faculty and rotation issues in other departments					
K5. The APD is approachable and respond to you whenever contacted.					
K6. The APD is Helpful and understands your problems.					
J7. The APD discuss with you to sort out your problems.					
Your overall rating of this module:	Unsatisfactory (Comment Why)			Satisfactory	
Additional comments					

Program Coordinator	Strongly disagree	Disagree	Unable to comment	Agree	Strongly agree
L1. PC is helpful and cooperative					
L2. PC always responds to issues and problems					
L3. Pc is reliable.					
L4. PC is efficient in dealing with your issues					
Additional comments					

Chief Resident	Strongly disagree	Disagree	Unable to comment	Agree	Strongly agree
M1. Is He Easily Approachable					
M2. Does he respond to you timely and efficiently when contacted					
M3. Does he cooperate with you					
M4. Does he represent you and raise your issues to PD/ APD and CF timely?					
M5. Do you think that he is perfectly doing what he is expected to do as CR					
Additional comment: (please write your expectations and issues you would like to raise)					

Core faculty	Strongly disagree	Disagree	Unable to comment	Agree	Strongly agree
N1. Is CF Easily Approachable					
N2. Do they respond to you timely and efficiently when contacted					
N3. Do they cooperate with you					
N4. Do they represent you and raise your issues to PD/ APD timely?					
N5. Do you think that they are perfectly doing what they are expected to do as CF.					
Additional Comment: (please write your expectations and issues you would like to raise)					
1 = Unable to comment, 2 strongly disagree, 3 Disagree, 4 agree, 5 strongly agree					

Table 1. Program evaluation form.

1. Your Mentor is approachable when required. Yes/No
2. Your Mentor is helpful in your educational tasks when asked for. Yes/No
3. Your Mentor is professional whenever you approach him. Yes/No
4. Your Mentor is helpful in the clinical teaching and training whenever you approach him. Yes/No
5. Your Mentor helps you in exam preparation and guidance whenever you approach him. Yes/No
6. Your Mentor has good teaching skills. Yes/No
7. Your mentor is helpful in research guidance. Yes/No
8. Your Mentor helps you in preparing lectures and didactic activities whenever you approach him. Yes/No
9. Your Mentor has done Case Based Discussions whenever you have approached him. Yes/No
10. Your Mentor has helped you in preparing and completing logbook. Yes/No
11. Your Mentor has helped you in completing the DOPS. Yes/No
12. Your Mentor has completed SDOT forms when asked for. Yes/No
Explain what are the good things about your mentor and why?
Explain what are the concerns which you want to be addressed?

Table 2. Mentor Evaluation by Mentee.

(institution-trainee-trainer). The trainers are given objectives and goals. There is a standardized assessment tool and the trainers are trained in using these tools to do assessment. The faculty development programs run by the institution make sure that the trainers are trained to do these assessments. This is a dynamic process which makes sure that there is a continuous environment for learning and training to have better outcome. Following are the different tools used to assess the trainee:

Domains		(July- Oct)	(Nov-Feb)	(Mar-June)
Log Book				
WBA	Mini-CEX			
	DOPS			
	SDOT			
	CBD			
Educational	Oral cases			
	Presentations			
	M&M			
	JC			
	Follow up cases			
MSF/360 evaluation				
Formative assessment				
Research				
Quality Projects				
Courses and Conferences				
Attendance				
Global Report				

Table 3. Mentee Evaluation by Mentor.

- Mini-Cex: [5, 7] the mini clinical evaluation exercise provides a 15-min snapshot of how you interact with patients in a secondary care setting. It covers major core competencies including history taking, examination skills, communication skills, clinical judgment, professionalism and overall clinical care. This is a snapshot of performance where in a short time, the assessor assesses the trainee's performance. There is no active participation from trainee and it is just observation of what trainee does. There is no argument or discussion over the case.

- SDOT: Refs. [8–12] the standardized direct observational assessment tool (SDOT) is a tool developed by Council of Emergency Medicine Residency Directors (CORD) to assess and evaluate the residents based on the core competencies as defined by the ACGME. They are: medical knowledge, patient care, professionalism, interpersonal and communication skills, practice-based learning, and system-based practice. The SDOT is based on a direct observation of the resident by a faculty member

  This assessment tool, the SDOT, is designed to obtain objective data through observation of residents during actual ED patient encounters. Each item should be judged as either: "Needs Improvement (**NI**)," "Meets Expectations (**ME**)," "Above Expected (**AE**)," or "Not Assessed (**NA**)" for level of training. This detailed assessment tool bounds assessor as well to have a detailed evaluation of trainee. It needs proper training and understanding of the assessor, which requires faculty development programs to make sure that all the trainers are on same page and they are trained to evaluate and assess the trainee.

- DOPS: [13–15] direct observation of procedural skills is a workplace-based assessment tool for trainees, which has been designed for the assessment of practical skills. It is an assessment of performance. All the important procedures can be taught and tested in controlled environment on models or phantoms, and this tool can be used to assess:
  - trainees' understanding of basics of subject including the anatomy and landmarks.
  - trainees' skills to perform the procedure and
  - trainees' depth of knowledge on the subject, including awareness of complications and ability to deal with them.

It provides an environment for one-to-one discussion and interaction.

- Formative Assessment: [17] this is an assessment of trainee at the end of each block or rotation. It is the snapshot of that rotation. The trainer is expected to complete this evaluation within the time frame offered by the program. Formative evaluation gives information about the performance of trainee during that block. It will reflect the performance of trainee during specialty rotation. Each rotation block will be given the objectives of rotation which are expected from the trainee and the trainer. The trainer will make sure that the trainee is given all the important skills which are required by the parent specialty. This will help in keeping the trainee focused.
- Summative Assessment: [18] this is the assessment of trainee at the end of each academic year or after completion of training. This will depend on overall performance of trainee during each rotation. It is a collective evaluation which will be based on multiple assessments done throughout the training sessions.
- Case-based assessment: [19–21] a case-based assessment or discussion involves a comprehensive review of clinical case(s) between an advanced trainee and an assessor. After the case-based discussion, the assessor provides valuable feedback to help the trainee improve and structure their future learning.

Aim of this exercise is to:

(I) Give a detailed and structured feedback on trainees' learning. This will be used as a guide to improve his learning. This is quick, instant and readily available.

(II) Improve clinical decision-making, clinical knowledge and patient management. The valuable advices of assessor which is based on his knowledge, expertise and experience will help in giving the best possible solution and also platform for healthy discussion where evidence-based problem solving is done.

(III) Provide a trainee with an opportunity to discuss their approach to the case and identify strategies to improve their practice.

(IV) Enable the assessor to share professional knowledge and experience.

2.6. Multisource feedback (360 evaluation)

Multisource feedback is one of the best ways to look at the overall personality and performance of the trainee [22]. It covers all the aspects including medical knowledge, attitude, behavior, communication skills and leadership qualities. This is done by the colleagues, seniors, paramedical staff, nurses as well as patients. Multisource feedback is one of the best ways to look at the minute details about the trainee physician which may impact the future performance as a leader.

2.7. Teaching assessment

- **Faculty and Trainee Teaching Assessment:** the program should provide opportunity and environment for teaching assessments to maintain the quality of program. All the presentations done by the trainee as well as the trainer are evaluated by the senior core faculty to have quality check of the program. The Core Faculty should give feedback to all presenters about their presentations These Feedbacks are given by completing a detailed form. The detailed form should focus on the contents of presentation, style, format, time management, audience engagement as well as the presentation skills.
- **Teaching Activity Evaluation:** the teaching activities must be evaluated to look at the outcomes and the targets achieved. The curriculum covered should be looked at. Comparison to international curriculum by curriculum mapping is done. Any deficiencies found must be addressed.

2.7.1. Rotation assessment

At the end of the rotation, the trainee must give feedback about his experience during the rotation. It will give information about the rotation if it is helpful in providing the required expertise and training. There are standard requirements and objectives for each rotation and these are mentioned in the program's letter of agreement (PLA). There is a PLA for each rotation which clearly says the objectives of this rotation, and it is expected that the department where the resident is rotating is respecting this requirement and make sure to do every effort to achieve this. The feedback given by the trainee during the rotation is a guide for the Program Director and the education team to decide how they should work to improve the system and make the rotation more effective for the trainee. We take this feedback at three stages. One is before starting the rotation where we discuss with trainee to know his awareness about the goals and objectives of his rotation. Second during the rotation when they have completed 50% of their rotation. Any issues highlighted by the trainee during this time are raised to the relevant department to take necessary steps to improve it. Third is after the completion of rotation when their input and feedback about their rotation helps us in planning to modify and rectify the rotation as per our requirements and take necessary steps which will benefit the other trainees in future.

2.7.2. Milestone assessment

Milestone Assessment is one of the ways to assess the trainee's progress in the program. [6, 23] Different milestones are assessed in the six core competencies, and residents' level is measured. The EM milestones are a matrix of the knowledge, skills, abilities, attitudes and experiences that should be acquired during specialty training in emergency medicine. The level which a trainee is demonstrating in each year helps us in assessing his performance and gives a comparison with his other colleagues. Before the trainee is promoted to the next stage, the level is recorded so that performance is monitored. There are standard milestones identified in the emergency medicine training program. These milestones focus on ACGME core competencies and also test the following important aspects of training:

- taking focused history and performing physical examination
- requesting investigations and diagnostic tests and interpretation of these investigations
- performing important tasks like managing airway
- emergency stabilization of patient
- pharmacotherapy
- observation and reassessment
- disposition of patient
- skills of multitasking
- general approach to procedures
- anesthesia and acute pain management
- other diagnostic and therapeutic procedures (goal-directed focused ultrasound-diagnostic and procedural)
- wound management
- vascular access
- medical knowledge
- patient care
- system-based management
- practice-based learning
- technology

- professionalism
- accountability
- interpersonal communication skills
- team management

The trainee is assessed to look for if he is at beginner level or at advanced level. There are five levels based on his performance. Each level identifies trainee's capability and performance. The trainer will mark the trainee's level which can be used to identify the deficiencies so that other faculty members can work on this. These milestone levels are not related to years of training. A trainee in year 2 may be at level 3 in history taking, whereas a trainee in year 3 may be at level 2.

2.8. Designing curriculum

Curriculum designing is the core of emergency medicine program [16]. The curriculum should address the standard emergency medicine requirements as well as should address the local area requirements to focus on those important topics which need special attention. This includes important diseases prevalent in that area as well as the local management protocols and procedures. The curriculum should include all the important topics and contents which are considered core of this specialty. There must be an annual review of curriculum and mapping with international curriculum to look for any modifications needed. The curriculum should focus on skills, procedures, scientific knowledge, quality and research, leadership and management skills, communication skills, awareness about cost-effectiveness and focus on new modalities and technology.

2.9. Empowering core faculty

The core faculty must be empowered to deliver the quality education and training. They must be given protected time and resources so that they can spend enough time in delivering the quality education and training. The core faculty must be given the leadership role in each committee so that they can make sure that each aspect of the program is given proper attention. The lead for program evaluation is responsible for quality of teaching and training. He gathers all the important information and data by taking feedbacks and doing surveys about the program. He writes a detailed independent report about the program and should give recommendations to the Program Director about the changes required. These recommendations are discussed in the quarterly program evaluation committee meeting for proper actions. Each committee lead should work independently to collect information and data about the program and these data should be used for program improvement.

2.10. Dedicated educational hours and different teaching methods

To have quality training, there must be a dedicated day for the didactic teaching and training [3]. All the important topics need to be covered. Different teaching methods and styles need to be adopted to make sure that relevant information is delivered to the trainee. The methods adopted should assure that trainee is given the skills of teaching and presentations, skills to learn evidence-based knowledge, skills to get familiar with system and protocols in the organization and skills to implement the evidence-based knowledge. We have divided our teaching activity into four basic components. One is didactic teaching which is done by junior residents (year 1 and 2); interactive lectures and workshops which is done by the senior residents (Year 3 and 4); oral scenarios, simulations and objectively structured clinical examination (OSCE) (for clinical and applied knowledge testing of trainee) and a session for mortality and morbidity meeting, grand rounds, journal clubs which are done once per month alternatively.

Academic teaching planner: the academic teaching planner is released at the start of each academic Year. Our academic calendar starts in July and ends in June. The topics are assigned before the start of academic year. There are four slots for the teaching day. One slot is given to junior resident (Year 1 or 2) with the name of the topic and supervising faculty. The second slot is interactive lecture or workshop with the name of faculty who is responsible to prepare this topic and names of two residents who will be conducting the show as a leader but supervised by the faculty. The third slot is for the OSCE, oral clinical scenario or simulation (one alternatively on each week), and fourth is for the sessions like mortality and morbidity conference, grand rounds and journal clubs which are attended by other members of the department. Each teaching component has goals and objectives which are discussed as follows:

2.10.1. Didactics

During this teaching day, the target is to train the trainee to improve their teaching and presentation skills. This is one of the foundational requirements. The trainee should be given chance and environment to improve this skill. This assignment is given to junior residents (Year 1 and 2) who are assigned topics at the start of academic calendar. All the important topics in emergency medicine curriculum are covered in this teaching slot. The lectures are prepared by junior trainee (Year 1 and 2). Each trainee is expected to do at least one presentation in 1 year. This is prepared with the help of a mentor. The objective of this exercise is to:

- improve the presentation skills of trainee;
- develop and improve his skills to do literature search for the given topic to look for the best treatment model available;
- discuss the practical approach to deal with the problem;
- discuss the local policies and protocols and learn the system-based practice in the institution; and
- improve the skills of preparing the presentation. He learns how to improve power point presentation preparation skills by getting help from his peers, seniors and faculty members.

The presentation is given by the resident, and at the end of his presentation, one of the senior trainees does critique which improves the skills of critiquing of trainee. Finally, the faculty member gives his evaluation which is used as a tool for residents' performance assessment.

2.10.2. Interactive lectures and workshops

One of the new ways of improved teaching is interactive lectures and workshops [24]. This is different from the traditional lecturing where faculty comes on the podium and give 30–40 min talk to a big group of trainees. In the interactive style lectures and workshops, the trainees are divided into small groups who interact with a senior faculty member. The topic is divided in such a way that each group discusses a certain aspect of topic. There is a clear learning objective of each station. The group should be kept as small as possible. Ideally, there should not be more than 8–10 trainees in each group. The faculty member does interactive style discussion in each station where there is a clear objective of discussion. This makes sure that the trainees are actively participating in the discussion. The face-to-face discussion keeps them engaged, and all the important messages are given in a much better style.

These topics are prepared by the faculty members as they understand the needs and requirements of the topic. The presentation must be evidence-based discussion with emphasis on important points and take-home messages. The faculty may prepare the topics and delegate it through the final year senior residents who can discuss these in interactive style with the junior group. Each topic can be split in to three subgroups (20–30 min each). Small group discussion ensures better chance of delivering important points. When done by senior residents under the supervision of trainee, it improves their presentation and communication skills. Thus, we achieve multiple objectives at a same time. We have seen a very positive impact of these interactive presentations on teaching and training. There is more friendly discussion between the faculty and trainee. The faculty gets the opportunity to assess the individual need of trainee and thus tailor his discussion according to the need of individuals. The small groups either have representation from all years of training or may be having all trainees from the same year. The faculty then decides what difficulty level he will adopt depending on the trainee level in the group. Mixing the groups is one way of doing it where representations from all the years of training will fulfill certain aspects of requirement. On the other hand, separating all the groups strictly based on their year of training will fulfill other requirements of training. The education lead and core faculty should decide what model he wants to adopt depending on the requirement of the workshop.

2.10.3. Skill stations

The skill station includes practical demonstration of all the important skills. All the important procedures are discussed on manikins, models, phantoms or biological models. The curriculum is looked at and all the required procedures and skills are highlighted and covered during this exercise. We have highlighted all the important procedures which are included in the curriculum of emergency medicine residency training. These procedures are given slots in the planner. The faculty who is assigned this workshop has two residents from the senior group (year 3 and 4) who conduct this workshop. The faculty member prepares the workshop in such a way that all the goals and objectives are defined. The objectives are to test the knowledge for that procedure. It includes knowledge of landmarks, anatomy, steps, techniques, complications and management of complications. There are hands-on training sessions which include testing of skills of the trainee on models. This gives excellent opportunity to deal with the trainee in small groups (not more than 8–10). Each station is 30–40 min where all the candidates are given chance to participate. The faculty also gets the opportunity to engage all the trainees and do one-to-one discussion.

2.10.4. *Objectively structured clinical examination*

Ref. [15] this is one of the most important ways of teaching the subject where the topic is prepared in such a way that important clinical point is taught. Multiple topics are tested in a short time. Each OSCE has a clear objective. This is one of the best modalities to test trainees' knowledge about the subject. The OSCE topics are selected from day-to-day clinical practice. We have a pool of OSCE cases which are collected over the period of last 15 years. The OSCE cases include ECGs, ultrasound findings, CT scan findings, X-ray findings, toxicology cases, important physical signs and findings. In each OSCE case, few questions are given to test the knowledge of the candidate. In each testing session, 20 cases are given which are projected on the projector, and each case is given 3 min where they have to answer the questions. This test their clinical approach and skills of identifying and diagnosing the case.

2.10.5. *Oral clinical scenarios*

Oral clinical scenarios are used to test in detail the approach of emergency medicine knowledge and lateral thinking. Emergency medicine field is challenging in a way that the true and real-time testing cannot be done on patients. Different methods are thus adopted to cover these aspects. One of the ways is to have oral clinical scenarios to test the approach and knowledge of trainees. The candidate is given a scenario and the length and depth of his knowledge is tested by asking questions related to the subject. The candidate can be challenged in knowledge by taking him to different directions, and examiner has the liberty and flexibility to test him in a more broader way. We have pool of important topics and scenarios. It includes trauma, resuscitation, toxicology, pediatrics, environmental as well as orthopedics. Some scenarios are developed to test the atypical or race presentation of a common emergency. Some scenarios are used to test the approach to manage undifferentiated emergency situation. Different aspects which are tested include art of history taking, approach to deal with the scenario, selection of suitable investigation, skill of interpreting ECG, X-ray findings or CT and US findings. It helps in testing the collateral thinking of candidate and gives a chance to test the evidence-based knowledge and familiarity with the new literature. The examiner prepares a key which defines the marking scheme and strategy and also points out the important red flags which are mandatory to pass. Trainee who fails to manage these red flags is failed considering it as a basic requirement to be a safe physician. Thus, we use this as a wonderful opportunity to test the very important aspects of training which are not possible in real-time situation. The cases are long cases (15 min) or short cases (7.5 min). After each case, there is a detailed discussion and feedback session which helps residents to know about their mistakes and deficiencies.

2.10.6. *Simulation-based teaching*

Refs. [26–29] simulation-based teaching and testing is also one of the new ways of educating the candidate where different skills of candidates are tested at a same time. The candidate is given a scenario and he is tested on high fidelity manikins. We test different skills like communication skills, leadership qualities, approach to critical information provided and response to clinical situation. [4]. This teaching model tests the multitasking capabilities of the candidate. The instructor tests the approach of the candidate toward a clinical presentation, his performance as a leader as well as a primary responder. The examiner tests his competency in gathering important information as well as his skills of timely intervention and management. The instructor also tests his knowledge of proper disposition and timely calling for help from subspecialties. It also tests the candidates' control over his team as a lead.

2.10.7. *Mortality and morbidity conference*

Refs. [30–32] these conferences are arranged once a month as a departmental learning conferences where all the important cases with mortality and morbidity issues are collected and discussed. The candidate is asked to prepare the case and look at the current evidence to support the management done or best management which should have been given. This gives a platform where the department and experienced staff give their feedback and input regarding the best possible management plan.

This is one of the best ways to teach the practice-based learning, system-based learning and evidence-based clinical approach and problem-based learning. We have a dedicated senior consultant who is lead for the mortality and morbidity cases. All the cases which fulfill the criteria to be presented are reviewed by the consultant, and it is selected for presentation. The physician involved in the case prepares the case and this is discussed in M&M conference which is arranged once a month. The case is presented by the physician and the session is opened for questions and answers and discussions. This gives opportunity to the trainee to learn from the mistakes and also to learn the skills of defending their decision and management. These cases help them in improving their management skills and learn the evidence-based management as well as the departmental protocols and policies. Mortality and morbidity conferences can be used to teach the ACGME core competencies like medical knowledge, patient care, system-based practice, practice-based learning and professionalism. These cases can be used to teach different competencies in different scenarios. As a member of education team, we have found that mortality and morbidity cases are wonderful teaching examples and experiences to train junior staff by covering the different aspects of ACGME competencies.

2.10.8. *Journal club*

Refs. [36–40] the JC meetings are a way of training the residents to look for the best evidence-based practice. Important topics related to the specialty are selected and candidates are asked to prepare and present them. This will train them to do critique and also chose the best evidence in support or against any particular management or practice. Journal clubs stimulate critical appraisal skills among medical students. These journal clubs can be very effective

http://dx.doi.org/10.5772/intechopen.75162

platforms where the students can gather first-hand knowledge on analyzing, evaluating, dissecting and utilizing the scientific literature. Journal clubs have also been shown to motivate reading behaviors of physicians in-training and also increase their knowledge of epidemiology and biostatistics. We feel that by making journal clubs part of the training curriculum will benefit the purpose of exposure of students to the world of frontline research and pave their way for future entry in the world of translational research. We make sure that all the senior residents present at least 3–4 articles during their residency training. They chose the article which is related to their working environment and specialty and appraise it. During the journal club presentations, the trainees are taught to do critical appraisal. They learn art of writing a research question and the abstracts. We started official research training in 2013 and as a result, multiple trainees published papers, wrote abstracts and presented in international conferences. It improved the scholarly activities in our department.

2.10.9. Grand rounds

Refs. [30, 33–35] the multidisciplinary grand rounds are used to discuss the subject where multiple specialties have stakes in management. This provides a platform where all the experts sit together and share their view point and expertise to manage the case in a best possible way and to agree on a standardized management plan agreed in the light of local policies and protocols. We have been inviting speakers from different specialties to give talks on their subjects related to emergency medicine practice. It has helped in bridging the gap between specialties and emergency department and improved the management and patient care. This platform is used to improve our understanding of the subject and to accept the common pathway accepted by both the departments.

2.10.10. Bedside teaching

Refs. [25, 41–44] bedside teaching is seen as one of the most important modalities in teaching a variety of skills important for the medical profession. Bedside teaching has shown to improve certain clinical diagnostic skills in medical students and residents. Several other skills essential for patient's contact can, for a great part, best be learned at the bedside. Bedside teaching gives an opportunity to faculty to assess the six core competencies of ACGME and different aspects of trainee's training including their communication skills, professionalism, system-based practice, medical knowledge, practical approach to patient's problems and critical thinking. The faculty members use this model of teaching to discuss the subject with evidence and also by using their experience as a teaching tool. This is the best opportunity to teach the competency of system-based practice and amalgamate it with the patient management. The faculty members assess the different qualities of trainee. They look at how they approach the patient, introduce themselves, how they take the detailed history and do proper physical examination, how they interact and communicate with patient, relatives and other staff, how they choose investigations and interpret the lab findings. They also assess the critical thinking of the trainee. Different work-based assessment (WBA) tools are used to get the detailed information about the trainee. The WBA tools include CBD, Mini-Cex and DOPS.

2.10.11. Defining learning objectives

There must be clearly defined learning objectives. All the topics should be taught in such a way that there are clear learning objectives which are conveyed and taught at the end of the teaching session. The learning objectives must include the local policies and protocols and evidence-based practice.

2.10.12. Defining rotation objectives

All rotations in emergency medicine have some objectives and goals. These objectives are defined on the basis of specialty requirement. With the passage of time and by the feedbacks provided by the trainee and the faculty, program evaluation committee and the clinical competency committee give their recommendations to improve the curriculum and the program. These recommendations must be forwarded to the Program Director who with his team should take necessary steps to improve the program. This is a dynamic process and must be repeated frequently.

2.10.13. Communication skills and leadership qualities

Emergency medicine teaching is incomplete without the communication and leadership skills. The nature of the specialty demands high level of communication skills from the trainee. The difficulty of work environment, the pressure of work and the dynamics of clinical work expect from the physician to be an expert in averting any issues or problems which arise at shop floor. Looking at the diversity of problems and conditions which are expected to use emergency department as a gateway to the hospital, lack of good communication skills and leadership qualities will add on the disposition time of patient and would add to length of the stay in the department.

2.10.14. Administration and management skills

These skills are important to be taught during the training program. We have seen that the emergency departments are getting bigger and busier all over the world. Emergency departments are used more and more as walk-in facility where patients come to get opinion about their problems and issues. Lack of rapidly expanding primary care setup, readily access to health information on internet and social media, improving public awareness about health are the reasons for more patients visiting emergency department. They need quick answer to their questions and they visit the emergency department with expectations and fixed ideas. This leads to overcrowding in the department. With the overcrowding, we face problems of space, delay and increased length of stay, diagnostic and therapeutic errors, improper disposition and unnecessary investigations. Thus, it is important that we teach administrative and management skills to our trainee to deal with all these issues.

Strong administrative and management qualities help the candidates to deal with issues of overcrowding, bed crisis, long waiting time, complaints and litigations and difficult and aggressive patients. This skill will help physicians to find out solutions for the problem.

3. Conclusion

To establish a good teaching program, all the important aspects of teaching and training need to be addressed. The trainer needs to be trained to deliver the best emergency medicine training and expertise to the trainer. It requires lot of faculty development programs and training of the trainer. Different tools need to be developed to keep a strict eye on the quality of the program so that timely interventions are done if there is any deficiency in the outcome.

Author details

Shahzad Anjum

Address all correspondence to: shahzad177@yahoo.com

Hamad Medical Corporation, Doha, Qatar

References

[1] Cooke KJ, Patt DA, Prabhu RS. The Road of Mentorship. American Society of Clinical Oncology Educational Book. 2017;**37**:788-792. DOI: 10.14694/EDBK_175193

[2] Yeung M, Nuth J, Stiell IG. Mentoring in emergency medicine: The art and the evidence. CJEM. 2010 Mar;**12**(2):143-149

[3] Shayne P, Heilpern K, Ander D, Palmer-Smith V. Protected clinical teaching time and a bedside clinical evaluation instrument in an emergency medicine training program. Emory University Department of Emergency Medicine Education Committee. Academic Emergency Medicine. 2002 Nov;**9**(11):1342-1349

[4] Okuda Y, Bryson EO, DeMaria S Jr, Jacobson L, Quinones J, Shen B, Levine AI. The utility of simulation in medical education: what is the evidence? Mount Sinai Journal of Medicine. 2009 Aug;**76**(4):330-343. DOI: 10.1002/msj.20127

[5] Mortaz Hejri S, Jalili M, Shirazi M, Masoomi R, Nedjat S, Norcini J. The utility of mini-clinical evaluation exercise (mini-CEX) in undergraduate and postgraduate medical education: Protocol for a systematic review. Systematic Review. 2017 Jul **18**;6(1):146. DOI: 10.1186/s13643-017-0539-y

[6] Hart D, Bond W, Siegelman JN, Miller D, Cassara M, Barker L, Anders S, Ahn J, Huang H, Strother C, Hui J. Simulation for Assessment of Milestones in Emergency Medicine Residents. Academic Emergency Medicine. 2017 Aug 20. DOI: 10.1111/acem.13296. [Epub ahead of print]

[7] Hejri SM, Jalili M, Shirazi M, Masoomi R, Nedjat S, Norcini J. The utility of mini-Clinical Evaluation Exercise (mini-CEX) in undergraduate and postgraduate medical education:

Protocol for a systematic review. Systematic Review. 2017;**6**:146. Published online 2017 Jul 18. DOI: 10.1186/s13643-017-0539-y

[8] Farook S, Chaudhry S, Al Kahlout B, Irfan FB, Pathan S. Acceptability and feasibility of the standardized direct observation assessment tool in the emergency department in Qatar. International Journal of Medical Education. 2017;**8**:428-429. Published online 2017 Dec 21. DOI: 10.5116/ijme.5a2e.7e16

[9] ACGME. Program requirements for graduate medical education. 2011 [cited 29 October 2017]; Available from: http://www.acgmei.org/Portals/0/FoundInternational03312016.pdf

[10] Shayne P, Gallahue F, Rinnert S, Anderson CL, Hern G, Katz E. Reliability of a core competency checklist assessment in the emergency department: the standardized direct observation assessment tool. Academic Emergency Medicine. 2006;**13**:727-732. DOI: 10.1197/j.aem.2006.01.030. [PubMed] [Cross Ref]

[11] LaMantia J, Kane B, Yarris L, Tadros A, Ward MF, Lesser M, Shayne P. Real-time inter-rater reliability of the Council of Emergency Medicine residency directors standardized direct observation assessment tool. Academic Emergency Medicine. 2009:51-57. DOI: 10.1111/j.1553-2712.2009.00593.x. [PubMed] [Cross Ref]

[12] Van Der Vleuten CP. The assessment of professional competence: developments, research and practical implications. Advance in Health Sciences Education Theory and Practice. 1996;**1**:41-67. DOI: 10.1007/BF00596229. [PubMed] [Cross Ref]

[13] Cobb KA, Brown G, Jaarsma DADC, Hammond RA. The educational impact of assessment: A comparison of DOPS and MCQs. Medical Teacher. 2013 Nov;**35**(11):e1598-e1607. Published online 2013 Jun 28. DOI: 10.3109/0142159X.2013.803061 PMCID: PMC3809925

[14] Morris A, Hewitt J, Roberts CM. Practical experience of using directly observed procedures, mini clinical evaluation examinations, and peer observation in pre-registration house officer (FY1) trainees. Postgraduate Medical Journal. 2006 Apr;**82**(966):285-288. DOI: 10.1136/pgmj.2005.040477 PMCID: PMC2579636

[15] Humphrey-Murto S, Varpio L. Teaching and assessing procedural skills: A qualitative study Claire Touchie. BMC Medical Education. 2013;**13**:69. Published online 2013 May 14. DOI: 10.1186/1472-6920-13-69 PMCID: PMC3658931

[16] Kilroy DA, Southworth SA. The Foundation Programme and the emergency department: A review of the curriculum and experience of a UK pilot. Emergency Medical Journal. 2006 Mar;**23**(3):167-171. DOI: 10.1136/emj.2005.029892 PMCID: PMC2464437

[17] MK Joshi, Singh T, Badyal DK. Acceptability and feasibility of mini-clinical evaluation exercise as a formative assessment tool for workplace-based assessment for surgical postgraduate students. Journal of Postgraduate Medicine. 2017 Apr-Jun;**63**(2): 100-105. DOI: 10.4103/0022-3859.201411 PMCID: PMC5414419

[18] Summative clinical competency assessment: A survey of ultrasound practitioners' views Gill Harrison. Ultrasound. 2015 Feb;**23**(1):11-17. Published online 2014 Sep 17. DOI: 10.1177/1742271X14550238. PMCID: PMC4760562

[19] Davies D, Ekeocha S, Kidd JM, MacDougall C, Matthews P. The effectiveness of case-based learning in health professional education. A BEME systematic review: BEME Guide No. 23. Jill Elizabeth Thistlethwaite. Published online: 11 May 2012

[20] Australian college of Physicians guidelines

[21] Williamson JML, Osborne AJ. Critical analysis of case based discussions. BJMP 2012; **5**(2):a514

[22] Ferguson J, Wakeling J, Bowie P. Factors influencing the effectiveness of multisource feedback in improving the professional practice of medical doctors: A systematic review. BMC Medical Education. 2014;**14**:76. Published online 2014 Apr 11. DOI: 10.1186/1472-6920-14-76 PMCID: PMC4011765

[23] Dehon E, Jones J, Puskarich M, Sandifer JP, Sikes K. Use of emergency medicine milestones as items on end-of-shift evaluations results in overestimates of residents' proficiency level. Journal of Graduate Medical Education. 2015 Jun;**7**(2):192-196. DOI: 10.4300/JGME-D-14-00438.1 PMCID: PMC4512788

[24] Sricharoen P, Yuksen C, Sittichanbuncha Y, Sawanyawisuth K. Teaching emergency medicine with workshops improved medical student satisfaction in emergency medicine education. Advance Medical Education Practice. 2015;**6**:77-81. Published online 2015 Feb 2. DOI: 10.2147/AMEP.S72887.PMCID: PMC4321415

[25] Celenza A, Rogers IR. Qualitative evaluation of a formal bedside clinical teaching programme in an emergency department. Emergency Medical Journal. 2006 Oct;**23**(10): 769-773. DOI:10.1136/emj.2006.037796. PMCID: PMC2579596

[26] Qayumi K, Pachev G, Zheng B, Ziv A, Koval V, Badiei S, Cheng A. Status of simulation in health care education: an international survey. Advance Medical Education Practice. 2014;**5**: 457-467. Published online 2014 Nov 28. DOI: 10.2147/AMEP.S65451 PMCID: PMC4257018

[27] Lin Y, Cheng A. The role of simulation in teaching pediatric resuscitation: Current perspectives. Advance Medical Education Practice. 2015;**6**:239-248.Published online 2015 mar 31. DOI: 10.2147/AMEP.S64178.PMCID: PMC4388005

[28] Stefan MS, Belforti RK, Gerard Langlois PA, Rothberg MB. A simulation-based program to train medical residents to lead and perform advanced cardiovascular life support. Hosp Pract. 1995). Author manuscript; available in PMC 2015 May 21. Published in final edited form as: Hosp Pract (1995), 2011 Oct;**39**(4):63-69. DOI: 10.3810/hp.2011.10.923. PMCID: PMC4440234.NIHMSID: NIHMS557580

[29] Semler MW, Keriwala RD, Clune JK, Rice TW, Pugh ME, Wheeler AP, Miller AN, Banerjee A, Terhune K, Bastarache JA. A randomized trial comparing didactics, demonstration, and simulation for teaching teamwork to medical residents. Annals of American Thoracic Society. 2015 Apr;**12**(4):512-519. DOI: 10.1513/AnnalsATS.201501-030OC. PMCID: PMC5466182

[30] Kravet SJ, Howell E, Wright SM. Morbidity and mortality conference, grand rounds, and the ACGME's Core Competencies. Journal of General Internal Medicine. 2006 Nov;**21**(11): 1192-1194. DOI: 10.1111/j.1525-1497.2006.00523. x. PMCID: PMC1831665

[31] Using the morbidity and mortality conference to teach and assess the ACGME general competencies. Rosenfeld JC, St. Luke's Hospital, Bethlehem, Pennsylvania. PlumX Metrics. DOI: https://DOI.org/10.1016/j.cursur.2005.06.009

[32] Epstein NE. Morbidity and mortality conferences: Their educational role and why we should be there. Surgical Neurology International. 2012;**3**(Suppl 5):S377-S388. Published online 2012 Nov 26. DOI: 10.4103/2152-7806.103872.PMCID: PMC3520073

[33] Hull AL, Cullen RJ, Hekelman FP. A retrospective analysis of grand rounds in continuing medical education. The Journal of Continuing Education in the Health Professions. 1989; **9**(4):257-266

[34] Richmond DE. The educational value of grand rounds. The New Zealand Medical Journal. 1985 Apr 24;**98**(777):280-282

[35] Lewkonia RM, Murray FR. Grand rounds: A paradox in medical education. CMAJ. 1995 Feb 1;**152**(3):371-376.PMCID: PMC1337535

[36] Biswas T. Role of journal clubs in undergraduate medical education. Indian Journal of Community Medicine. 2011 Oct-Dec;**36**(4):309-310. DOI: 10.4103/0970-0218.91422. PMCID: PMC3263155

[37] Alguire PC. A review of journal clubs in postgraduate medical education. Journal of General Internal Medicine. 1998 May;**13**(5):347-353. DOI: 10.1046/j.1525-1497.1998.00102.x.PMCID: PMC1496950

[38] Linzer M. The journal club and medical education: over one hundred years of unrecorded history. Postgraduate Medical Journal. 1987 Jun;**63**(740):475-478.PMCID: PMC2428317

[39] Afifi Y, Davis J, Khan K, Publicover M, Gee H. The journal club: a modern model for better service.and training. The Obstetrician & Gynaecologist Education. 2006;**8**:186-189

[40] Kleinpell RM. Rediscovering the value of the journal club. American Journal of Critical Care. 2002;**11**:42

[41] Max Peters and Olle ten Cate. Bedside teaching in medical education: A literature review. Perspective Medical Education. 2014 Apr;**3**(2):76-88. Published online 2013 Sep 19. DOI: 10.1007/s40037-013-0083-y.PMCID: PMC3976479

[42] Garout M, Nuqali A, Alhazmi A, Almoallim H. Bedside teaching: An underutilized tool in medical education. International Journal of Medical Education. 2016;**7**:261-262. DOI: 10.5116/ijme.5780.bdba

[43] Alpert JS. Some thoughts on bedside teaching. The American Journal of Medicine. 2009; **122**:203-204

[44] Subharamani Boston University School of Medicine, Boston, USA. Twelve tips to improve bedside teaching. Medical Teacher. 2003;**25**(2):pp. 112-115

www.ingramcontent.com/pod-product-compliance
Lightning Source LLC
Chambersburg PA
CBHW080737061126
54393CB00051B/543
* 9 7 8 1 7 8 9 8 4 8 3 2 8 *